Neurological Physiotherapy

For Churchill Livingstone

Editorial Director: Mary Law
Project Manager: Valerie Burgess
Project Editor: Dinah Thom
Copy Editor: Sue Beasley
Project Controller: Derek Robertson/Pat Miller
Design Direction: Judith Wright
Sales Promotion Executive: Maria O'Connor

Neurological Physiotherapy

A Problem-solving Approach

Edited by

Susan Edwards FCSP
Lead Professional Adviser for Physiotherapy,
National Hospital for Neurology and Neurosurgery, London, UK

Foreword by

Alan J. Thompson MD FRCP FRCPI
Consultant Neurologist in Neuro-rehabilitation,
The National Hospital for Neurology and Neurosurgery, London, UK

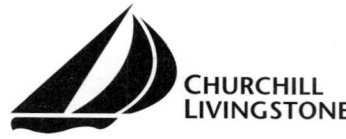

CHURCHILL
LIVINGSTONE

NEW YORK   EDINBURGH   LONDON   MADRID   MELBOURNE   SAN FRANCISCO   TOKYO 1996

CHURCHILL LIVINGSTONE
Medical Division of Pearson Professional Limited

Distributed in the United States of America by Churchill
Livingstone Inc., 650 Avenue of the Americas, New York,
N.Y. 10011, and by associated companies, branches and
representatives throughout the world.

First published 1996
    Reprinted 1997

ISBN 0 443 048878

British Library of Cataloguing in Publication Data
A catalogue record for this book is available from the
British Library.

Library of Congress Cataloging in Publication Data
A catalogue record for this book is available from the
Library of Congress.

The
publisher's
policy is to use
**paper manufactured
from sustainable forests**

Produced by Longman Singapore Publishers (Pte) Ltd.
Printed in Singapore.

Contents

Contributors **vii**

Foreword **ix**

Preface **xi**

Introduction **1**
Susan Edwards

1. Physiotherapy approaches to the treatment of
   neurological conditions – an historical
   perspective **3**
   Cecily J. Partridge

2. An analysis of normal movement as the basis for
   the development of treatment techniques **15**
   Susan Edwards

3. Neuropsychological problems and solutions **41**
   Dawn Wendy Langdon

4. Abnormal tone and movement as a result of
   neurological impairment: considerations for
   treatment **63**
   Susan Edwards

5. General principles of treatment **87**
   Philippa Carter, Susan Edwards

6. Case histories **115**
   Susan Edwards

7. Postural management and special seating **135**
   Pauline M. Pope

8. Splinting and the use of orthoses in the
   management of patients with neurological
   disorders **161**
   Susan Edwards, Paul Charlton

9. Longer-term management for patients with
   residual or progressive disability **189**
   Susan Edwards

Index 207

Contributors

Philippa Carter MCSP
Superintendent Physiotherapist, King's College
Hospital, London

Paul Thomas Charlton DipOrthotics DipOTC
Senior Orthotist specialising in Neurology,
J. C. Peacock & Son Ltd, Orthotic Services,
Newcastle upon Tyne

Susan Edwards FCSP
Lead Professional Adviser for Physiotherapy, National
Hospital for Neurology and Neurosurgery, London

Dawn Wendy Langdon MA MPhil PhD CClinPsychol
AFBPS
Clinical Neuropsychologist in Neurological
Rehabilitation, National Hospital for Neurology and
Neurosurgery, London

Cecily J. Partridge PhD FCSP
Honorary Reader in Physiotherapy, Centre for Health
Services Studies, University of Kent, Canterbury

Pauline M. Pope FCSP MSc
Consultant in Disability Therapy, Mary Marlborough
Centre, Nuffield Orthopaedic Centre, Oxford

Foreword

While the role of the physiotherapist in managing disability resulting from neurological disorders is much appreciated, the approach and methodology used are often shrouded in mystery. This tends to result in an underestimation of the contribution of the therapist. In this book Sue Edwards, an acknowledged neurophysiotherapist with a well-founded international reputation, brings all her clinical expertise and experience to address the complex and variable disability resulting from neurological disease. She adopts a problem-solving approach, the basis of which is set firmly in the analysis of normal movement. The text covers a wide range of areas, including neuropsychological aspects of management and case histories from carefully selected conditions to illustrate the main issues. It is above all a clinically orientated text which crosses the 'discipline' divide and may therefore be useful not just for physiotherapists in training but also for the many other professions involved in the management of neurological disability.

A.J.T.

Preface

The purpose of this book is to provide both undergraduate and qualified therapists with an improved understanding of problems commonly encountered in their work with people with neurological disability. It is based on the analysis of movement as a means of evaluating the disability arising from a wide variety of neurological conditions.

I wish to emphasise that the perspective is clinical and arises from clinical experience. I recognise the need for evidence-based practice and wherever possible references are given to support the text. However, I have not been constrained by lack of references in making assertions about treatment approaches. The challenge is to substantiate the constructive and functional changes demonstrated by patients treated in this manner.

There are many people who have provided invaluable support and assistance to me in compiling this manuscript. Jon Marsden, senior physiotherapist at the National Hospital for Neurology and Neurosurgery provided a constant supply of articles and books, without which, this text would never have been written. Cecily Partridge has been stalwart in reading and correcting many of the chapters, and my grateful thanks also go to the other authors of this book for their contributions.

I wish to acknowledge all the members of staff in the Directorate of Neurorehabilitation and Therapy Services at the National Hospital for their assistance in critically appraising many of the chapters and for taking part in the photographic sessions. The managers, too, have been extremely supportive in granting me study leave when overloaded with the work of writing. I am grateful, also, to the staff in the Audiovisual Department at the National Hospital for their support during the production of this book, particularly George Kaim – for his humour and patience and for his excellent photography.

Finally, my grateful thanks go to the Consultant medical staff at the National Hospital who, within their busy schedules, found time to read the chapters in their particular specialities. The most significant help was from Dr Alan Thompson and Professor Anita Harding. Tragically Professor Harding died as this book went into production. Her loss is immeasurable.

London 1996   S.E.

Introduction

Susan Edwards

The purpose of this book is to describe aspects of normal movement and difficulties which may arise as a result of neurological damage. The emphasis is on the analysis of the abnormal pathology which prevails and determining appropriate treatment interventions.

The ability to solve problems has been described as an integral part of physiotherapy practice (Newman Henry 1985). 'Problem solving' is a term often used in the management and treatment of patients with a variety of disabilities, and particularly for those with neurological dysfunction. Patients with neurological disability may present with complex and extensive movement disorders in addition to cognitive and sensory impairments. Analysing these deficits and determining the most appropriate course of treatment is the aim of all staff working in this field.

Problem solving may be considered in the context of both the physiotherapist identifying the patient's problems and adopting an appropriate treatment approach and the patient himself learning to contend with the movement deficit through compensatory strategies. Much has been written with respect to the former, the terms 'clinical reasoning' and 'problem solving' often being used synonymously (Higgs 1992). The concept of the patient being a problem solver is perhaps less well recognised.

The physiotherapist as a problem solver is dependent upon an accurate and extensive knowledge of movement, taking into consideration all aspects of the impairment which may contribute to the movement deficit. The patient, unable to function in the same way as before the onset of his neurological deficit, must determine the most efficient way to contend with his disability. Function is the ultimate goal for both parties but the means by which this is attained raises several issues.

The current clinical environment requires that the therapist makes judgements that weigh the advantages and disadvantages of each intervention (Shewchuk & Francis 1988). While quality of movement is imperative for optimal function, it must be recognised that restoration of normal movement is often an unattainable goal for the majority of patients with neurological disability. There must be a balance between re-education of more normal movement patterns and acceptance – and indeed promotion – of necessary and desirable compensation. Patients, therefore, must be involved in the decision-making process. 'In essence, they have a PhD in their own uniqueness that is very powerful in solving complex problems' (Weed & Zimny 1989).

REFERENCES

Higgs J 1992 Developing clinical reasoning competencies. Physiotherapy 78: 575–581

Newman Henry J 1985 Identifying problems in clinical problem solving. Perceptions and interventions with nonproblem-solving behaviors. Physical Therapy 65(7): 1071–1074

Shewchuk R M, Francis K T 1988 Principles of clinical decision making–an introduction to decision analysis. Physical Therapy 68(3): 357–359

Weed L L, Zimny N J 1989 The problem-orientated system, problem knowledge coupling and clinical decision making. Physical Therapy 69(7): 565–568

CHAPTER CONTENTS

Introduction   3

Treatment approaches   4
  Rood   4
  Proprioceptive neuromuscular facilitation   5
  Brunnström   5
  Bobath   5
  Motor relearning programme: Carr &
    Shepherd   6
  Conductive education   7
  Affolter   8
  Sensory integration: Ayres   9
  The human sandwich: Hare   9
  Johnstone   10
  Educational programmes: Holmqvist &
    Wrethagen   10

Discussion   10

References   13

1

Physiotherapy approaches to the treatment of neurological conditions – an historical perspective

Cecily J. Partridge

INTRODUCTION

In this chapter there are two aims. The first is to provide a brief review of the origins of some of the most frequently used physiotherapy approaches to the treatment and management of neurological conditions; wherever possible citing the original authors. The second is to examine the evidence for the comparative effectiveness of the different approaches. The art of neurological physiotherapy is constantly changing in the light of experience and new information, and the reader is referred to other chapters in this book to guide clinical practice. The most recent work within each named approach is recommended to provide constant updating.

During the first half of this century there was little specialisation in neurological physiotherapy and a similar approach was used for most patients with disabling conditions. Few theories were put forward to explain the basis of treatment, which was often directed towards regaining lost function as quickly as possible by any means. Patients with stroke, for example, were encouraged to regain function by compensating for the paralysis of the affected side by using the unaffected side. This is thought to have led to lasting imbalance in movement and posture, often with contractures in the arm and leg on the affected side. Though research evidence is not available to support this direct link, now, four decades later, it is relatively rare to see stroke patients with severe contracture in Britain.

During the 1940s, physiotherapists and others started to develop new approaches to the treatment of neurological conditions. For some years these methods were spread mainly through the medium of courses and lectures; publication followed later. The uniqueness of each new approach was stressed by the author and its adherents, which was necessary initially to distinguish it from other approaches. However, common themes are apparent in many of them. Quality in the performance of movement started to become an important aim, with more normal movement and posture as the eventual goal; a considerable change in emphasis from the earlier years.

The key concepts and characteristics of the different methods will be described in roughly chronological order. As practice often preceded publication by some years, the actual starting point for each approach is not always clear.

TREATMENT APPROACHES

The methods of treatment first introduced during late 1940s and early 1950s represented a major change in treatment and management, and initiated the development of the speciality of neurological physiotherapy. The earlier approaches included the work of Rood (1954) Kabat & Knott (1954) Brunnström (1956) and Bobath (1969). These authors mainly cited references from neurophysiology to provide a theoretical basis for their work.

Rood

Key words: Ontogenetic sequences, postural stability, joint and cutaneous receptors, Golgi tendon organs, abnormal tone, normal patterns of movement.

The original author of this approach, Margaret Rood (1954), did not write extensively and we have to rely on Goff (1969) and Stockmeyer (1967) for much of the information. Rood's approach to neuromuscular dysfunction represented a philosophy of treatment which was concerned with 'the interaction of somatic, autonomic, and psychic factors, and their role in regulation of motor behaviour'. Motor functions were seen as inseparable from sensory mechanisms, which introduced a new emphasis at the time. The treatment sought to activate movement and the postural responses of the patient in the same automatic way that they occurred in the normal. Stress was placed on the sequence of movement from most basic to most complex.

An understanding of the seven stages of ontogenetic sequence of movement was considered to be essential; they were listed as:

1. Lying supine
2. Rolling over in lying
3. Pivoting in prone lying
4. Supporting on the elbows in prone lying
5. Supporting on all-fours (hands and knees)
6. Standing
7. Walking.

Rood (1954) identified four stages which were to be followed in order to achieve controlled free movement:

1. Total movement patterns elicited
2. Postural stability gained
3. Once stability was achieved the body was moved over the supporting distal segment (weight shift)
4. More normal patterns of free movement usually possible.

Sensory stimulation was a central concept; input to the skin was through techniques such as brushing and icing, maintained slow stretching of muscle and compression of joints. The starting point for planning treatment was seen as assessment of basic function, disability, and abnormalities of posture and tone. Motor disabilities were classified into the three main groups of hypokinesia, hyperkinesia and hypertonus. Muscle work patterns were described but the approach was not essentially prescriptive.

The rationale for this treatment method was said by Stockmeyer (1967) to be 'the application of neurophysiology in physiotherapy practice'; she quotes Sherrington (1906) to support this statement. Goff cites the work of Matthews (1968) on muscle receptors, Buller (1968) on spinal reflex action, and Bowden (1968) on the structure and function of striated muscle as supporting Margaret Rood's treatment approach.

Proprioceptive neuromuscular facilitation

Key words: Patterns of movement, stretch and postural reflexes, manual pressure, isometric and isotonic contraction, approximation of joint surfaces, afferent input.

Knott & Kabat (1954) developed this approach at the Kaiser Foundation in Vallejo California during the 1950s. It was originally known as proprioceptive facilitation, but is now more widely known as proprioceptive neuromuscular facilitation (PNF), the term used by Voss (1967). This approach was initially developed with children, but was soon widely used in the treatment of both adults and children with a wide range of neurological and orthopaedic conditions.

Active muscle contractions were intended to stimulate afferent proprioceptive discharges into the central nervous system. This increased excitation and the recruitment of additional motor units (Kabat & Knott 1954).

The concepts of diagonal and spiral patterns of active and passive movement were introduced and were an innovation at the time. They replaced the somewhat stereotyped patterns of Swedish Remedial Exercises, which then dominated practice. Stretch reflexes were superimposed on the patterns of movement to increase muscle activity. A quick stretch at the lengthened range of a movement pattern was given to produce a contraction following relaxation. Maximal resistance was used to promote 'irradiation patterns', and the patient's voluntary movement was encouraged wherever possible. The therapist's tone of voice was used together with very specific placement of the hands to encourage purposeful movements. Isotonic and isometric contractions, traction, and approximation of joint surfaces were all used to stimulate postural reflexes.

The classical experiments of Mott & Sherrington (1895) on unilateral limb deafferentiation were cited to explain the basis of this approach.

Brunnström

Key words: Normal development, sensory cues, synergies, tonic neck reflexes, associated reactions, assessment, movement patterns.

The neglect of the often useless upper extremity in the ambulant stroke patient was the starting point for Signe Brunnström's interest. As with most other approaches, Brunnström recommends starting with critical evaluation of the patient to assess the stage of recovery. These stages in recovery were seen as similar to normal development, following a definite sequence, though it was recognised that hemiplegic patients may plateau at any stage of the sequence (Brunnström 1956).

The aim of treatment was to take the patient's present level of function as the starting point and, with reflex training, allow progress from the subcortical to cortical control of muscle function. Elicitation of the motor synergy was employed until the patient had 'captured' the reflex, then conditioning of the reflex was attempted (Brunnström 1956).

Sensory cues were used in this approach with tapping or stroking. Resistance was also used on both the affected and the unaffected side to encourage movement. Perry (1967) described four stages in Brunnström's approach:

1. At a reflex level, elicit major synergies.
2. Establish voluntary control of the synergies.
3. Break away from flexor and extensor synergies by mixing components from antagonist synergies.
4. Voluntary function is elicited.

The theoretical basis for this approach to treatment relied on early work by Riddock & Buzzard (1921) on reflex movements and postural reactions in animals, and by Magnus on tonic neck reflexes and tonic labyrinthine reflexes in hemiplegic patients.

Bobath

Key words: Abnormal postural reflex activity, abnormal tonus, sensory deficit, balance, normal movement, postural control.

Berta Bobath worked with both children and adults from the 1940s until her death in 1991. Her work has spanned nearly five decades and she continued to develop her methods of treatment throughout this time. Her work has also been adapted and refined by Davies (1985) and other authors, such as Carr & Shepherd (1982), have referred to her influence on their work. Bobath (1970) maintained that activity of individual muscles and muscle groups was secondary to their coordination in patterns of activity. Patterns of coordination were 'patterns of normal and abnormal postural control against gravity'. The fundamental problems of patients were seen in terms of this and of reciprocal innervation. Treatment aimed to help the patient to develop and increase control over the dis-inhibited action of tonic reflex activity by the use of patterns which inhibited spasticity. Thus, more normal patterns of function were facilitated and the patient gained control over released abnormal, non-functional motor patterns.

In the earlier years of this approach Bobath (1969) emphasised the use of mat exercises, with reflex inhibiting postures (RIPs) to inhibit abnormal tonus. Later, Bobath (1990) identified the changes that had occurred over time in her treatment methods. Static work had been discarded, with active patient participation becoming a central part of all treatment. Functional everyday goals were emphasised which involved the whole patient, including sensory, perceptual, and adaptive behaviour as well as the patient's motor problems. However, she maintained that the central concept had not changed over the years, but had remained with the focus on poor coordination and lack of control of muscle function as the main problems. It was only the techniques which had been refined and developed.

The Bobath concept has had a major influence on the treatment and management of neurological patients in Britain today, though what is practised within the overall concept can vary considerably.

The theoretical basis of this approach was put forward mainly by Karel Bobath (1959, 1966). Sherrington (1931) was cited on reflex inhibition as a factor in the coordination of movement and posture, Magoun & Rhines (1946) on inhibitory mechanisms in the bulbar reticular formation, and (1948) on spasticity, the stretch reflex and the extrapyramidal system. Gatev (1972) was cited by Bobath at a later stage (1990) on the role of inhibition in the development of motor coordination in early childhood.

Motor relearning programme: Carr & Shepherd

Key words: Motor control, relearning programmes, feedback, practice, problem solving, positive reinforcement, environment.

As with so many of the developers of new approaches, the impetus for the work of Carr & Shepherd came from their perceptions of deficiences in the current treatment methods (Carr & Shepherd 1982). They maintained that 'the end result of patients' lengthy rehabilitation process is frequently disabilities which may have, to some extent, been augmented by the very procedures intended to overcome these disabilities'.

The authors considered motor control as a key concept and essential to every aspect of performance. This, together with an understanding of normal movement and an ability to analyse motor dysfunction, formed the basis of the Motor Relearning Programme (MRP). Three factors deemed essential for the learning of a motor skill were:

1. the elimination of unnecessary muscle activity
2. feedback of information about performance
3. practice.

The main aim in motor training with MRP was not muscle strength but muscle control, with adjustment to gravity and the preservation of a balanced alignment during movement. Relearning the everyday activities contained in the MRP involved patients in remembering the movements in which they were skilled prior to the neurological impairment; this triggered off previously learned motor programmes called 'engrams'.

The use of cognitive functions in the initial stages of learning was stressed, progressing to practice at a more automatic level. The need for the therapist to develop problem-solving skills was emphasised. These, together with an advanced knowledge of movement, enabled analysis of patient problems, and their solution.

The MRP was made up of seven sections representing essential functions of everyday life:

1. Upper limb function
2. Orofacial function
3. Sitting up from supine
4. Standing up
5. Sitting down
6. Standing
7. Walking.

A description of normal function was given in each of these sections with instructions for treatment. Detailed steps were provided for the therapist. Instructions followed on how to elicit muscle activity and stimulate movement. Practice was stressed and when the activity had been learned there were instructions on how to transfer the skill to everyday life.

Creating the right environment was considered essential and included the development of a rehabilitation plan with consistent goals. The patient should experience success in treatment sessions, and positive reinforcement should be given. An educational programme for relatives and carers, and careful planning for discharge were also considered essential features.

Studies of human movement, motor skill acquisition, and psychological theories of learning and motivation provide the theoretical framework. Considerable emphasis was placed on the brain's capacity for reorganisation and adaptation following injury. Authors cited include Rosner (1970) on redundancy theory, Goldberger (1980) on denervation supersensitivity, Lawrence & Stein (1978) on neural sprouting, and Luria (1963) on behavioural strategy change.

Conductive education

Key words: Education, dysfunctionals, ortho-

functionals, independence, mobility, integrated system, group work.

The Institute for Conductive Education of the Motor Disabled in Budapest was founded on the work of András Petö, a physician with training in rehabilitation and psychiatry, to deal with the problems of motor disabled children. Because he perceived the problems of interprofessional conflict as detrimental to the child's progress, he set up a new method of teaching and training with the emphasis on functional development. The work of Petö has not been widely translated and we have to rely on other authors such as Cotton & Kinsman (1983).

A new professional, a conductor, was trained for 4 years in education, to take on the task of dealing with all the problems of the child with neurological deficits. The task of the conductor was essentially educational rather than therapeutic. Conductive Education (CE) represented a totally integrated system, where the conductor aimed to develop adaptive and learning abilities. Petö likened his methods to those of the conductor of the orchestra who aimed to evoke sequences of harmonious movement in the players, the patients (Cotton & Kinsman 1983).

Group, rather than individual, work was the norm in this approach. It was thought to help the development of effective interpersonal relationships, initiative, drive, motivation and learning. Within the group, a 'task series' was worked out for each individual and used as small steps for progression, to be discarded when redundant. A common group goal was also built up which allowed for individual variations. Chanting a 'rhythmical intention' considered an integral part of the learning process. While attempting to perform the appropriate movement, the patient is encouraged chant things such as 'I clasp my hands', or up my hands'.

This approach relied on literature from cation, medicine and orthotics. The training course for the conductors now included principles of the basic medical sciences, therapy, and speech (Robinson et al Though primarily developed for use children, both Cotton & Kinsman (19

Kinsman (1989) have reported work with a range of adults with neurological conditions such as Parkinson's disease.

Affolter

Key words: Perception, assimilation, complex human performance.

In contrast to most others, this approach started from within a theoretical framework, rather than arising from clinical practice. Félice Affolter put forward the hypothesis that the adequacy of perceptual processes was a prerequisite for complex human performance, and this formed the basis of her treatment methods.

A learning model was proposed for relearning following neurological damage. The importance of the interaction between the individual and the environment was considered a fundamental part of this learning. Perception here included all the mechanisms used in processing the stimuli of the actual situation. They included the 'different sensory modalities, supramodal organisation levels, respective storage systems and retrieval and recognition performances' (Affolter 1980).

Perception was seen as having an essential in the cycle of learning, and, as it could not observed directly, inferences were made perceptual processes from observation of ance. Three examples of performance in are used to illustrate different levels of tor development: object manipulation, signals and events. By manipulating baby uses tactile kinaesthetic infor- earn about objects. As vision is nvolved, the child learns through als about relationships between . Once a repertoire of functional established, the child starts to n as a sequence leading to a nt.

dults who failed in language complex performances also in their perceptual pro- hem was aimed at stimu- processes, with all three The use of 'repertoires'

was stressed, where incoming information was compared with past experience, a process Affolter (1980) called assimilation (based on the work of Piaget 1936). The assimilation of actual stimuli with past experience led to anticipatory behaviour. These concepts were considered basic for planning and for the performance of complex movements. Feedback of information was also an important part of this therapeutic approach.

Five levels are suggested:

1. Starting at an elementary level, there will be no anticipation.
2. The patient is starting to initiate more steps.
3. There is increased anticipation of the steps to be taken. As experience increases, the patient will start to search for missing objects.
4. The patient is able to plan more than one stage ahead and can perform new sequences if functional signals are familiar.
5. Not only can the patient think ahead but is able to check all steps of the event/task in advance.

The example of polishing shoes was given, providing a sequence of steps. The starting point was dirty shoes and a container of polish; this must first be opened before the next stage of cleaning could be undertaken and the goal of clean shoes achieved. It was considered necessary for patients to experience the success of following a correct sequence and attaining a desired goal as part of rehabilitation.

This approach, which started in Switzerland, is more widely used in continental Europe than in Britain. It seems particularly appropriate for those with speech disturbances and perceptual problems. The theoretical background comes from psychology. The author suggested that information from a number of sources supported the hypothesis of perceptual prerequisites for the attainment of complex verbal and non-verbal human performance. Sources included normative data, sensorily deprived children and children, such as those with dyslexia, who fail in complex performance. The work of Piaget (1947), Chomsky (1969) and Carterette & Friedman (1973) were cited to support this hypothesis.

Sensory integration: Ayres

Key words: Sensory and perceptual impairment, behavioural goals, feedback, repetition, adaptive response.

Ayres' (1972) main thesis was that functional limitations in many brain-damaged people were compounded by sensory and perceptual impairment. Sensory integration was said to be based on neurobehavioural theories, and standardised tests were developed to investigate disorders (Ayres 1975). The aim was to identify problems in 'space and form perception, dyspraxia, tactile defensiveness, auditory language problems and vestibular processing disorders'. This approach is perhaps more widely used by occupational therapists than physiotherapists at present.

Ayres (1972) hypothesised that understanding how the brain processes sensation, especially vestibular and somatosensory input, would provide the basis for treatment of conditions with underlying perceptual dysfunction. The initial focus was on children with learning disabilities. She proposed (1972) that somatosensory and vestibular functions were the underpinnings of normal development. Sensory feedback and repetition were seen as important principles of motor learning. Behavioural goals were set by the patient, and treatment aimed to meet the patient's sensory needs.

The term 'adaptive response' was used to refer to active participation in treatment. Sensory information was organised by the individual in order to complete a task, solve a problem or plan a movement. The theoretical basis of this approach, as that of the last author Félice Affolter, relied heavily on the field of perception within psychology.

The human sandwich: Hare

Key words: Postural competence, physical performance, physical ability, base of support.

The concept of the human sandwich and the Physical Ability Scale are the work of Noreen Hare and were developed initially for work with children with cerebral palsy. But, as with so many other concepts of treatment that were developed initially with one neurological condition, it also has wider implications for treatment of other conditions. In one respect it is similar to the work of Ayres (1972), as published work in both focuses on assessment scales. The Physical Ability Scale was designed to assess the child's capability to assume the positions listed below (Hallett et al 1987) as a starting point for movement:

1. Supine
2. Right and left side-lying
3. Sitting on the floor
4. Sitting on a box
5. Standing against a wall
6. Free standing.

Ability in each position was divided into levels and rated on a scale of 0 to 5:

0 = unable to conform to base of support
1 = able to conform to position when placed
2 = able to maintain position when placed
3 = able to move head and limbs within position when placed
4 = able to move out of position
5 = able to assume position, this pre-supposes that the abilities of 1, 2, 3, and 4 have already been established.

The scale is an assessment tool and considered as both the starting point and an integral part of the approach. The development of the scale resulted from the author's questioning of current methods of measurement of posture, movement and motor development (Hallett et al 1987). Hare claimed that the central features of her approach were the interrelationship between the body, gravity, and the supporting surface, hence the term 'sandwich' (Hallett et al 1987). The emphasis was mainly on the interface between the body part and the supporting surface and the extent to which they conformed. There may also be movement at this interface with weight adjustment and the ability to displace.

The measurement was of the child's ability rather than disability, and ability was broadly classified into four stages, which are given in descending order:

1. Able to stand, learning to walk
2. Able to sit, learning to stand
3. Able to lie, learning to sit
4. Unable to lie (for the most severely disabled).

The author sees this approach as complementing those already available rather than replacing them. The key principles to guide clinical work are seen as listening, observation, explanation and application.

Johnstone

Key words: Muscle tone, pressure splints, reflex inhibition, tonic neck reflex, pressure splints, positioning, anti-gravity patterns.

Margaret Johnstone (1989) described her approach as sensorimotor in origin, and based on a concept which aimed to deal with 'the finely balanced facilitatory–inhibitory principles of the neuromuscular system'. The need to inhibit abnormal patterns (called excessive tonal patterns) of movement was central, and positioning was used at all times to influence the distribution of tone following the neurological damage. The most distinctive features of this approach are the orally inflatable splints that are used to give limb stability during rehabilitation sessions. Different types of splint have been developed for different parts of the body. They include a full arm splint, a half arm splint, an inflatable boot, and a leg gaiter, which is a two-chamber splint (Johnstone 1989). The air splints were designed to apply even, deep pressure to the soft tissues to address sensory dysfunction (Johnstone 1989).

This work has been used mainly for patients with stroke, where the problems were seen as an imbalance of muscle tone and the presence of disabling postures from loss of control from the central nervous system. During the early stages of recovery, the stroke patient was positioned in side-lying on the unaffected side, with the affected arm in an air splint and supported on a pillow.

This approach relies on a normal developmental model, with recovery occurring from proximal to distal. The aim is to achieve central stability with gross motor performance, before progressing to more skilled movements. With the use of the splints and pressure techniques in a planned exercise programme, the author claims successful rehabilitation can be achieved.

Educational programmes: Holmqvist & Wrethagen

Key words: Educational programmes, consistency, involvement of all care staff.

Holmqvist & Wrethagen (1986) moved the emphasis away from the therapist's manual skills to educational programmes for all those involved in the overall management of the patient. They saw inconsistency in the methods and goals of different professionals, and a general pessimism about recovery as mitigating any beneficial effects of treatment.

Educational programmes were included for all those involved in day-to-day patient care. For nursing aides and assistants, they started with description and explanation of the basic pathology of the condition, and an analysis of sitting and standing up. For nursing staff, the programme included more in-depth pathophysiology, and included symptoms of stroke, course of onset, recovery and prognosis. This was followed by sessions on motor and sensory dysfunction and body mechanics. Later, detailed descriptions of posture and movement and how to assist patients to correct their positions and movements were undertaken. Perceptual dysfunction was also targeted, with screening and educational programmes for staff and relatives.

The authors used references from medical rehabilitation to support their work. They included Mykyta et al (1976) on including relatives in a stroke programme, and Feigenson et al (1977) on factors influencing outcome and length of stay in a stroke rehabilitation unit. They also cited Taub (1980) from behavioural psychology, on somatosensory deafferentation.

DISCUSSION

Exploring similarities and differences between approaches is not always straightforward and there is some semantic confusion. New words have been invented by some authors to describe aspects of their work, while others use different words to describe similar phenomena. However, an aim common to most is a striving, albeit by different means, to regain more normal posture and movement, with treatment aiming to reduce abnormality in muscle tone and posture. All stress the importance of careful assessment of the patient as the starting point for treatment.

Looking more closely at the content of the approaches, other similarities can be identified. Perceptual problems are a salient feature of the work of Affolter and Ayres, but they are also mentioned by Bobath, Holmqvist & Wrethagen, and Carr & Shepherd. Sensory cues are central to the approaches of Rood, Kabat, Brunnström and Johnstone, and are mentioned by Bobath and others. Feedback of information and knowledge of results play a key role in Carr & Shepherd's MRP programme, as they do in the approaches of Brunnström and Affolter. The importance of the environment in which treatment takes place and the consistency of all professionals dealing with the patient are stressed by both Carr & Shepherd, and Holmqvist & Wrethagen. They are also central concepts of Conductive Education.

Some approaches have placed more emphasis on the therapist's manual skills; these include Brunnström, Bobath, Rood and Kabat, whilst in Conductive Education, manual skills are hardly mentioned. Developmental stages in recovery are an integral part of the approaches of Rood, Kabat, Affolter and Bobath, and are also mentioned by Johnstone.

Though the authors of the different approaches to treatment and management claim success in achieving their stated aims, either implicitly or explicitly, this is based mainly on clinical evidence rather than research. Overall there has been little research into the effectiveness of neurological physiotherapy for any condition and there are problems in interpreting the results of studies that have been undertaken.

In recent reviews of physiotherapy for stroke, the condition where most research work has been undertaken to date, Ernst (1990) and

Ashburn et al (1993) concluded that many of the published studies have the following shortcomings:

- results difficult to generalise because of small patient numbers
- the introduction of bias because of lack of random patient allocation to treatment groups
- sparse information about the details of different treatment schedules
- a dearth of appropriate outcome measures related to the aims of physiotherapy.

This means that practice in neurological physiotherapy is not yet evidence based.

Despite the current scarcity of scientific evidence of its efficacy, neurological physiotherapy is seen to be successful in that it is in great demand. Doctors frequently refer patients for physiotherapy, patients and their families request it and most physiotherapists are convinced of its effectiveness. It is also generally agreed that physiotherapists should be part of the rehabilitation teams (Langhorne et al 1993).

The comparative effectiveness of the different approaches has been investigated but no study has been able to provide unequivocal evidence of substantial benefit of any one treatment over others. Again, most work comparing the outcome of different approaches has been undertaken in the treatment of patients with stroke. A brief review of some of the more rigorous work in this field shows similar results.

Stern et al (1970) compared two groups of 31 patients treated by either 'proprioceptive neuromuscular facilitation of Knott and Voss, or Brunnström' with conventional physiotherapy. The authors found most patients in each group made some recovery, but did not find any significant differences in recovery of function, mobility or leg strength in patients in the different groups on completion of the study treatments. Few details were given about the actual treatments received by patients in each group.

Loggigian et al (1983) examined the outcome where 42 patients were randomly assigned to two different treatment programmes for the upper limb. The treatment was based on either 'a traditional programme according to Rood's principles', or 'a facilitation approach based on Bobath'. Scores on the Barthel Index and the Kendall muscle test (motor performance) showed significant changes in all patients over the study period, but no significant intergroup differences were found. Basmajian et al (1987) also reported a study of treatment for the upper limb. They compared the use of the Bobath concept with a programme of electromyographic feedback, but again, no statistically significant differences were found between patients in the two groups.

Dickstein et al (1986) undertook a clinical trial and investigated a larger sample of 131 patients who were assigned to three treatment groups, conventional treatment, PNF, and Bobath. Some details of the treatments given were provided in this study. However, at 6 weeks, scores on the Barthel Index did not reveal significant intergroup differences.

Finally, Wagenaar et al (1990) used a single case study B–C–B–C design (which assesses pre-test and post-test reponse patterns to alternating treatments) with a series of seven patients. A neurodevelopmental Bobath approach and Brunnström methods were alternated. The treatments were said to be given by specially trained therapists. The authors used a battery of tests each week but could not find any overall differences. One of the problems here is that carry-over between alternating treatments may have occurred. In addition, generalisation would not have been justified with this small sample size.

The lack of significant intergroup differences in outcome between the treatments may reflect a number of factors. Methodological flaws mentioned earlier, such as those identified by Ashburn et al (1993), may have complicated evaluation, particularly the use of inappropriate or insensitive outcome measures. The treatment received by patients in each group may not have been mutually exclusive, as detailed descriptions of treatment methods were often lacking. Treatments designated as conventional or traditional without further details have little meaning beyond the institutions in which they are practised. Also what is done under the title of Brunnström, Bobath, Rood, or any other named

approach may differ considerably. These results could also suggest that treatment given by a skilled physiotherapist working within a number of different treatment approaches may be equally effective. Only further rigorous research will help to clarify these issues.

This picture of a lack of research and general agreement on the most effective approach to treatment is not surprising as physiotherapy is a relatively young profession. Looking at the history of the development of science within disciplines, Kuhn (1965) noted that, at the beginning, scientific disciplines consist of little more than descriptive lists. A number of competing theories then emerge, indicating an early stage of scientific development. This stage continues for a long time and it is often centuries before a discipline becomes a fully mature science. It took around four centuries for mathematics and biology to become mature paradigm sciences. It helps to put things into perspective to realise that much of medicine has not yet reached the stage of a mature science, in Kuhn's terms, and much medical practice is not evidence based.

Because of this diversity there is at present little evidence for any generally agreed standard physiotherapy for people with neurological conditions; rather both the literature and observation of practice suggest that there is considerable diversity, even when the same named approach is being used. Some physiotherapists choose to adhere strictly to the tenets of one particular school of thought, a so-called 'purist' attitude. These followers often interpret the originators' views with even greater rigidity. It seems likely, however, that as they become more experienced, many physiotherapists, while staying broadly within one overall philosophy, may study a number of different treatment methods. These therapists are then able to choose from a wider armamentarium when faced with a patient with complex neurological symptoms. The practice of more experienced physiotherapists may also reflect their own individual interpretations of the different methods.

It is interesting to note that authors who have previously promoted only their own approach are now starting to refer to a range of different treatment methods which may be beneficial in the treatment of neurological patients. Davies (1994) refers to Butler (1991) on adverse mechanical tension, Maitland (1986) on manipulation, and Affolter (1980) on object manipulation.

The work of the last 50 years or so has been to develop new methods of treatment, and explain their theoretical base. The challenge of the next 50 years is to provide unequivocal evidence of the extent to which each approach actually achieves its stated aims and to explain the underlying mechanisms.

REFERENCES

Affolter F 1980 Perceptual processes as prerequisites for complex human behaviour. International Rehabilitation Medicine 3: 3–9

Ashburn A, Partridge C J, De Souza L 1993 Physiotherapy in the rehabilitation of stroke: a review. Clinical Rehabilitation 7: 337–345

Ayres A J 1972 Sensory integration and learning disorders. Western Psychological Services, Los Angeles CA

Ayres A J 1975 Southern California postrotatory nystagmus test. Western Psychological Services, Los Angeles CA

Basmajian J V, Gowland C A, Finlayson A J et al 1987 Stroke treatment: comparison of integrated behavioural physical therapy versus traditional physical therapy programs. Archives of Physical Medicine and Rehabilitation 68: 267–272

Bobath B 1969 The treatment of neuromuscular disorders by improving patterns of coordination. Physiotherapy 55: 18–22

Bobath B 1970 Adult hemiplegia: evaluation and treatment, 1st edn. Heinemann Medical Books, London

Bobath B 1990 Adult hemiplegia: evaluation and treatment, 3rd edn. Heinemann Medical Books, London

Bobath K 1959 The effect of treatment by reflex inhibition and facilitation in cerebral palsy. Folia Psychiatrica, Neurologica et Neurochirugica Neerlandica 62: 448–450

Bobath K 1966 Motor deficits in patients with cerebral palsy. Clinics in Developmental Medicine 23: 24–25

Bowden R E M 1968 The structure and function of striated muscle. Physiotherapy 6: 190–195

Brunnström S 1956 Associated reactions of the upper extremity in adult patients with hemiplegia. An approach to training. Physical Therapy 45: 17–32

Buller A J 1968 Spinal reflex action. Physiotherapy 6: 208–211

Butler B S 1991 Mobilisation of the nervous system. Churchill Livingstone, London

Carr J H, Shepherd R B 1980 Physiotherapy in disorders of the brain. Heinemann Medical Books, London

Carr J H, Shepherd R B 1982 A motor relearning programme for stroke. Heinemann Medical Books, London

Carterette E C, Friedman M P 1973 Handbook of perception. Academic Press, New York

Chomsky N 1969 The acquisition of syntax in children from 5–10. MIT Press, Cambridge

Cotton E, Kinsman R 1983 Conductive education and adult hemiplegia. Churchill Livingstone, Edinburgh

Davies P M 1985 Steps to follow: a guide to the treatment of adult hemiplegia. Springer-Verlag, Berlin

Davies P M 1994 Starting again: early rehabilitation after traumatic brain injury or other severe brain lesions. Springer-Verlag, London

Dickstein R, Hocherman S, Pillar T, Shaham R 1986 Stroke rehabilitation. Three exercise approaches. Physical Therapy 66: 1233–1238

Ernst E 1990 A review of stroke rehabilitation and physiotherapy. Stroke 21: 1081–1085

Feigenson J S, McDowell F H, Meese P et al 1977 Factors influencing outcome and length of stay in a stroke rehabilitation unit. Stroke 8: 651–656

Gatev V 1972 The role of inhibition in the development of motor coordination in childhood. Developmental Medicine and Child Neurology 6: 251–259

Goff B 1969 Appropriate afferent stimulation. Physiotherapy 51: 9–17

Goldberger M 1980 Motor recovery after lesions. Trends in Neuroscience 2: 288–291

Hallett R, Hare N, Milner A D 1987 Description and evaluation of an assessment form. Physiotherapy 73(5): 220–225

Holmqvist L W, Wrethagen N 1986 Educational programmes for those involved in total care of the stroke patient. In Banks M (ed) Stroke. Longman, Singapore

Johnstone M 1987 Restoration of motor function in the stroke patient; a physiotherapist's approach. Churchill Livingstone, New York

Johnstone M 1989 Current advances in the use of pressure splints in the management of adult hemiplegia. Physiotherapy 75(7): 381–384

Kabat H, Knott M 1954 Proprioceptive facilitation therapy for paralysis. Physiotherapy 40: 171–176

Kinsman R 1989 A conductive education approach to stroke patients at Barnet General Hospital. Physiotherapy 75: 418–421

Kuhn T S 1965 The structure of scientific revolutions. University of Chicago Press, Chicago

Kurtzke J F 1983 Rating neurologic impairment in multiple sclerosis: an expanded disability status scale (EDSS). Neurology 33: 1444–1452

Langhorne P, Williams B O, Gilchrist W, Howie K 1993 Do stroke units save lives? Lancet 342: 395–398

Lawrence S, Stein D G 1978 Recovery after brain damage and the concept of localisation of function. In: Finger S (ed) Recovery from brain damage. Plenum Press, London

Loggigian M, Samuels M, Falconer J 1983 Clinical exercise for stroke patients. Archives of Physical Medicine and Rehabilitation 64: 364–367

Luria A R 1963 The role of speech in the regulation of normal and abnormal behaviour. Pergamon, Oxford

Magnus R 1926 Some results of studies in the physiology of posture. Lancet ii: 531–536, 585–588

Magoun H W, Rhines H 1946 Inhibitory mechanisms in bulbar reticular formation. Neurophysiology 9: 163–171

Magoun H W, Rhines H 1948 Spasticity, the stretch reflex and the extrapyramidal system. C C Thomas, Springfield Illinois

Mahoney F, Barthel D 1965 Functional evaluation: the Barthel Index. Maryland (State) Medical Journal 14: 61–65

Maitland G D 1986 Vertebral manipulation, 5th edn. Butterworths, London

Mathews P B C 1968 Receptors in muscle. Physiotherapy 6: 204–208

Mott F W, Sherrington C S 1895 Experiments upon the influence of sensory nerves upon movement and nutrition of the limb. Proceedings of the Royal Society 57: 481–488

Mykyta L J, Bowling J H, Nelson D A, Lloyd D J 1976 Caring for relatives of stroke patients. Age and Ageing 5: 87–90

Perry C E 1967 Principles and techniques of the Brunnström approach to the treatment of hemiplegia. American Journal of Physical Medicine 46(1): 719–815

Piaget J 1936 Origins of intelligence in children. (Reprinted 1952) International Universities Press, New York

Piaget J 1947 Plays dreams and imitation in childhood. (Republished 1960) Norton, New York

Riddock G, Buzzard E F 1921 Reflex movements and postural reactions in quadriplegia and hemiplegia with special reference to those of the upper limb. Brain 44: 397–489

Robinson R O, McCarthy G T, Little T M 1989 Conductive education at the Petö Institute. British Medical Journal 299: 1145–1149

Rood M S 1954 Neurophysiologic reactions: a basis for physical therapy. Physical Therapy Review 34: 444–449

Rosner B S 1970 Brain functions. Annual Reviews in Psychology 21: 555–594

Sawner K A, LaVigne J M 1992 Brunnström's movement therapy in hemiplegia. J B Lippincott, Philadelphia

Sherrington C 1906 The integrative action of the nervous system. University Press, New Haven

Sherrington C S 1931 Reflex inhibition as a factor in the coordination of movements and postures. Quarterly Journal of Experimental Physiology 6: 251–259

Stern P, McDowell F, Miller J M et al 1970 Effects of facilitation exercise techniques in stroke rehabilitation. Archives of Physical Medicine and Rehabilitation 51: 526–531

Stockmeyer S A 1967 An interpretation of the approach of Rood to the treatment of neuromuscular dysfunction. American Journal of Physical Medicine 46(1): 900–955

Taub E 1980 Somatosensory deafferentiation research with monkeys: implications for rehabilitation medicine. In: Ince L P (ed) Behavioural psychology in rehabilitation medicine: clinical implication. Williams & Wilkins, Baltimore

Voss D E 1967 Proprioceptive neuromuscular facilitation. American Journal of Physical Medicine 46: 838–898

Wagenaar R C, Meijer O G, Wieringen P C W, Kuik D J, Hazenberg G J, Lindeboom J, Wichers F, Rijswijk H 1990 The functional recovery of stroke: a comparison between neurodevelopmental treatment and the Brunnström method. Scandinavian Journal of Rehabilitation Medicine 22: 1–8

CHAPTER CONTENTS

Introduction   15

Features of normal movement   16
    Normal postural tone   16
    Reciprocal innervation   16
    Sensory-motor feedback and feedforward   18
    Balance: equilibrium, righting and protective
        reactions   19
    Biomechanical properties of muscles   20

An approach to the analysis of posture and
    movement   22
    Rotation of body segments   22
    Postural sets   22
    Key points of control   23
    Midline – the alignment of body segments   24

Analysis of specific positions   24
    Supine lying   24
    Prone lying   25
    Side-lying   26
    Sitting   26
    Standing   28

Analysis of movement sequences   29
    Moving from supine lying to sitting   29
    Moving from sitting to standing   31
    Walking   32
    Upper limb function   36

Conclusion   38

References   38

2

An analysis of normal movement as the basis for the development of treatment techniques

Susan Edwards

INTRODUCTION

The purpose of this chapter is to describe aspects of posture and movement which relate to the normal adult population. Many components of movement are consistent, and these form the basis of this analysis of normal behaviour. Similarities and differences which arise within the normal adult population will be discussed throughout this chapter as they relate to specific positions or movement components.

Normal movement has been described by many authors as a basis for treatment of the neurologically damaged patient (Bobath 1990, Carr & Shepherd 1986, Davies 1985, 1990, Galley & Forster 1987, Lynch & Grisogono 1991). A wide range of different clinical presentations exist in patients with neurological dysfunction and, consequently, different aspects of movement impairment will be demonstrated. For example, a patient following head injury or one with multiple sclerosis may present with spasticity or ataxia or indeed a combination of the two. The clinical presentation and appropriate treatment intervention may only be accurately assessed on the basis of an extensive knowledge of normal movement. The main remit of physiotherapy is to enable patients to attain their optimal level of function with regard to effectiveness and economy of movement.

It is not within the context of this chapter to discuss the neuro-psychological impairment which may be an integral component of the patient's disability. The implications of behavioural, perceptual, cognitive or memory dysfunction are described in Chapter 3, and movement cannot be considered to be a separate entity from these aspects. Lack of emphasis on these neuro-psychological aspects in this chapter in no way reflects any lack of recognition of their importance in the total picture of neurological rehabilitation.

FEATURES OF NORMAL MOVEMENT

Normal movement is dependent upon a neuromuscular system which can receive, integrate and respond appropriately to multiple intrinsic and extrinsic stimuli. It is controlled, not only by central commands and spinal activity, but also by functional and behavioural aspects which influence posture and movement. The central and peripheral systems interact extensively during the execution of motor plans and comprise sets of feedforward commands for complex motor actions. These are learned from successful, previous motor performance (Brooks 1986).

In order for this interaction to be effective in producing normal movement, key components should be considered.

Normal postural tone

In the assessment of patients with neurological impairment, neurologists define muscle tone in an operational manner as the resistance to movement when the patient is in a state of voluntary relaxation (Davidoff 1992). However, in a broader context, postural tone has been described as the state of readiness of the body musculature in preparation for the maintenance of a posture or the performance of a movement (Bernstein 1967). Normal postural tone enables an individual to:

- maintain an upright posture against the force of gravity
- adapt to a varying and often changing base of support
- allow selective movement to attain functional skills.

Postural tone is adaptable and varies throughout different parts of the body in response to

desired goals. Brooks (1986) describes the intricacy of the golf swing to illustrate the synchronous coordination of posture and movement. The stance of the golfer must be such as to afford stability during the arm swing by setting the stance muscles at the proper steady tensions, whilst at the same time setting the readiness to respond to stretch of contracting muscles. The tone of the trunk and lower limbs must provide adequate postural support for the moving parts before a successful swing can be accomplished.

From this example of a golf swing, it can be seen that the distribution and intensity of postural tone can be influenced by the size of the base of support. This is the area within the boundaries of each point of contact with the supporting surface. The larger the base of support and the lower the centre of mass in relation to the supporting surface, the less effort is required to maintain position and stability. For example, lying provides a far greater base of support than does standing and therefore is the more stable position. Postural tone is therefore normally lower in lying than in standing.

Clinical application

These factors are relevant in the choice of position in which to treat a patient. Many patients following neurological damage spend a considerable proportion of time in lying and, depending on the extent of their disability, may be unable to stand independently. Recruitment of muscle activity in lying, particularly for patients with low tone, is often difficult. Considerable effort is required to overcome the force of gravity and, in functional terms, it is a position which, in normal circumstances, is rarely used for activities of daily living. For this reason, it is often more appropriate for the patient to be placed in a more upright position with a reduced base of support and the centre of mass higher in relation to the supporting surface.

Reciprocal innervation

Reciprocal innervation is the graded and synchronous interaction of agonists, antagonists and synergists throughout the body (Bobath 1990). Marsden (1982) describes this interaction when:

starting from an initial posture, the limb or digit is repositioned in space by activation of the prime moving muscle, the agonist; at the same time, the activity of antagonists must be adjusted, and the actions of both the agonists and antagonists around a joint must be complemented by appropriate changes in activity in synergistic muscles. Not only do simple synergies fixate a joint to allow action of the prime movers, there must also be appropriate contraction of proximal fixating muscles so as to adjust the trunk to maintain balance.

Reciprocal innervation occurs during discrete, selective movements, for example of the fingers during fine manipulation, and also in postural control.

Postural adjustments occur automatically in response to the functional goal. Postural adjustments which accompany voluntary movement provide:

- equilibrium by maintaining the centre of gravity within the base of support; these adjustments occur during the performance of a selective movement such as reaching forwards with the arm and when there is an application of an external force to the body (a perturbation)
- body stability; that is, the postural adjustments govern the position of given segments such as the head or trunk (Soechting & Flanders 1992, Massion 1992).

Reciprocal innervation is an integral part of balance. The constant postural adjustments and interaction between muscle groups provides the automatic adaptation of the body to changes in the environment.

When standing, the interaction of muscle groups, primarily those of the pelvis, trunk and legs, is of a dynamic nature with constant adjustments occurring to enable mobility within the base of support. This dynamic feature frees the arms for selective movement.

Fractionation of movement, the ability to make specific movements at a single joint without also moving other joints, is described by Musa (1986) in relation to the stability afforded

by the interaction of the knee flexors and extensors during the stance phase of gait. This is a further example of reciprocal innervation.

Clinical application

Patients with abnormal tone following neurological damage, illustrate impaired reciprocal innervation. This may be as a result of hypotonus causing inadequate stability due to reduced activity, or of hypertonus where there is excessive and stereotyped activity preventing these tonal adaptations. In the latter case, co-contraction may become static and constant. Dominance of the hypertonic muscles prevents interaction between the opposing and complementary muscle groups, resulting in a static fixation rather than a dynamic stability (Massion 1984).

Reciprocal innervation is important in terms of trunk control. Basic functional tasks such as eating and dressing require constant adaptation of muscular activity with regard to the trunk and pelvis. Reaching to pick up a cup from a table requires stability within the trunk and of the pelvis in order to transfer weight and accomplish the task most efficiently (Moore et al 1992). A disabled person with a neurological impairment adversely affecting trunk and pelvic stability, may be able to perform the function, but the effort required may be substantially greater and compensatory strategies may be used.

Altered reciprocal innervation is a feature in patients with cerebellar lesions. Complex motor programmes involving postural adjustment in support of the focal movement of the limb are impaired (Diener et al 1990, 1992). This is illustrated in the finger–nose test which is used to determine the severity of ataxia. It is often considerably easier for the patient to coordinate arm movement with the body supported and the elbow resting on a firm surface than with the body and arm unsupported (Haggard et al 1994). In this way, the movement is broken down to the more simple task of elbow flexion and extension and is therefore less dependent on proximal stability.

Sensory-motor feedback and feedforward

Postures and movements are guided by a mixture of motor programmes and sensory feedback. Motor programmes have been described as a set of muscle commands that are structured before a movement sequence begins and that allow the entire sequence to be carried out uninfluenced by peripheral feedback (Keele 1968). Feedback brings the programme commands up to date with their execution and corrects errors (Brooks 1986) (Fig. 2.1).

'Until recently we thought the cortex behaved like a dictatorship, governing every move we made. But now some people think the central nervous system may have more in common with a democracy' (Altman & Kien 1993).

Control of posture and movement requires initiation and planning at the highest level, control and updating from the middle level and execution and regulation of the task at the lowest level. However, it must be stressed that interaction between these levels is constant and ongoing, providing information in both directions.

Movement skills are constantly reinforced and refined by repetition, the CNS being ever sensi-

tive to both intrinsic and extrinsic sensory information, which is assimilated to produce effective activity. Motor learning is therefore an active process. This is of particular relevance in the treatment of patients with neurological disability. Patients who are unable to move cannot reinforce their motor programmes through repetition and the maxim 'use it or lose it' may therefore apply.

Everyday activities such as walking and getting out of bed require little conscious effort once they become established movement patterns. The objective is to achieve a functional goal, as opposed to having to consider how one accomplishes each stage of the task. In contrast, the learning of new skills, such as how to drive a car, will initially involve considerable concentration until the movement patterns become established, after which time the task becomes relatively automatic (Schmidt 1991a).

Normal movement is dependent upon constant interaction of neural structures within the CNS. This neural activity may be considered a cyclical event during the performance of normal movement which reinforces movement patterns. Any interruption in this cycle of events will affect the outcome. If there is abnormal postural tone as a result of neurological damage, there

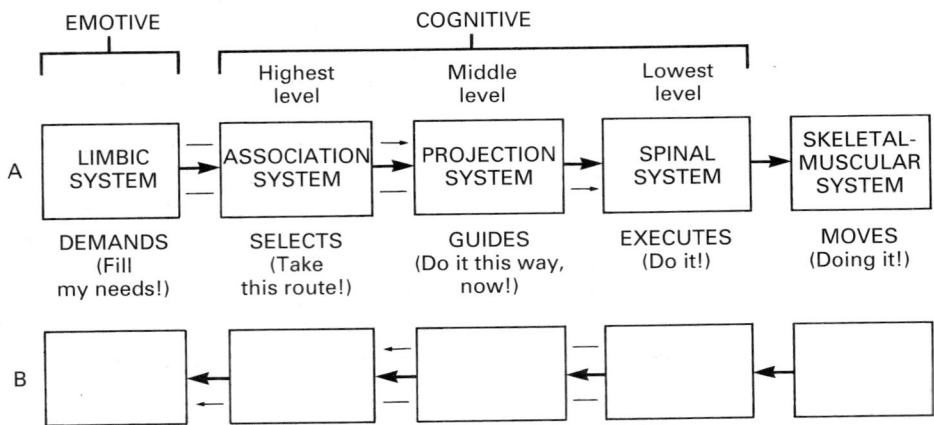

Figure 2.1 Cartoon summary highlighting the motivational function of the limbic system in motor control. Direct connections are indicated by heavy arrows and indirect connections by light arrows. Feedforward connections are represented in (A) and feedback between equivalent systems in (B). (Reproduced from Brooks 1986 The neural basis of motor control, Oxford University Press, with kind permission.)

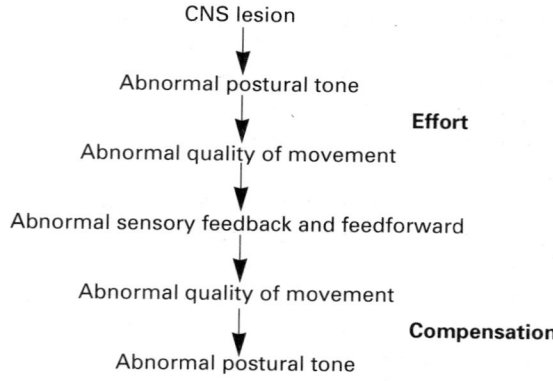

CNS lesion

↓

Abnormal postural tone

↓ **Effort**

Abnormal quality of movement

↓

Abnormal sensory feedback and feedforward

↓

Abnormal quality of movement

↓ **Compensation**

Abnormal postural tone

Figure 2.2   Pattern of response following CNS lesion (Bryce 1989).

may be disordered movement or a limited movement repertoire, producing an abnormal sensory input to the CNS. This may give rise to a response which is produced by effort and/or compensation which in turn produces abnormal movement and abnormal postural adaptation (Fig. 2.2).

Established patterns of spasticity may create new motor programmes that are dictated by the stereotyped activity. The purpose of therapy is to inhibit these undesirable responses by facilitating more normal postures and movements and re-establishing the memory of purposeful movement.

Sensory-motor integration in terms of continual feedback and feedforward is essential in the learning experience of any individual. By enabling the patient to move in a more normal way, effective motor programmes may be regained.

Motor learning is a set of processes associated with practice or experience leading to relatively permanent changes in the capability for skilled performance (Schmidt 1991b). The only way motor learning may be clinically observed is in a change in the patient's functional capability. The performance at the end of practice is not an indicator of the degree of learning. In fact certain factors which improve performance at the end of practice do not necessarily lead to long-term learning or carry-over (Schmidt 1988).

Balance: equilibrium, righting and protective reactions

These reactions described by Bobath (1990) refer to the postural adjustments and adaptations which occur consistently in everyday life to maintain alignment of body posture and the centre of gravity within the base of support.

Equilibrium reactions

Equilibrium reactions are synonymous with the postural adjustments which occur throughout daily life and as such they may be considered as one with reciprocal innervation. Balance is maintained by constant adaptation of muscular activity throughout the body. When a movement is performed, equilibrium control is provided by the displacement of segments which compensate for the displacement of the centre of gravity caused by the moving segments (Massion 1992). Changes in the location of the centre of gravity necessitate continuous postural adjustments during any movement, and even the smallest alteration has to be countered by modifications of tone throughout the body musculature (Bobath 1990). In standing, for example, these reactions are particularly noticeable in the feet, especially when standing on one leg. It is only when the body mass is displaced outside the base of support that balance is compromised and righting or protective reactions are called into action.

Equilibrium reactions require a high level of reciprocal innervation through the coordinated response of neuromuscular excitatory and inhibitory control. This graded response produces selective activity to counter the effects of gravity and allow acceptance of the base of support. The interaction between opposing and complementary muscle groups is the basis for the maintenance of posture and the performance of selective movement. The ability to maintain equilibrium in a great variety of positions provides the basis for all the skilled movements that are required for self-care, work and recreation (Davies 1985).

Righting reactions

The righting reactions are balance reactions which are activated on displacement of the body's centre of gravity outside of its base of support.

Righting reactions also refer to the relationship of the head, trunk and limbs with each other and with the environment. These reactions develop from birth and serve to maintain body alignment appropriate to a task or position. For example, when reversing a car, the head is turned to the right or left, with the trunk responding to accommodate the head position in order to minimise the strain taken on the neck. In spite of this adaptation, it is not a position which can be maintained for any length of time. The head rights itself in respect of its alignment with the trunk at the earliest opportunity. Any individual who has sustained injury to either the neck or back appreciates the difficulty in accomplishing this supposedly simple task.

Righting reactions are observed in virtually all sequences of movement such as rolling, sitting up from lying, and turning round in standing. In rolling, the movement is often initiated from the head but always in conjunction with postural adaptation throughout the body. The limbs and trunk respond appropriately to bring the body once more into its position of relative symmetry. Although the limbs frequently adopt a position of asymmetry in relation to each other, there is invariably predominant symmetry of the trunk, pelvis and shoulder girdles. It is important to recognise that, although many positions are asymmetrical in normal movement, this asymmetry is transient and interchangeable through symmetry.

In contrast, patients with neurological disability are observed to have asymmetry imposed by abnormal movement. For example, if a patient with a dense left hemiplegia attempts to roll towards the right side, the affected side may be unable to initiate or participate in the movement and tends to be left behind. Realignment of body segments on completion of the movement is often impaired.

Protective reactions

These reactions are activated when the centre of gravity is displaced outside of the base of support and the righting and equilibrium reactions are unable to regain balance. These protective reactions include stepping in the direction of displacement and the parachute response of putting the hands out to protect the face when falling.

Summary

Balance may be considered to be a holistic motor activity which will be influenced by any alteration in neuromuscular control. The equilibrium reactions may be considered as the first line of defence in the maintenance of balance with the fine postural adjustments occurring constantly and automatically. Movement of the centre of gravity outside of the base of support will require a righting response or, if this proves to be inadequate due to the extent of displacement, protective reactions will be activated. However, in everyday life these reactions often occur concurrently, the perfect example being that of walking.

Biomechanical properties of muscles

The nervous system cannot be considered in isolation from the musculoskeletal system in the control of movement. This section discusses some of the biomechanical properties of muscle which may be affected by neurological impairment.

Different types of skeletal muscle are referred to as slow oxidative (SO), fast glycolytic (FG) and fast oxidative glycolytic (FOG).

The characteristics of these muscles are summarised in Table 2.1.

Table 2.1 The characteristics of different types of skeletal muscles (from Rothwell 1994, Table 3.1, with kind permission)

Fibre type	I	IIA	IIB
	SO	FOG	FG
Motor unit type	Slow (S)	Fast fatigue resistant (FR)	Fast fatiguable (FF)
Fibre diameter	Small	Medium–small	Large

An excess of one type of motor unit gives the muscle its characteristic properties.

Henneman et al (1956), as cited by Rothwell (1994), postulated that the recruitment order of a motor unit depends on the size of its motoneurone. Axons with small action potentials are recruited before those with large action potentials; that is, in the order SO, FOG, FG. Therefore postural muscles, which are predominantly slow oxidative and participate in long-lasting but relatively weak contractions, are recruited before those which are predominantly fast glycolytic and generate large forces but are more readily fatigued. For example, soleus is used almost continuously during walking and standing whereas gastrocnemius comes into action for the more explosive movements of running and jumping.

Muscles may alter their characteristics depending upon their usage (Dietz 1992). FG muscles will readily hypertrophy when they are recruited and overloaded during sustained exercise training, as under normal circumstances, compared to the SO muscles, they are recruited relatively infrequently. Conversely, although the SO muscles may also hypertrophy, this will be to a lesser extent as they already participate to a more maximal degree in postural control (Rothwell 1994).

Changes in function imposed through neurological impairment will produce changes in muscle type. It is the pattern of activity imposed on the muscle, rather than trophic substances coming from the nerve, that regulates the expression of gene coding for proteins responsible for slow contractile properties (Jones & Round 1990). Hufschmidt & Mauritz (1985) proposed that 'elastic and velocity-independent plastic resistance are enhanced in long standing spasticity' and support the hypothesis of secondary tonic transformation of muscles as an additional component of increased muscle tone.

Skeletal muscle may be considered basically in terms of:

- the active contractile element
- a passive series elastic component, which transmits the force of contraction
- a parallel elastic component, which both distributes the forces associated with passive stretch and maintains the relative position of the fibres (Goldspink & Williams 1990).

The elastic compliance of muscle is dependent upon the concentration of collagen, this being a major component of intramuscular connective tissue. This concentration is higher in slow, as opposed to fast, muscle and is reflected in the passive length–tension curves which show that fast muscle has a higher compliance. Therefore, if muscles alter their properties to become predominantly SO, their elastic compliance will be diminished.

The force developed by a muscle is dependent upon the number of cross-bridges which can be engaged between actin and myosin filaments and this in turn depends on the overlap of these filaments in the sarcomere (Goldspink & Williams 1990). The number of sarcomeres in series determines the distance through which a muscle can shorten, and regulation of the sarcomere number is considered to be an adaptation to changes in the functional length of muscle. If a muscle is immobilised in a shortened position, there is a reduction in the number of sarcomeres and, conversely, if the muscle is immobilised in a lengthened position, there is an increase in the number of sarcomeres.

For patients with neurological impairment, muscles may be constrained in either shortened or lengthened positions due to the prevalence of abnormal tone. The resultant decreased or increased number of sarcomeres enables the muscle to develop its maximum tension in the immobilised position. For example, the posterior crural muscle group may become shortened when the patient is dominated by severe extensor spasticity of the lower limbs. There is a loss of sarcomeres and a reduction in muscle fibre length which is accompanied by an increased resistance to passive stretch (Goldspink & Williams 1990). In this way the impaired supraspinal input leads to changes in the mechanical properties of muscle fibres (Dietz 1992). It is postulated that muscle shortening potentiates the stretch reflex and a vicious circle develops whereby spasticity leads to muscle contracture and muscle contracture in turn increases spasticity (Nash et al 1989).

AN APPROACH TO THE ANALYSIS OF POSTURE AND MOVEMENT

This section aims to identify key components relating to the analysis of positions and movement sequences which have been observed and developed from clinical practice. Many of these components are based on the Bobath concept.

Rotation of body segments

Rotation may be described as the coordinated response between flexion and extension in all planes of movement. The importance of rotation in the maintenance of posture and performance of movement is discussed by many authors (Bobath 1990, Galley & Forster 1987, Knott & Voss 1968). Certainly, loss of rotation and arm swing are noticeable aspects of impaired movement, characterised in, for example, the patient with Parkinson's disease (Rogers 1991, Marsden 1984).

This interplay between flexion and extension can be illustrated when observing the development of rolling in children. At birth, the child is predominantly flexed, with some extension at the neck allowing for rotation of the head. Slowly over a period of 3–4 months, the child learns to lift his head when in prone, support on his forearms and, by 6 months, push up on to extended arms, developing extensor activity throughout the body. The initial movements of the child from prone to supine is a crude, gross movement rather than a controlled activity. As the child becomes more confident in pushing up on to extended arms, he begins to look around, and in so doing transfers his weight from side to side. Over-exuberance takes the centre of gravity outside of the base of support and he falls on to his back. This first experience of movement from prone to supine is an illustration of the innate lack of coordination between extension and flexion. Over the succeeding months, rolling from prone to supine and from supine to prone, is refined as a direct integration of extensor and flexor activity. The weight-bearing side actively works against the surface as the body rotates around its axis, providing stability for the movement (Alexander et al 1993). The more intricate skill, of getting from lying into sitting, is only achieved when the child has developed the necessary level of neuromuscular control.

Rotation within the trunk and of the prime movers in the limbs is fundamental for the performance of functional skills such as eating, dressing, writing and walking. Any alteration in the distribution of tone, either excessive flexion or extension, will result in impaired rotation and subsequent impoverishment of movement.

Postural sets

'Postural sets' is a term used by Bobath (1990) to describe adaptations of posture or adjustments which precede and accompany a movement. They can be viewed as anticipatory postural adjustments which occur prior to the disturbance of posture and equilibrium resulting from the movement (Massion 1992).

When considering these responses in relation to activity of the arm, Cordo & Nashner (1982) observed that, with a voluntary arm movement, the leg muscles involved in postural control are activated prior to the prime movers. The duration of the anticipatory postural adjustments increases with the load to be raised by the arm (Lee et al 1987). These authors suggest that the preparatory adjustments are not specifically related to balance control but that they also directly provide additional force for performing the movement. These anticipatory postural adjustments also serve to stabilise the position of segments such as the head, trunk or limbs during movement performance (Massion 1992).

A practical example of this preparation for movement and the control during performance of the movement is in jumping into the deep end as opposed to the shallow end of a swimming pool. When jumping into deep water, contact with the bottom is cushioned by the volume and depth of the water. The legs tend to be held straight as the feet search for the bottom of the pool. Conversely, when jumping into shallow water, the legs remain slightly flexed in preparation for the impact of hitting the bottom. On making contact with the bottom of the pool, the knees give, cushioning the effects of the impact. Providing the individual is aware of the depth of the water, the body is pre-programmed to respond appropriately. However, if an individual jumps into shallow water thinking it to be considerably deeper, then the correct adjustments are not made and injury may result.

There are an infinite number of postural sets relating to both the posture which an individual assumes and the preparatory adjustments made in advance of movement. For example, no one individual will consistently assume or maintain repeatable positions in standing. Equally, the means by which a person attains the standing position will vary according to the starting position and the reason for standing. For any given task from a given position, postural adjustments are considered to be uniform but flexible to change with changing task (Horak et al 1994, Hansen et al 1988).

Key points of control

Key points of control are described as areas of the body from which movement may be most effectively controlled (Edwards 1991). The main key points are identified by Bobath as being both proximal and distal. The proximal key points are the trunk, head, shoulder girdles and pelvis, and the distal key points, the hands and feet. Clinical observation has shown that posture and movement within the trunk may be effectively controlled by manual guidance provided from a central point on a diagonal and rotational plane between the xiphisternum and the T8 vertebra. This is described as the central key point (Edwards 1991). This is one means of assessing stability and alignment within the trunk. Postural adjustment within the trunk may be effectively assessed, in respect of the sagittal, coronal and horizontal planes, from these key points.

A key point from which to influence movement is determined by the ability of the individual to respond to facilitation of movement

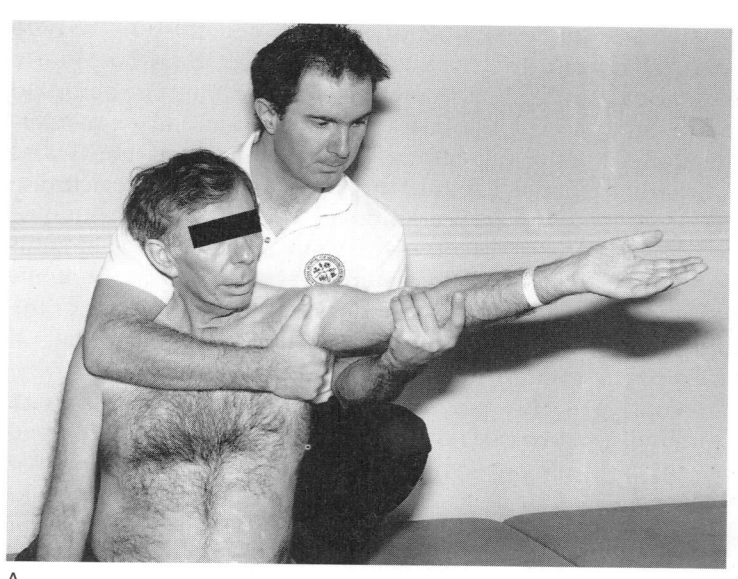

A

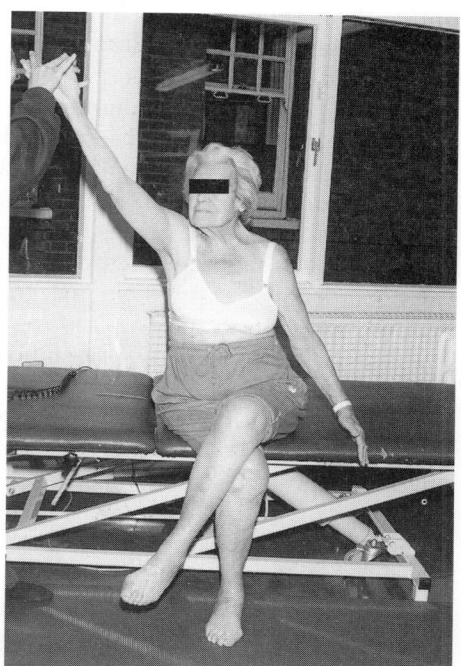

B

Figure 2.3   (A) Proximal key point control. (B) Distal key point control.

(Fig. 2.3A & B). For example, if the therapist facilitates movement using the patient's hand as a key point, there must be adequate postural tone within the trunk to make an appropriate response. If proximal control is lacking, attempts to bring the patient forwards from this key point may traumatise the shoulder joint. It is for this reason that the proximal key points tend to be utilised more frequently to ensure stability within the trunk prior to facilitating movement of the limbs.

Midline – the alignment of body segments

The midline is an abstract reference point against which alignment of the aforementioned key points, particularly the shoulder girdles, pelvis and the central key point can be compared. It may be considered a dividing line that serves as a point of reference for analysing body alignment and movement in either the sagittal, coronal or horizontal planes. Taylor et al (1994) describe the midline as an imaginary line that bisects the body into a right and left sector in the sagittal plane. This definition, which is limited to one plane, enables the physiotherapist to assess and describe body alignment in terms of lateral symmetry when observing the patient from in front or behind. The midline should also be considered as a point of reference in the coronal and transverse planes which provides a means of describing the anteroposterior relationships of body structures and alignment with regard to rotation.

The perception of body orientation in space depends on multisensory evaluation of visual, vestibular and proprioceptive sensory input (Karnath et al 1994). The concept of midline has physiological significance as it seems, at least for the upper limb, that some movements are programmed to occur relative to the midline (Soechting & Flanders 1992).

ANALYSIS OF SPECIFIC POSITIONS

It is useful to analyse positions because it provides a baseline for determining differences which may arise due to pathology. It is important to recognise that very few normal subjects demonstrate the exact characteristics identified in this analysis. Many will show variability such as excessive flexion at the shoulders, an increased lumbar lordosis in supine or a greater degree of lateral rotation in one leg than the other. This variability may ultimately prove to be irrelevant but one may question whether there is a reason for this discrepancy.

The analysis of tonal influences in certain positions may be based on observation of the relationship between the central key point with the proximal key points and the limbs. It can be used to determine the overall influence of extension or flexion in each particular position. This approach to analysis, which is based on clinical observation, enables the therapist to identify the normal characteristics of different postures and to utilise this knowledge to select appropriate treatment positions.

Supine lying

An individual generally adopts a symmetrical position in relation to the supporting surface (Fig. 2.4).

When lying supine, the influence of gravity and the reduction in the level of postural activity result in the shoulder girdles falling posteriorly in relation to the central key point. The ability to accept the base of support will vary considerably, depending upon the level of tonus and biomechanical properties of soft tissue structures.

The upper limbs tend to adopt a position of lateral rotation with some abduction, the amount of which is determined by the individual's inherent level of postural tone. In general, the lower the tonus, the greater the degree of lateral rotation and abduction.

The pelvis tends to tilt posteriorly with increased extension at the hips. The extent of this pelvic movement is determined by the anatomical structure of the individual, in particular the alignment of the pelvis with the lumbar spine and the bulk of the gluteal region. The legs usually adopt a position of lateral rotation with some degree of abduction.

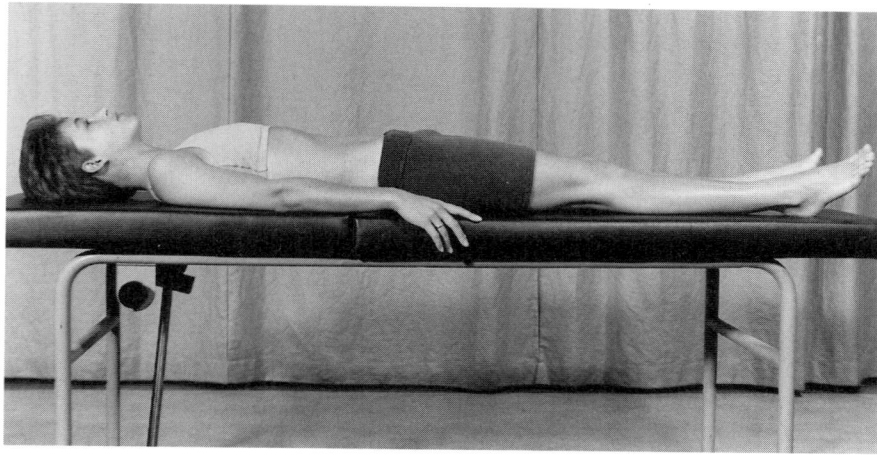

Figure 2.4 Supine lying.

The proximal key points of the shoulder girdles and pelvis are posterior in relation to the central key point which is indicative of this being a position of predominant extension. Movement out of this position demands flexor activity, most commonly observed in conjunction with rotation.

Prone lying

The individual generally adopts a symmetrical position in relation to the supporting surface, but with the head turned laterally (Fig. 2.5).

When prone, the shoulder girdles fall forwards in relation to the central key point. The upper limbs rest in a position of flexion, medial rotation and adduction with the degree of adduction being determined by the amount of flexion.

The pelvis tends to tilt anteriorly, producing a degree of flexion at the hips. The legs are extended, adducted and medially rotated and the feet plantar flexed.

The proximal key points are anterior in relation to the central key point which is indicative of a position of predominant flexion. Movement out of this position requires extensor

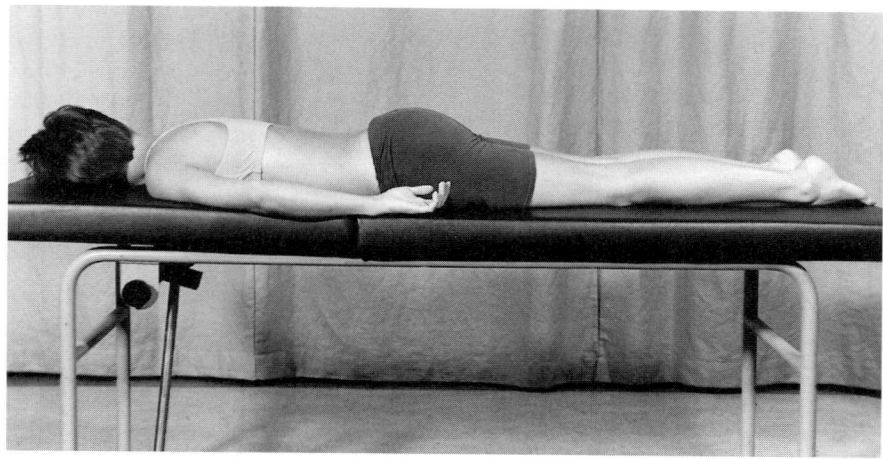

Figure 2.5 Prone lying.

activity with a rotational component determined by the side to which the head is turned.

As prone is a position with a predominant flexor influence, it is not necessarily the position of choice for preventing or correcting flexion contractures, such as those of the hips. Standing, which has a greater influence of extension, may be more effective in managing this problem.

Side-lying

This is a position in which a degree of asymmetry between the two sides of the body is invariably present. Figure 2.6 illustrates one posture which may be adopted by an individual when asked to assume this position.

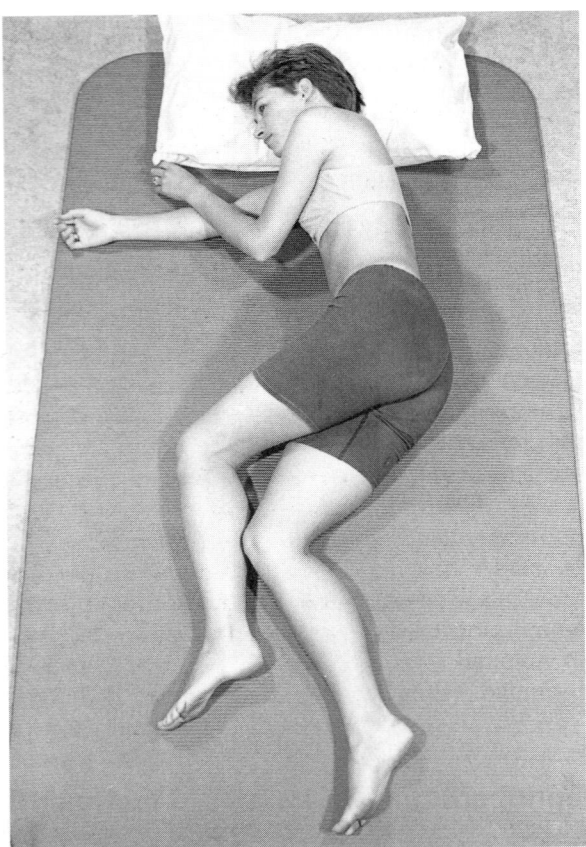

Figure 2.6   Side-lying.

Certain characteristics may be noted. The weight-bearing side of the body is more extended and elongated than the non-weight-bearing side which is side flexed. This position is influenced by the anatomical structure of the individual; the greater the pelvic girth, the greater is the side flexion of the non-weight-bearing side.

There are many variations of the side-lying position. One such variation is bilateral flexion of the legs where the individual takes up a modified foetal position.

The position of the shoulder is determined by the tendency to lie towards prone or supine. Only those with bilateral leg flexion will lie with one side of the body virtually in alignment with the other. People who lie towards supine tend to protract the supporting shoulder whereas those who lie towards prone tend to lie with the supporting shoulder retracted. Accordingly, the degree of trunk rotation varies in respect of the position of the shoulders and their relationship with the pelvis.

The weight-bearing side provides stability, through its acceptance of and interaction with the base of support, to allow for selective movement of the non-weight-bearing side. Impairment resulting in inactivity or inappropriate activity of the weight-bearing side may disrupt or prevent functional movement of the non-weight-bearing side.

This is a position widely used and recommended in the positioning of patients with neurological disability (Bobath 1990, Davies 1994). The relative asymmetry of this position enables 'the break up' of either predominant flexor or extensor spasticity and thereby helps to normalise tone. It is also recommended as a position whereby coordination, postural control and sensory reintegration of the weight-bearing side may be facilitated through functional movement of the non-weight-bearing side.

Sitting

Analysis of this position is complex due to the varying amount and type of support offered. This posture is described in terms of unsupported and supported sitting.

Unsupported sitting with the hips and knees at 90 degrees

Anti-gravity control in unsupported sitting (Fig. 2.7) is recruited primarily through extensor activity at the pelvis and lumbar spine. In the absence of full support this anti-gravity, extensor activity is essential for dynamic maintenance of an upright posture. Consideration of the base of support in relation to the feet is discussed when analysing moving from sitting to standing.

The shoulder girdles are protracted with medial rotation and adduction of the shoulders. This reflects the relative lack of activity required by the upper limbs to maintain this posture.

The position of the pelvis depends upon the degree of upright or slumped sitting assumed by the individual. There is an element of extensor activity observed primarily at the lumbar spine and reflected in the degree of anterior pelvic tilt.

The degree of pelvic tilt influences the position of the lower limbs. It is observed that the starting position affects associated limb movements. With the hips and knees at 90 degrees or more flexion, the greater the anterior tilt, the more pronounced will be the degree of lateral rotation and abduction. However, if the subject is seated on a higher chair with the hips and knees at an angle of less than 90 degrees, an increase in the anterior pelvic tilt tends to produce medial rotation and adduction.

Unsupported sitting is a position predominantly of flexion but with recruitment of extensor activity arising primarily at the pelvis/lumbar spine.

Supported sitting

The amount and type of support offered varies considerably between, for example, a dining chair and a lounge chair. The dining chair is a more rigid structure and therefore most individuals are less likely to relax and depend on it for full support. In many respects, the posture taken up by an individual sitting on a dining chair is no different from that of unsupported sitting. Conversely, the lounge chair, depending upon the degree of comfort, the angle of recline and the provision or otherwise of a head support, affords more support to the individual (Fig. 2.8). The body conforms to the chair with the upper limbs supported forwards of the central key point and the pelvis tilted posteriorly. The arms and legs rest in various and diverse positions. Movement away from this position of full support initially requires flexor activity closely followed by extension to provide the proximal stability essential for the achievement of function such as reaching for a cup or preparing to stand.

Supported sitting in a lounge chair is a position of predominant flexion, there being no necessity to recruit anti-gravity activity, given the extended base of support offered by the chair back and arms.

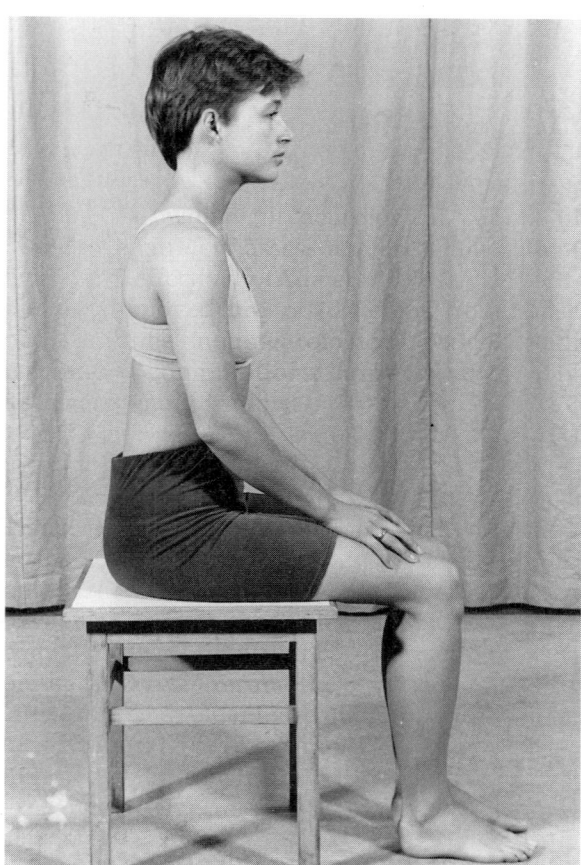

Figure 2.7 Unsupported sitting.

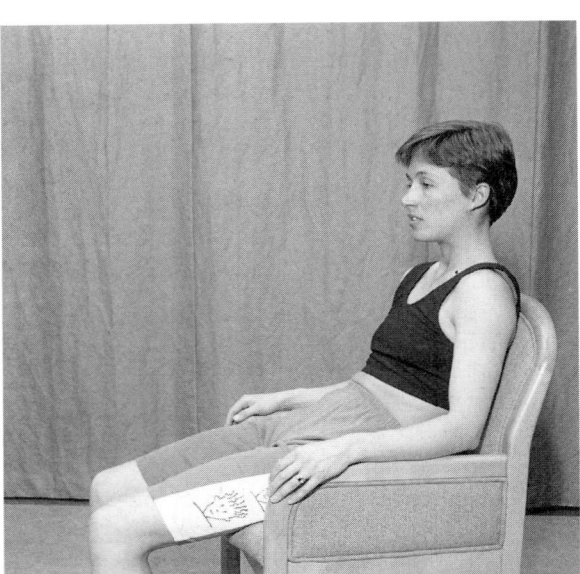

Figure 2.8 Supported sitting.

In contrast, the amount of activity when sitting on a dining chair depends upon the position of the pelvis; the degree of anterior or posterior tilt and whether it is forwards on the edge of the chair or positioned at the back of the chair. The distribution of tone is also dependent on the extent of support. This support is substantially increased if the individual leans forward, resting the arms on a table such as when writing. In this posture there is a marked reduction in the anti-gravity activity within the trunk and pelvis. The size and distribution of the base of support are changed significantly with more weight being taken through the upper limbs, and hence the requirement for dynamic postural stability within the trunk and pelvis is reduced.

Clinical application

This analysis of sitting assists with the planning of treatment interventions. For example, trunk mobilisations may aim to provide a greater or lesser degree of support depending upon the treatment goal. Inhibition of hypertonus by mobilisation of the trunk is more successful if the therapist increases the base of support of the patient by fully supporting him. Alternatively, if the aim of treatment is to increase tonus, less support should be provided by the therapist, thereby facilitating extensor activity within the trunk. This analysis is also relevant to the provision of wheelchairs and the correct positioning of the patient in the chair. The position of the pelvis will have a direct influence on the posture of the lower limbs. Equally, the use of upper limb support, such as a tray attached to a wheelchair, will have a direct effect on trunk and pelvic activity.

Standing

Standing requires extensive anti-gravity activity to sustain the upright position over a relatively small base of support.

Muscle relaxation tends to accentuate the lumbar, thoracic and cervical curvatures and the pelvis tilts anteriorly. This posture may be seen in particularly lethargic individuals and in women in the later stages of pregnancy (Kapandji 1980).

Normal subjects demonstrate flattening of spinal curvatures commensurate with their level of tonus (Fig. 2.9). This is initiated at the level of the pelvis. The anterior tilt of the pelvis is counterbalanced by the activity, primarily of gluteus maximus and the hamstrings, restoring the horizontal alignment of the interspinous line between the anterior superior iliac spine and the posterior superior iliac spine. The abdominal muscles contract in conjunction with the gluteus maximus to flatten the lumbar curvature. From this position the paravertebral muscles can act effectively to pull back the upper lumbar vertebrae and extend the vertebral column (Kapandji 1980).

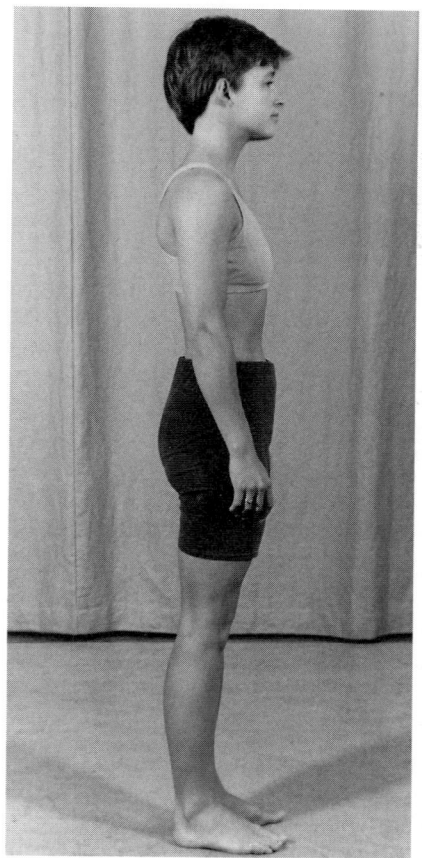

Figure 2.9   Standing.

In standing, the upper limbs adopt a position of medial rotation with the shoulder girdles forwards of the central key point. Providing the centre of gravity remains within the base of support, the upper limbs are not essential for the maintenance of balance. This state of relative inactivity enables freedom of movement of the arms for the performance of functional tasks.

It may be postulated that the position of the pelvis determines the extent of activity at the shoulder girdles and upper limbs. An anterior pelvic tilt introduces an element of flexion at the hips counteracted by increased extensor activity in the trunk, shoulder girdles and upper limbs. A neutral position of the pelvis or a slight posterior tilt produces a more mechanically efficient position as the iliofemoral ligament provides

anterior stability which complements the extensor activity at the hips and pelvis.

Activity within the foot musculature varies according to the size of the base of support. There is less activity in stride standing than when standing with a smaller base of support when the feet are closer together. The constant adjustments by the lower limbs and feet in response to any change in weight distribution serve to maintain the centre of gravity within the supporting surface. For this activity to be effective, adequate mobility within the feet is essential.

In clinical practice it is observed that the majority of patients with abnormal tone affecting the feet lose some and, in severe cases, all of this mobility and as a result their balance in standing is compromised. Unless the problem of immobility of the feet is first addressed, rehabilitation of standing balance will be severely affected.

ANALYSIS OF MOVEMENT SEQUENCES

Although adults may be consistent in their performance, they have the ability to vary the movement patterns used in order to accomplish the task. It is this potential for variability that characterises normality (VanSant 1990a).

Analysis of movement in clinical practice is based primarily on observation and knowledge of what is considered to be within normal limits. The movements of lying to sitting, sitting to standing, and walking are discussed in a clinical perspective to identify certain features of these movement sequences. Although there will be significant variability in these movement sequences depending upon age, gender, body build, the height of the bed and the firmness of the supporting surface, the characteristics described are those which may be considered to be within normal limits.

Moving from supine lying to sitting

Initiation of movements from supine have been discussed in part in the previous analysis of the position of supine lying. The biomechanical effects of the large base of support and low centre of mass demand significant effort on the part of the individual to move away from this position. The movement sequence will differ significantly between sitting up from lying on the floor and sitting up and placing the legs over the side of a bed. For relevance to treatment, it is the latter sequence which will be analysed. An assumption is made that the height of the bed is such that the individual can sit with the hips and knees at 90 degrees on completion of the movement and the surface of the bed is firm.

As with all movement, the speed at which the sequence is carried out influences the coordination and degree of effort entailed. Young agile individuals will move more quickly and fluently than those of an older age group. The slower the speed at which the movement is carried out, the greater the effort required and the greater the likelihood of dependence on the arms.

How is this movement from lying initiated? Bobath (1990) states that turning commences with the upper part of the body. It is observed that the majority of individuals flex forwards at the head and shoulders with a varying degrees of rotation towards the side to which they are moving. However, others may initiate the movement with propulsion from the leg opposite to the side to which they are moving. Here the initial movement is one of flexion prior to pushing through the limb to generate the movement. The movement of the leg is then followed almost simultaneously by flexion of the head and trunk.

The fulcrum of movement is at the pelvis. As the individual brings the upper trunk forwards off the bed, the legs move towards the side of the bed. As the subject pivots over the pelvis to sit with the legs over the side of the bed, the weight-bearing side is elongated with contralateral side flexion of the opposite side of the trunk. During the course of the movement, the pelvis tends to be in a position of posterior tilt, but this will vary depending on the strength and control of the abdominals. Having attained this end position, the trunk is then realigned with more equal weight-bearing over the ischial tuberosities and the pelvis moving towards a position of anterior tilt.

To move from lying into sitting requires that the abdominal muscles move or hold the weight of the trunk against the pull of gravity and control the speed at which it moves (Davies 1990). The strength and power of the abdominals determine the ease at which the movement is accomplished. Many young adults with good abdominal control move from lying to sitting in one fluid movement using minimal, if any, arm support. On the other hand, people of an older age group, with weaker abdominals, rely increasingly on their arms to assist in the movement sequence.

Clinical application

In clinical practice, impairment of this sequence of events is observed in a wide variety of cases. For example, in patients following surgery to the lumbar spine, pain inhibits movement and there is a loss of flexibility at the operation site. This disturbs the balance of activity and grading of movement within the trunk, most noticeably, through the relative inactivity of the abdominals. Characteristically, these patients break up the movement sequence into specific components with an absence of rotation to minimise movement at the operation site. They first turn on to their side, often initiating the movement with one or both legs. They then move the legs over the side of the bed at virtually the same moment as they push up on their arms with little or no interplay within the trunk and pelvis as described above. The psoas muscle seems to be more active, compensating for the inhibition of the abdominals, in that the pelvis is held in a position of anterior tilt throughout the movement. A further illustration of the relationship between abdominal control and arm support is in people with a high thoracic cord lesion with paralysis of the abdominals. They are only able to attain the sitting position independently by means of a forced ballistic type movement of the upper limbs to initiate movement out of supine, and arm support to maintain themselves once in sitting.

Moving from sitting to standing

Standing from sitting is an activity which is performed frequently in daily life. In a review of the literature, Kerr et al (1991) categorised the research relating to rising from a chair into four major areas:

- biomechanical investigations
- kinematic studies
- investigations of muscle activity
- general studies of the functional aspects of seating for disabled people.

Many variables have been shown to influence getting up from a chair. These include the height of the chair, use of the arms, speed of movement, the direction of movement, placement of the feet and the age and sex of the individual. An example of the complexity of analysis of this movement sequence may be found in a study which demonstrated that in a sample of 10 young adults, five different arm patterns, three different head and trunk patterns and three different leg patterns were found to occur (Francis et al 1988, as cited by VanSant 1990b).

While producing definitive numerical data on moments of force generated at the joints and muscles of the lower extremity during rising, many of the biomechanical studies have demonstrated substantial complexity in study design, involving highly sophisticated technical equipment and considerable manipulation of subjects. This may preclude the application of such procedures to large samples of disabled subjects (Kerr et al 1991). The following analysis discusses the key components of sitting to standing and their significance to clinical practice.

The initial base of support is relatively large and includes the surface area of the chair with which the body is in contact, the floor area within the base of the chair and the area within and posterior to the foot position. A key component of this movement is the transference of weight from a relatively large base of support to one which is significantly smaller – the feet alone.

Many studies identify two distinct phases in moving from sitting into standing, those of initial forward trunk lean and upward extension (Schenkman et al 1990, Nuzik et al 1986).

On clinical observation, the movement forwards of the trunk varies. In some individuals the trunk moves forwards on the pelvis prior to the pelvis tilting anteriorly, whereas in others the trunk is held more rigidly and the trunk and pelvis move forwards simultaneously. This trunk and pelvic movement enables the weight to be transferred forwards over the feet. It may also be necessary for the individual to move the buttocks forwards, depending upon the initial position in the chair.

As the trunk and pelvis move forwards, the head extends and the knees move forwards over the feet so as to facilitate the transference of weight during upward extension. The knees move forwards over the feet producing dorsiflexion at the ankle, the maximum range of dorsiflexion occurring as the buttocks are lifted from the seat of the chair. The legs extend as the individual moves into the upright position with a decreasing amount of activity in quadriceps as the knee angle approaches zero (Schuldt et al 1983). The anterior tilt of the pelvis is at its maximum as the buttocks are lifted off the chair and reduces as the sequence progresses, with extension of the hips on completion of the movement. Similarly, the position of the head adjusts relative to the trunk throughout the sequence, moving from a more extended position at the beginning of the movement to one of relative flexion.

Clinical application

Many people with neurological disability have difficulty with this complex movement sequence. Treatment strategies vary depending on the different reasons for the problem. Such problems may include restricted joint range at the foot and ankle or abnormal tone within the trunk and pelvis, both of which may preclude or impair the initial forward lean.

In clinical practice, the height of the chair or plinth is seen to be a critical factor in performance of the activity. Increasing seat height and the use of arms decreases muscle and joint forces at the hips and knees (Burdett et al 1985, Arborelius et al 1992) and also decreases energy expenditure (Didier et al 1993). Many patients benefit from first practising the movement from a higher seat and gradually reducing the height as they become more proficient.

Walking

The purpose of this analysis is to consider aspects of normal gait in relationship to pathological gait of neurological origin. Throughout this section the terms 'walking' and 'gait' are used interchangeably although Whittle (1991) defines gait as the manner or style of walking rather than the walking process itself. There are many definitions of gait, which include:

- a series of controlled falls (Rose et al 1982)
- a method of locomotion involving the use of the two legs, alternately, to provide both support and propulsion, at least one foot being in contact with the ground at all times (Whittle 1991)
- a highly coordinated series of events in which balance is being constantly challenged and regained continuously (Galley & Forster 1987).

There are numerous studies which have described aspects of gait in detail. These include Saunders et al (1953), Murray et al (1964) and Whittle (1991). Saunders et al (1953) identified the primary determinants of human locomotion in respect of the behaviour of the centre of gravity of the body. In normal level walking, this follows a smooth, regular sinusoidal curve in the plane of progression which enables the human body to conserve energy. Murray et al (1964) recorded the displacements associated with locomotion and established the ranges of normal values for many components of the walking cycle. These were considered in respect of the speed and timing of gait and stride dimensions; sagittal rotation of the pelvis, hip, knee and ankle and vertical, lateral and forward movement of the trunk and the transverse rotation of the pelvis and thorax.

The gait cycle

The gait cycle is the time interval between two successive occurrences of one of the repetitive events of walking (Whittle 1991). The cycle comprises two component parts, the stance and swing phases. The stance phase is the portion of the cycle where the foot is in contact with the floor and the swing phase is where the leg is off the ground moving forwards to take a step. There are two periods during the cycle when both feet are in contact with the ground. The proportion as a percentage of the walking cycle is 60% stance and 40% swing. The durations of the supportive phases of the walking cycle decrease with increased walking speeds (Smidt 1990).

Common characteristics of gait

Step and stride length. The step length is the distance between successive points of floor-to-floor contact of alternate feet; the stride length is the linear distance between successive points of floor-to-floor contact of the same foot. The step and stride length are related to the height of the individual, shorter subjects taking shorter steps and taller subjects longer steps, and to age, subjects over 60 having a shorter step length than those of a younger age group (Murray et al 1964).

The stride width or walking base. This is the side-to-side distance between the line of the two feet, usually measured at the midpoint of the heel (Whittle 1991). It is directly related to the lateral displacement of the pelvis produced by the horizontal shift of the pelvis or relative adduction of the hip (Saunders et al 1953). This allows the stride width to remain within the pelvic circumference throughout the gait cycle, and Murray et al (1964) observed that the midpoint of one foot may even cross over the other. The stride width is not related to age or height nor does it correlate significantly with foot length, bi-acromial or bi-iliac measures (Murray et al 1964). Murray et al (1964) identified an increase in the foot angle (outward placement) of subjects over 60 years of age and suggested

Table 2.2 Normal ranges for gait parameters

Approximate range (95%) limits for general gait parameters in free-speed walking by normal *female* subjects of different ages (reproduced from Whittle 1991 with kind permission)

Age (years)	Cadence (steps/min)	Stride length (m)	Velocity (m/s)
13–14	103–150	0.99–1.55	0.90–1.62
15–17	100–144	1.03–1.57	0.92–1.64
18–49	98–138	1.06–1.58`	0.94–1.66
50–64	97–137	1.04–1.56	0.91–1.63
65–80	96–136	0.94–1.46	0.80–1.52

Approximate range (95%) limits for general gait parameters in free-speed walking by normal *male* subjects of different ages

Age (years)	Cadence (steps/min)	Stride length (m)	Velocity (m/s)
13–14	100–149	1.06–1.64	0.95–1.67
15–17	96–142	1.15–1.75	1.03–1.75
18–49	91–135	1.25–1.85	1.10–1.82
50–64	82–126	1.22–1.82	0.96–1.68
65–80	81–125	1.11–1.71	0.81–1.61

this to be their means of achieving additional lateral stability as the neuromuscular system begins to decline. The foot angle is also increased at slower walking speeds. An increase in the stride width is a notable feature in people with impaired balance. The degree to which it occurs depends on the extent of the damage to the CNS.

Cadence and velocity. The cadence is the number of steps taken in a given time and the velocity of walking is the distance covered in a given time. The normal ranges for gait parameters are given in Table 2.2.

Greater velocities of locomotion are achieved by the lengthening of the stride rather than by an increase in cadence (Saunders et al 1953) and this depends to a great extent on the functional objective. For example, strolling along the promenade is more leisurely than walking quickly knowing one is late for an appointment. Balance modification is directly related to speed; enforced reduction in the natural cadence will require increased postural adaptation. The muscle activity required to step forwards differs in accordance with the speed of movement. For example, a step from a standing position requires

greater hip flexor activity than a step taken as part of the gait cycle at the individual's natural cadence. Similarly, the initiation of a step from a standing position produces a backward displacement of the body to counter the extended lever anteriorly, whereas the body is more upright in the natural gait cycle. These are important considerations for the physiotherapist when re-educating gait. In many instances, treatment of necessity takes the form of re-education of the component parts, but it must be appreciated that fluidity and economy of movement are dependent upon the many factors associated with the gait cycle, not least cadence and speed.

Rotation. The pelvis and thorax rotate simultaneously in the transverse plane during each cycle of gait, the pelvis and shoulders rotating in opposite directions. Murray (1967) suggested that one of the functions of arm swing is to counteract excessive trunk rotation in the transverse plane. Maximum rotation occurs at the time of heel contact and the greater the speed, the greater the degree of rotation and subsequent arm swing. The enhanced amplitude of rotation is achieved mainly by increased shoulder extension on the backward end of the arm swing (Murray 1967). There is a decreased amplitude of rotation in the elderly which may be related to a more flexed posture (Elble et al 1991).

With increasing speed, either walking as quickly as possible or when running, the arm swing becomes more vigorous to help in both generating pace and in maintaining balance. An example is that of a sprinter in action. As the speed increases, so to does the pumping action of the arms combined with increased extension of the thoracic spine, perfectly illustrated as the athlete crosses the finishing line.

Disability resulting in an imbalance of the inter-reaction between flexor and extensor activity may impair rotation. An example of this is illustrated in the person with Parkinson's disease (Rogers 1991). The main observable features are those of increased flexion and lack of rotation with the characteristic shuffling gait. In the past, therapists were taught to work for improved rotation by facilitating arm swing.

Little attention was paid to the inherent loss of extensor activity. It is now widely accepted in clinical practice that rotation can only be facilitated on the basis of appropriate inter-reaction between flexion and extension within the trunk. Hence, in this instance, improving extension must occur before rotation is possible.

Vertical displacement. This occurs twice during the gait cycle and is approximately 50 mm (Whittle 1991). The summit of these oscillations occurs during the middle of stance phase and the centre of gravity falls to its lowest level during double stance when both feet are in contact with the ground (Saunders et al 1953). The magnitude of the vertical excursion cor-relates with the length of stride because when the step lengths are longer the lower limbs are more obliquely situated (Murray et al 1964). This characteristic ascent and descent of the body mass is altered in patients with hemiplegia. The movement is dependent upon sufficient muscle activity to maintain stability of the pelvis and hip joint during stance phase. Patients with hemiplegia often have inadequate or inappro-priate activity to provide this stability. This gives rise to the characteristic unilateral Trendelenburg gait whereby the vertical displacement occurs only during stance phase of the unaffected leg (Wagenaar & Beek 1992).

Joint range and muscle activity associated with gait

The joint angles of the lower limbs and the typical muscle activity which occurs during gait are illustrated in Figures 2.10 and 2.11.

The foot and ankle

Efficient transfer of weight from one leg to the other is partly dependent upon the ability of the feet to respond and adjust effectively to the base of support, be it a firm surface or rough ground. The ankle and intrinsic foot musculature make constant adjustments to adapt appropriately to provide the dynamic stability, essential for this acceptance of, and movement over, the base of support. The mobility of the foot and ankle is

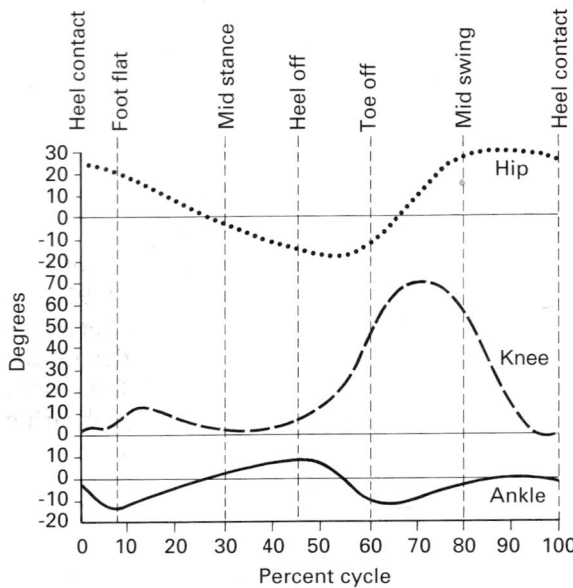

Figure 2.10 Angles during a single gait cycle (reproduced from Whittle 1991 with kind permission).

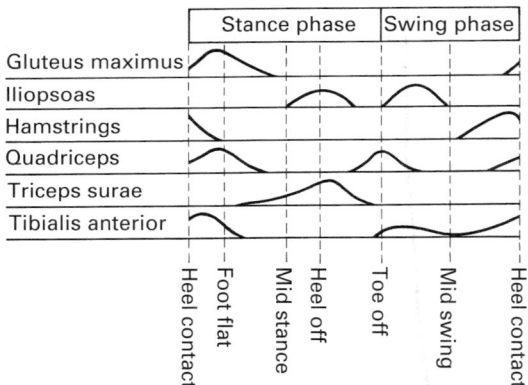

Figure 2.11 Typical activity of major muscles during the gait cycle (reproduced from Whittle 1991 with kind permission).

therefore essential for effective transfer of weight. The total range of dorsiflexion and plantar flexion varies between about 20 and 35 degrees. Any restriction in this mobility will necessitate compensatory adjustments particu-larly of the knee (Saunders et al 1953).

The muscle action occurring at the ankle is primarily that of dorsiflexion controlling the placing of the foot on the supporting surface following heel strike and plantar flexion to propel the body forwards (Winter 1987, Kameyama et al 1990).

The knee

The range of movement at the knees is between approximately 70 degrees during the swing phase and full extension at the moment of heel strike and in mid-stance (Whittle 1991). In normal locomotion, the body moves forwards over the leg while the knee joint is flexed, the knee extending during stance and then once more flexing to carry the non-weight-bearing limb forwards. Saunders et al (1953) refer to the knee being 'locked in extension' during heel strike and during mid-stance but, on clinical observation, it would seem that this only occurs with pathology.

The hip

Movement at the hip is between approximately 30 degrees flexion and 20 degrees extension (Whittle 1991). The predominant activity during stance phase is that of extension and abduction as the body moves forwards over the supporting foot. Prior to initiation of swing phase, the extended position at the hips is dependent upon the ability of the hip flexors to lengthen, thereby allowing this transference of weight. During swing phase, the primary activity is again that of extension acting as a deceleration force as the leg moves forwards under its own momentum prior to heel strike (Whittle 1991). The leg initially flexes, with adduction and medial rotation at the hips. As the knee begins to extend in preparation for heel contact, the leg becomes more laterally rotated.

The pelvis

The pelvis provides the dynamic stability essential for coordinating the activity of the lower limbs and the control and alignment of the trunk. Many authors refer to rotation of the pelvis although it may be more appropriate, as the pelvis is a rigid structure, to consider rotation in relation to the hips and the thoracolumbar spine. Palpating the anterior superior iliac spines while walking at one's natural pace, reveals little discernible movement, the rotational movement being approximately 4 degrees on either side of the central axis, the lateral movement approximately 5 degrees (Saunders et al 1953) and the anterior/posterior movement approximately 3 degrees (Murray et al 1964).

As the body moves forwards over the supporting leg, the pelvis maintains its stability predominantly through the action of gluteus maximus and medius. The maintenance of a neutral or slight posterior tilt of the pelvis is also determined by this activity.

Neural control

Locomotion, like many postural reactions, does not require control by the cerebral cortex; it is managed by subcortical and spinal centres, which are subject to cortical intervention (Brooks 1986). Walking may therefore be considered to be an automatic function. The importance of this cannot be overestimated in rehabilitation. For normal subjects, walking is goal-oriented and automatic with no consideration given to the component parts necessary to propel them on their way. In contrast, many patients with neurological impairment may have to consider every aspect of movement in walking. Conscious thought of how to put one foot forward in front of the other and maintain balance in order to achieve a functional goal is both physically and mentally demanding. If patients are to walk functionally and for pleasure, their walking must be safe, automatic and not require too great an expenditure of energy (Davies 1990).

This analysis of gait is largely based on the individual walking over even ground and in a straight line. This is somewhat inconsistent with everyday life. Walking over uneven ground, up or down inclines, avoiding objects, climbing stairs, walking backwards or sideways will all produce appropriate adaptations in response to these changes in demand and of the environment. From a functional perspective, consideration must also be given to the purpose of the movement: walking with the intention of picking up an object from the floor; walking to straighten a picture on the wall; or walking whilst carrying a tray with several pints of beer towards a table in a crowded pub. Each of these functional objectives adds additional considerations to the analysis of gait and to rehabilitation following neurological damage.

Summary

In summary, gait is an holistic motor goal of enormous complexity. There is only partial agreement between investigators as to what is the 'normal' pattern of muscle usage during gait (Whittle 1991). It is an automatic function whereby there is continual adaptation of postural tone in response to the constantly changing base of support. Any impairment, particularly of the trunk, pelvis or lower limbs, may produce compensatory strategies, thereby disturbing the rhythm and economy of movement.

Upper limb function

Selective movement of the upper limb is dependent upon, not only normal neuromuscular innervation of the muscles of the arm but also that of the musculature of the shoulder girdle, trunk and legs. The shoulder has been described as being the most mobile joint of the body, being dependent primarily on muscle activity for its stability (Lippitt & Matsen 1993). Following neurological impairment, weakness and abnormal tonus result in impaired coordination of movement of the shoulder girdle musculature. This has a devastating effect on the glenohumeral joint, which is so dependent on its musculature for stability. It is for this reason that it is so vulnerable to trauma.

In order to fully understand the functional problems which occur as a result of neurological impairment, it is first important to review the anatomy of the shoulder girdle. For this purpose, the shoulder mechanism is best considered in the context of thoracoscapular–humeral arti-

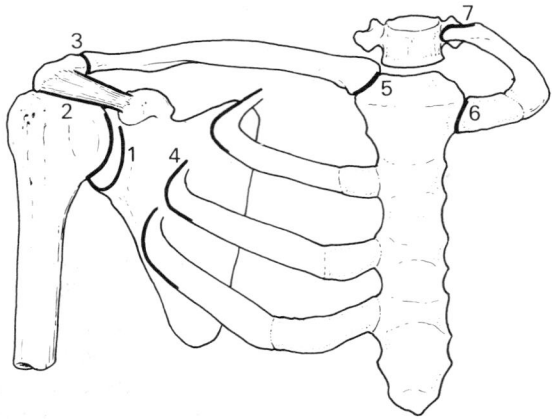

Figure 2.12 Composite drawing of the shoulder girdle (reproduced from Cailliet 1980 with kind permission). Key: 1 = glenohumeral; 2 = suprahumeral; 3 = acromioclavicular; 4 = scapulocostal; 5 = sternoclavicular; 6 = costosternal; 7 = costovertebral.

culation. There are seven joints which provide this articulation (Fig. 2.12):

- glenohumeral
- suprahumeral (a functional joint as opposed to a true articulation)
- acromioclavicular
- scapulocostal
- sternoclavicular
- costosternal
- costovertebral.

Relationship between shoulder girdle structures

Each joint is dependent on the others for the stability and control required in the performance of selective movement.

The angular alignment of the glenoid fossa and its resultant position in relation to the head of humerus, provides a degree of stability described by Basmajian (1979) as 'the locking mechanism' of the shoulder.

The positioning of the scapula is of importance in providing the degree of stability described by Basmajian. In normal subjects, if the arm is slightly abducted and then displaced downwards, there is greater laxity at the glenohumeral joint than when this force is applied with the arm close in to the side of the body. Conversely, if the scapula rests in a more medially rotated position around the chest wall, this produces an increased range of abduction at the glenohumeral joint with the potential for instability in the same way as that described above.

Prevost et al (1987) dispute Basmajian's description of the scapula position in producing 'a locking mechanism'. In their study of 50 subjects following cerebrovascular accident (CVA), they found that there was a greater degree of downward facing of the glenoid fossa in the non-affected arm of these subjects than in the affected arm. They concluded that 'the glenoid fossa has a downward orientation in most normal shoulders and that Basmajian's generalisation that the normal angle faces upward and the suggestion of a 'locking mechanism' should be questioned'.

It may be hypothesised that following CVA the sound side becomes stronger to compensate for the impaired movement of the affected side. On observation, it seems that the greater the development of the shoulder girdle musculature, the greater the degree of medial rotation of the scapula.

Functional movement of the upper limb is also dependent upon thoracic joint motion. Increased thoracic mobility in younger subjects is related to a large range of arm elevation, whereas an increased kyphosis in older subjects is related to a reduced range of arm elevation (Crawford & Jull 1993). O'Gorman & Jull (1987) also revealed significant changes in the angle of kyphosis after the fifth decade and that the range of thoracic spine movement decreased with age. This relationship between thoracic and glenohumeral movement is of significance when treating patients who are wheelchair dependent. The constant adoption of a flexed posture will consequently reduce extensor activity within the trunk.

When sitting or standing, anti-gravity muscle activity is recruited primarily in the trunk, pelvis and lower limbs; the shoulder girdles being relatively inactive in the maintenance of balance. This anti-gravity activity is seen to be essential in the provision of proximal stability for the performance of upper limb function.

Prehension/reaching and grasping

A prehensile act can be considered as two coordinated functional components that allow the hand to eventually establish the required contact with the object for manipulation to ensue.

The *transport component* is responsible for bringing the hand/wrist system into the vicinity of the object to be grasped, and the *grasp component* is responsible for the formation of the grip (Bootsma et al 1994). The transport component is that of a high-velocity, ballistic movement, involving primarily the proximal musculature of the shoulder and elbow to place the hand in the correct spatial location. The grasp component, the low-velocity phase, involves the musculature of the hand and forearm and serves to:

- orientate the hand and fingers to the structural characteristics of the object
- ready the hand by forming an appropriate grasping shape
- capture the object by closing the fingers about it (Marteniuk et al 1990).

These components occur at the same time and are thought to be independently programmed processes with visuomotor links (Jeannerod 1984). The theory of independence of the transport and grasp components is strengthened by the different times at which they develop (Rosenbaum 1991, Gordon 1994), the fact that each can be solely affected by brain insult (Jeannerod 1994) and the different reaction times of the two components to a perturbation (Jeannerod et al 1991).

Inevitably the two components must be coordinated in some way in that the hand must open before contact with the object if prehension is to be achieved (Marteniuk et al 1990). This coordination is felt to be task specific, the exact temporal relationship between the two depending on the requirements of the task (Wier 1994, Marteniuk et al 1990, van Vliet 1993).

The velocity of the transport component is asymmetrical, there being a sharp rise to its peak and then a less-steep deceleration. There is a break point in the deceleration after approximately 70–80% of the movement where the velocity becomes constant.

The grasp component occurs at the same time as the transport component. The grip size rapidly increases to a maximum aperture, the fingers then flex and the grip size decreases to match the size of the object. The finger grip opens wider than required so that the index finger can turn around the object to achieve the proper orientation of the grip. The index finger seems to contribute most to the grip formation with the thumb position remaining constant (Jeannerod 1984).

Prehension is influenced by many factors. These include:

- vision (Jeannerod 1984, Marteniuk et al 1990)
- proprioception (Gentilucci et al 1994, Jeannerod 1984)
- touch (Wier 1994)
- object properties relating to:
  - substance: size and width (Jeannerod 1984, Bootsma et al 1994, Marteniuk et al 1987)
  - structure: weight, texture and fragility (Wier 1994, Marteniuk et al 1987)
- function (van Vliet 1993, Ada et al 1994).

In the context of re-education of upper limb function it is important to take these factors into account. Retraining should be functional, as information about the environment and the task appears to influence movement organisation (van Vliet 1993). The postural adjustments accompanying reaching and grasping, either in sitting (Moore et al 1992) or standing (Lee 1980, Horak et al 1984, Freidli et al 1984) must also be addressed (Shepherd 1992). Brain-damaged patients may have difficulty eliciting any muscle activity in the early stages (Ada et al 1994, Shepherd 1992) or in controlling that activity in the presence of increased tone.

Compensatory motor patterns may emerge as a result of several factors which include:

- the effects of the lesion
- the mechanical characteristics of the musculoskeletal linkage
- the environment in which the action is performed (Shepherd 1992).

These must be considered in respect of positioning and appropriate treatment strategies to modify the demands placed upon the neuromuscular system when attempting to re-educate prehension.

CONCLUSION

Analysis of 'normal movement' is recognised as an essential prerequisite for the assessment of patients with impairment of movement. It is this analysis that provides the basis for the problem-solving approach to treatment. Improved understanding and awareness of movement enables the therapist to identify how a posture or movement differs from the normal and why an individual may have difficulty with functional skills.

It is inappropriate to imply that individuals must move or take up positions in a certain way to be considered normal. People with physical disability resent the implication that they are in some way abnormal merely because, through necessity, they use compensatory strategies and no longer function in the way they did before the onset of their disability.

Subsequent chapters will use this analysis in determining appropriate treatment strategies which may be adopted in the management of patients with neurological disability.

REFERENCES

Ada L, Canning C, Carr J, Kilbreath S, Shepherd R 1994 Task-specific training of reaching and manipulation. In: Bennett K, Castiello U (eds) Insights into reach and grasp movement. Elsevier Science, London

Alexander R, Boehme R, Cupps B 1993 Normal development of functional motor skills. Therapy Skill Builders, Arizona

Altman J, Kien J 1993 Many neurones make light work? New Scientist 139(1885): 34–38

Arborelius U, Wretenberg P, Lindberg F 1992 The effects of arm rests and high seat heights on lower-limb joint load and muscular activity during sitting and rising. Ergonomics 35(11): 1377–1391

Basmajian V J 1979 Muscles alive: their function revealed by electromyography, 4th edn. Williams & Wilkins, London

Bernstein N 1967 The co-ordination and regulation of movements. Pergamon, Oxford

Bobath B 1990 Adult hemiplegia: evaluation and treatment, 3rd edn. Heinemann Medical Books, London

Bootsma R, Marteniuk R, MacKenzie C, Zaal F 1994 The speed accuracy trade-off in manual prehension: effects of movement amplitude, object size and object width on kinematic characteristics. Experimental Brain Research 98: 535–541

Brooks V 1986 The neural basis of motor control. Oxford University Press, Oxford

Bryce J 1989 Lecture: the Bobath concept. International Bobath Tutors' Meeting, Nijmegen, Holland

Burdett R, Habasevich R, Pisciotta J, Simon S 1985 Biomechanical comparison of rising from two types of chairs. Physical Therapy 65(8): 1177–1183

Cailliet R 1980 The shoulder in hemiplegia, 5th edn. F A Davis, Philadelphia

Carr J H, Shepherd R B 1986 Motor training following stroke. In: Banks M (ed) Stroke. Churchill Livingstone, London

Cordo P J, Nashner L M 1982 Properties of postural adjustments associated with rapid arm movements. Journal of Neurophysiology 47: 287–302

Crawford H J, Jull G A 1993 The influence of thoracic posture and movement on range of arm elevation. Physiotherapy Theory and Practice 9(3): 143–148

Davidoff R A 1992 Skeletal muscle tone and the misunderstood stretch reflex. Neurology 42: 951–963

Davies P M 1985 Steps to follow: a guide to the treatment of adult hemiplegia. Springer-Verlag, Berlin

Davies P M 1990 Right in the middle. Springer-Verlag, Berlin

Davies P M 1994 Starting again: early rehabilitation after traumatic brain injury or other severe brain lesions. Springer-Verlag, London

Didier J, Mourey F, Brondel L, Marcer I, Milan C, Casillas J, Verges B, Winsland J 1993 The energetic cost of some daily activities: a comparison in a young and old population. Age and Ageing 22: 90–96

Diener H-C, Dichgans J, Guschlbauer B, Bacher M, Rapp H, Klockgether T 1992 The coordination of posture and voluntary movement in patients with cerebellar dysfunction. Movement Disorders 7(1): 14–17

Diener H-C, Dichgans J, Guschlbauer B, Bacher M, Rapp H, Langenbach P 1990 Associated postural adjustments with body movements in normal subjects and patients with parkinsonism and cerebellar disease. Revue Neurologique (Paris) 146: 555–563

Dietz V 1992 Human neuronal control of automatic functional movements: interaction between central programs and afferent input. Physiological Reviews 72(1): 33–69

Edwards S 1991 The incomplete spinal lesion. In: Bromley I (ed) Tetraplegia and paraplegia: a guide for physiotherapists. Churchill Livingstone, Edinburgh

Elble R J, Sienko Thomas S, Higgins C, Colliver J 1991 Stride-dependent changes in gait of older people. Journal of Neurology 238: 1–5

Friedli W, Hallett M, Simon S 1984 Postural adjustments associated with rapid voluntary arm movements 1. Electromyographic data. Journal of Neurology, Neurosurgery and Psychiatry 47: 611–622

Galley P M, Forster A L 1987 Human movement: an introductory text for physiotherapy students, 2nd edn. Churchill Livingstone, London

Gentilucci M, Toni I, Chieffi S, Pavesi G 1994 The role of proprioception in the control of prehension movements: a kinematic study in a peripherally deafferented patient and in normal subjects. Experimental Brain Research 99: 483–500

Goldspink G, Williams P 1990 Muscle fibre and connective tissue changes associated with use and disuse. In: Ada L, Canning C (eds) Key issues in neurological physiotherapy: physiotherapy foundations for practice. Butterworth-Heinemann, Oxford

Gordon J 1994 The development of the reach to grasp movement. In: Bennett K, Castiello U (eds) Insights into reach and grasp movement. Elsevier Science, London

Haggard P, Jenner J, Wing A 1994 Coordination of aimed movements in a case of unilateral cerebellar damage. Neuropsychologia 32(7): 827–846

Hansen P, Woollacott M, Debu B 1988 Postural responses to changing task conditions. Experimental Brain Research 73: 627–636

Horak F, Esselman P, Anderson M, Lynch M 1984 The effects of movement velocity, mass displaced and task certainty on associated postural adjustments made by normal and hemiplegic individuals. Journal of Neurology, Neurosurgery and Psychiatry 47: 1020–1028

Horak F, Shupert C, Dietz V, Horstmann G 1994 Vestibular and somatosensory contributions to responses to head and body displacements in stance. Experimental Brain Research 100: 93–106

Hufschmidt A, Mauritz K-H 1985 Chronic transformation of muscle in spasticity: a peripheral contribution to increased muscle tone. Journal of Neurology, Neurosurgery and Psychiatry 48: 676–685

Jeannerod M 1984 The timing of natural prehension movements. Journal of Motor Behaviour 16(3): 235–254

Jeannerod M 1994 Object orientated action. In: Bennett K, Castiello U (eds). Insights into reach and grasp movement. Elsevier Science, London

Jeannerod M, Paulignan Y, MacKenzie C, Marteniuk R 1991 Parallel visuomotor processing in human prehension movements. Experimental Brain Research Suppl. 16: 27–44

Jones D A, Round J M 1990 Histochemistry, contractile properties and motor control. In: (eds) Skeletal muscle in health and disease: a textbook of muscle physiology. Manchester University Press, Manchester

Kameyama O, Ogawa R, Okamoto T, Kumamoto M 1990 Electric discharge patterns of ankle muscles during the normal gait cycle. Archives of Physical Medicine and Rehabilitation 71: 969–974

Kapandji I A 1980 The physiology of joints. Volume 3 The trunk and the vertebral column. Churchill Livingstone, London

Karnath H-O, Sievering D, Fetter M 1994 The interactive contribution of neck muscle proprioception and vestibular stimulation to subjective 'straight-ahead' orientation in man. Experimental Brain Research 101: 140–146

Keele S W 1968 Movement control in skilled motor performance. Psychological Bulletin 70: 387–403

Kerr K M, White J A, Mollan R, Baird H E 1991 Rising from a chair: a review of the literature. Physiotherapy 77(1): 15–19

Knott M, Voss D 1968 Proprioceptive neuromuscular facilitation. Harper & Row, New York

Lee W 1980 Anticipatory control of posture and task muscles during rapid arm flexion. Journal of Motor Behaviour 12(3): 185–196

Lee W A, Buchanan T S, Rogers M W 1987 Affect of arm acceleration and behavioural conditions on the organisation of postural adjustments during arm flexion. Experimental Brain Research 66: 257–270

Lippitt S, Matsen F 1993 Mechanisms of glenohumeral joint stability. Clinical Orthopaedics and Related Research 291: 20–28

Lynch M, Grisogono V 1991 Strokes and head injuries. John Murray, London

Marsden C D 1982 The mysterious motor function of the basal ganglia: the Robert Wartenberg lecture. Neurology 32: 514–539

Marsden C D 1984 Motor disorders in basal ganglia disease. Human Neurobiology 2: 245–250

Marteniuk R, Leavitt J, MacKenzie C, Athenes S 1990 Functional relationships between grasp and transport components in a prehension task. Human Movement Science 9: 149–176

Marteniuk R, MacKenzie C, Jeannerod M, Athenes S, Dugas C 1987 Constraints on human arm movement trajectories. Canadian Journal of Psychology 41: 365–378

Massion J 1984 Postural changes accompanying voluntary movements. Normal and pathological aspects. Human Neurobiology 2: 261–267

Massion J 1992 Movement, posture and equilibrium: interaction and coordination. Progress in Neurobiology 38; 35–56

Moore S, Brunt D, Nesbitt M, Juarez T 1992 Investigation of evidence for anticipatory postural adjustments in seated subjects who performed a reaching task. Physical Therapy 72(5): 335–343

Murray M P 1967 Patterns of sagittal rotation of the upper limbs in walking. Physical Therapy 47(4): 272–284

Murray M P, Drought A B, Kory R C 1964 Walking patterns of normal men. Journal of Bone and Joint Surgery 46A(2): 335–359

Musa I 1986 Recent findings on the neural control of locomotion: implications for the rehabilitation of gait. In: Banks M (ed) Stroke. Churchill Livingstone, London

Nash J, Neilson P D, O'Dwyer N J 1989 Reducing spasticity to control muscle contracture of children with cerebral palsy. Developmental Medicine and Child Neurology 31(4): 471–480

Nuzik S, Lamb R, VanSant A, Hirt S 1986 Sit to stand movement pattern. Physical Therapy 66(11): 1708–1713

O'Gorman H J, Jull G A 1987 Thoracic kyphosis and mobility: the effect of age. Physiotherapy Practice 3: 154–162

Prevost R, Arsenault A B, Dutil E, Drouin G 1987 Rotation of the scapula and shoulder subluxation in hemiplegia. Archives of Physical Medicine and Rehabilitation

68: 786–790

Rogers M 1991 Motor control problems in Parkinson's disease. In: Lister M (ed) Contemporary management of motor control problems. Foundation for Physical Therapy, Alexandria VA

Rose G K, Butler P, Stallard J 1982 Gait: principles, biomechanics and assessment. Orlau Publishing, Oswestry

Rosenbaum D 1991 Human motor control. Academic Press, London

Rothwell J 1994 Control of human voluntary movement, 2nd edn. Chapman & Hall, London

Saunders J, Inman V, Eberhart H 1953 The major determinants in normal and pathological gait. Journal of Bone and Joint Surgery 35A(3): 543–558

Schenkman M, Berger R, O'Riley P, Mann R, Hodge W 1990 Whole-body movements during rising to standing from sitting. Physical Therapy 70(10): 638–648

Schmidt R A 1988 Motor control and learning: a behavioural emphasis, 2nd edn. Human Kinetics Publishers, Leeds

Schmidt R A 1991a Motor learning and performance: from principles to practice. Human Kinetics Publishers, Leeds

Schmidt R A 1991b Motor learning principles for physical therapy. In: Lister M (ed) Contemporary management of motor control problems. Foundation for Physical Therapy, Alexandria VA

Schuldt K, Ekholm J, Nemeth G, Arborelius U, Harms-Ringdahlk K 1983 Knee load and muscle activity during exercises in rising. Scandinavian Journal of Rehabilitation Medicine 9 (Suppl.): 174–188

Shepherd R B 1992 Adaptive motor behaviour in response to perturbations of balance. Physiotherapy Theory and Practice 8: 137–143

Smidt G 1990 Rudiments of gait. In: Smidt (ed) Clinics in physical therapy. Gait in rehabilitation. Churchill Livingstone, London

Soechting T F, Flanders M 1992 Moving in three dimensional space: frames of reference, vectors and coordinate systems. Annual Reviews of Neuroscience 15: 167–191

Taylor D, Ashburn A, Ward C D 1994 Asymmetrical trunk posture, unilateral neglect and motor performance following stroke. Clinical Rehabilitation 8: 48–53

van Vliet P 1993 An investigation of the task specificity of reaching: implications for retraining. Physiotherapy Theory and Practice 9: 69–76

VanSant A F 1990a Life span development in functional tasks. Physical Therapy 70(12): 788–798

VanSant A F 1990b Commentary. Physical Therapy 70(10): 648–649

Wagenaar R C, Beek W J 1992 Hemiplegic gait: a kinematic analysis using walking speed as a basis. Journal of Biomechanics 25(9): 1007–1015

Whittle M 1991 Gait analysis: an introduction. Butterworth-Heinemann, Oxford

Wier P L 1994 Object property and task effects on prehension. In: Bennett K, Castiello U (eds) Insights into reach and grasp movement. Elsevier Science, London

Winter D A 1987 The biomechanics and motor control of human gait. University of Waterloo Press, Waterloo, Ontario

CHAPTER CONTENTS

General intellectual function   42
  Neuropsychological tests of general intellectual
    impairment   42
  Clinical observations of general intellectual
    loss   44
  Treatment strategies for patients with general
    intellectual loss   44

Memory function   45
  Neuropsychological tests of memory function   45
  Clinical observations of memory dysfunction   45
  Treatment strategies for patients with memory
    dysfunction   47

Attention   48
  Neurological tests of attention   48
  Clinical observations of attentional deficits   48
  Treatment strategies for patients with attentional
    deficits   49

Language function   49
  Neuropsychological tests of language   49
  Clinical observation of language dysfunction   50
  Treatment strategies for patients with language
    dysfunction   50

Visual perception   50
  Neuropsychological tests of visual perception   50
  Clinical observations of visual perceptual
    deficits   51
  Treatment strategies for patients with visual
    perceptual deficits   51

Spatial processing   51
  Neuropsychological tests of spatial processing   51
  Clinical observations of patients with spatial
    impairments   52
  Treatment strategies for patients with spatial
    impairments   53

Executive functions   54
  Neuropsychological tests of executive function   54
  Clinical observation of dysexecutive syndrome   54
  Treatment strategies for patients with dysexecutive
    syndrome   55

Insight   55
  Neuropsychological testing of insight   55
  Clinical observation of insight   56
  Treatment strategies for patients with poor
    insight   56

Emotional distress   56
  Neuropsychological tests of emotional distress   56
  Clinical observations of emotional distress   57
  Treatment strategies for emotionally distressed
    patients   58

Conclusions   59
  Neuropsychological tests   59
  Clinical observation   60
  Treatment strategies   60

References   60

3

Neuropsychological problems and solutions

Dawn Wendy Langdon

Many neurological conditions involve the cerebral hemispheres and thus have an impact on higher cortical function. A patient's cognitive function can have a great influence on the efficiency and success of a physiotherapy treatment. Sometimes this can be at a basic level, for example where a patient's memory dysfunction or inability to initiate action means that she cannot present herself for treatment appointments and on a busy inpatient unit the physiotherapist must escort her to and from the treatment area, which uses up clinical time in escort duties. On other occasions the influence of cognitive dysfunction might be at a more complex level, where, for example, a patient with multiple sclerosis (MS) who has the physical potential to walk is nevertheless unsafe to do so, because of a marked disinhibition and impulsivity in his actions, and thus physiotherapy may target wheelchair techniques because they provide a safer form of mobility.

Neuropsychology attempts to understand the relationship between brain and behaviour. In a clinical setting, this means determining the pattern of neuropsychological impairment that a patient has suffered. The consequent cognitive profile is then related to clinical observations of the patient's disability. Behaviours to be targeted in treatment are identified and agreed. A treatment programme is designed taking account of the patient's cognitive profile. Lastly, mechanisms for the evaluation of treatment and for making programme adjustments are put in place. Thus the approach does not differ substantially in structure from that of a physiotherapist except, understandably, cognitive functions is considered in a more explicit and detailed manner and, correspondingly, physical aspects receive much less attention. These differences in emphasis and experience between the two disciplines make collaborative work essential with many neurological patients.

Neuropsychologists are very fortunate in having a wealth of validated measures and research findings to inform their clinical work. However, the purpose of this chapter is not to explore theoretical aspects in detail and copious referencing has been avoided. Similarly, no consideration is given to diagnostic groups or anatomical correlates. There are many excellent neuropsychology texts that cover this ground admirably. The clearest and probably the best is McCarthy & Warrington (1990). A good introductory text is Ellis & Young (1988). For child neuropsychology, there are two volumes edited by Obrzut (1986).

Interested readers are advised to consult these authors for discussion of cognitive models of neuropsychological syndromes, anatomical considerations and for standard references. This chapter will focus on how acquired neuropsychological deficits affect the function of adult neurological patients and ways in which these deficits can be identified and overcome in therapy. This is a less-well researched area and is therefore approached from a clinical context.

The remainder of this chapter is arranged under nine main headings: general intellectual function; memory function; attention; language function; visual perception; spatial processing; executive functions; insight and emotional distress; finishing with some brief conclusions. These sections reflect the areas that might concern a neuropsychologist in the assessment and treatment of a patient. Each section is divided into three parts. First, one or two measures devised by neuropsychologists to delineate the deficit are described. In order for an aspect of a patient's cognitive function to be assessed in a valid and quantitative way, standard instructions, procedures and scoring must be used. The test must have certain psychometric properties

that make it valid and reliable. For a detailed introduction to these aspects of test theory, see Kline (1993). This part aims to give a flavour of neuropsychological testing and also a clearer impression of the impairment under consideration. Secondly, clinical observations and therapeutic problems that typically relate to the cognitive deficit are described. If you can call on the assistance of a neuropsychologist, then the clinical observations can be related to test findings and a clear profile of the patient's cognitive abilities may emerge. If you are relying on your own professional skill to determine cognitive impairment, impairment, then the part on clinical observation offers a brief description of how the cognitive deficit might manifest itself in therapy and a few pointers towards clinical assessment. Thirdly, some basic treatment strategies and options are discussed in relation to the cognitive deficit.

Admittedly, in most clinical practices it is rare to see patients with a single, or 'focal', cognitive deficit. However, this way of considering neuropsychological dysfunction tends to be the clearest. It is also the most convenient arrangement for those seeking to locate specific information relevant to a particular clinical problem.

GENERAL INTELLECTUAL FUNCTION

Neuropsychological tests of general intellectual impairment

The most widely used test of individual general intellectual level is the Wechsler Adult Intelligence Scale - Revised (WAIS-R; Wechsler 1981). It comprises 11 subtests which are divided into verbal and performance subscales. The verbal subtests are:

- Information, which tests general knowledge
- Comprehension, which examines common sense and social competence
- Vocabulary, which requires the subject to define a graded list of words
- Similarities, which asks the subject to say how pairs of words are alike
- Arithmetic, a graded set of arithmetic problems

- Digit Span, requiring the repetition of strings of digits either forwards or backwards.

The five performance subtests utilise pictorial and spatial materials:

- Digit Symbol, a recoding task which requires the subject to write appropriate abstract symbols under printed numbers
- Picture Completion, where the subject must indicate which important part is missing from each of 21 line drawings
- Picture Arrangement, where small groups of drawings are laid on a desk in scrambled order and the subject must rearrange them to make a sensible story
- Object Assembly, where the subject must assemble a complete two-dimensional object from the several flat fragments scattered before her on the desk.

The six verbal subtest scores are summed as part of the calculation of the Verbal IQ and, similarly, the five performance subtests are added together to obtain the Performance IQ. The Verbal, Performance and Full Scale IQs are derived by reference to normative data. As well as for the three IQs, age-referenced norms are also tabulated for each of the 11 subtests. The standardisation includes 1880 people, stratified by age (16–75 years), sex, region, urban or rural residence, race, occupation and years of education. The classification and distribution of IQ scores are given in Table 3.1.

Table 3.1 The classification and distribution of IQ scores. From the manual of the Wechsler Adult Intelligence Scale - Revised. Copyright © 1981 by The Psychological Corporation. Reproduced by permission. All rights reserved.

IQ	Classification	% included	
		Theoretical normal curve	Control sample
130 and above	Very superior	2.2	2.6
120–129	Superior	6.7	6.9
110–119	High average	16.1	16.6
90–109	Average	50.0	49.1
80–89	Low average	16.1	16.1
70–79	Borderline	6.7	6.4
69 and below	Mentally retarded	2.2	2.3

The WAIS-R gives a good indication of the patient's current level of intellectual function, a cognitive 'snapshot'. However, in order to detect intellectual deterioration, it is necessary to compare current function with how good a person's intellect has been in the past, which is termed their pre-morbid optimum. For some patients, their educational or occupational history will provide a pointer to their pre-morbid optimum, but this can at best only give a broad indication. A more precise estimate of pre-morbid intellect can be obtained from a patient's reading, for example on the National Adult Reading Test - Revised (NART-R; Nelson & Willison 1992). Reading scores are less affected in dementia than other cognitive skills (Nelson & O'Connell 1978, Nelson & McKenna 1975).

The NART-R consists of 50 printed words whose correct pronunciation is irregular, in the sense that the usual English spelling-to-sound rules do not apply. For example, a person who was to read the word 'debt' for the first time would probably sound the 'b' as part of the word and thus read it aloud incorrectly. However, people familiar with the word 'debt' pronounce it 'det'. Their previous knowledge of the word allows them to pronounce it. Because all of the words in the NART-R are similarly irregular, they are unlikely to be guessed correctly. Only words already in a patient's reading vocabulary will be accurately read aloud. By comparing a patient's current IQ with the NART-R, it is possible to determine whether any significant loss of general intellectual function has occurred.

Tests of cognitive ability which were originally developed for general population use, such as the WAIS-R, often include materials and task demands which can be inappropriate for neurological patients. For example, the Picture Arrangement subtest requires the patient to study between three and six cards, each of which carries a detailed line drawing (none greater than 5 cm square) and then rearrange them so that they tell a story. Good manual dexterity and visual acuity are required, in addition to reasoning skills. Clearly, peripheral neurological dysfunction can handicap a patient on this subtest. If a patient with poor acuity and poor dexterity does badly, it is not clear whether peripheral deficits, cognitive deficits, or some mixture of both are to blame. The interpretation of the test result becomes problematic.

Many tests have been developed especially for neurological populations, although none have attained the dominance of the WAIS-R. An example of one designed to assess the general intellectual level of neurological patients is the Verbal and Spatial Reasoning Test (VESPAR; Langdon & Warrington 1995). The VESPAR tests three types of inductive reasoning: categorisation, analogy and series completion. The problems are arranged in three matched sets of 25 verbal and 25 spatial items. The matched design allows fairly clear conclusions to be drawn if either verbal or spatial stimuli lead to poor performance, because the difference is unlikely to be due to different test procedures or task demands and most likely to be due to a specific deficit in either verbal or spatial processing.

The stimuli were selected for their appropriateness for neurological patients. The verbal items use common, or high frequency, words which are less vulnerable to acquired language deficits. The spatial items are all clearly drawn and their solution does not depend on fine visual acuity or shape discrimination, faculties which may be compromised by neurological disease (see Fig. 3.1). No manual dexterity is required of the patient. The forced choice format means that a variety of output modalities are possible. There are no penalties for slow performance. Thus the VESPAR attempts to minimise the effects of peripheral neurological deficits that may confound patients' performance on traditional reasoning tests, which attempt to measure central cognitive processes.

Clinical observations of general intellectual loss

The clinical detection of a dementia can often be problematic, particularly in the early stages. This is especially true of Alzheimer's disease, where typically social skills are preserved and a casual conversation will not reveal anything amiss; or of MS, where typically language skills are unaffected and even an in-depth conversation will not reveal anything untoward. In general, patients who have suffered a widespread cognitive deterioration will find new information difficult to absorb and retain. They may require a great deal of prompting and repetition. Their powers of abstraction will be weakened and they will tend to see the world (and themselves) in rather concrete terms. This may result in their failing to bring problems to your attention or realise the implications of medical or treatment developments.

Their reduced cognitive capacity may have forced them to withdraw from established activities, although patients may explain the change in terms of peripheral, physical causes. For example, a patient whose reasoning powers fell to a level where they could no longer carry her through a knitting pattern, explained that she had given up knitting due to failing eyesight. A self-employed painter and decorator, who presented with pain in the back and legs which prevented him from climbing ladders, was no longer able to calculate the pattern repeats of wallpaper and thus could no longer paper a room. Enquiring which newspaper a patient used to enjoy reading can often provide the clinician with a rough guide to the patient's pre-morbid optimum.

A AMERICA GERMANY COUNTRY ENGLAND

B

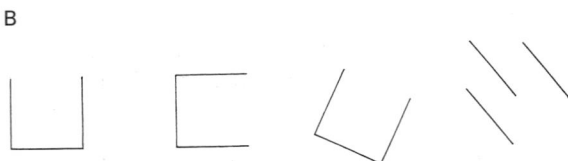

Figure 3.1 Sample items from the (A) verbal and (B) spatial odd-one out sections of the VESPAR. (From Langdon D W, Warrington E K 1995 The VESPAR: a verbal and spatial reasoning test. Reprinted by permission of Lawrence Erlbaum Associates Ltd., Hove, UK.)

Treatment strategies for patients with general intellectual loss

A good recent summary of psychological treatment approaches to patients with dementia can be found in Holden & Woods (1995). In general, the poor abstracting abilities of these patients make it necessary for the reasons for treatment to be described in clear, concrete terms. It is best to use short sentences and everyday words. For example a patient with a significant intellectual loss, who spends most of the day in a wheelchair and long periods immobile in bed, may not appreciate the need for a pressure care regime. The reasons why a pressure care regime will prevent pressure areas developing may not be obvious to the patient. Similarly, the results of developing a pressure sore may need to be spelt out in graphic detail, because the logical outcome of failing to implement pressure care may well escape the patient. A written account, again in clear, concrete terms, can pay dividends both as a prompt and as an aid to understanding.

It is usually a good idea to give this patient group as much structure as possible in their physiotherapy programme and follow-up. They may need to be oriented at the start of each therapy session as to its purpose and content. They may need reminding of this and their progress summarised at regular intervals. They may need help, perhaps explicit practice, in transferring techniques to new settings. If they have a home exercise programme to follow, a diary or weekly chart to follow can be very helpful.

MEMORY FUNCTION

Neuropsychological tests of memory function

Memory function is the registration and retrieval of information of all kinds. A detailed review of the neuropsychology of memory in clinical practice may be found in Kapur (1988). The basic principles of assessing memory function require a valid and systematic procedure in which a person remembers certain pieces of information in response to standard instructions. A memory test in widespread clinical use is the Recognition Memory Test (RMT; Warrington 1984). 50 everyday words are presented to the patient at a rate of one every

3 seconds. The patient is required to say whether she likes each word, as a way of ensuring her attention. Next the patient is shown 50 pairs of everyday words. Each pair includes one word from the original single showing. The patient must say which of the two words she has just seen. A visual version, using photographs of male faces, follows the same procedure. The standardisation sample comprised 310 volunteers, mainly inpatients with extracerebral disease, aged between 18 and 70 years. The RMT is a relatively pure test of memory function, in that the test procedure places few demands on other cognitive skills. It was designed as a diagnostic test, to detect minor degrees of memory dysfunction across a wide range of the adult population.

Wilson et al (1985) devised a test to evaluate everyday memory function. It includes a number of procedures:

- remembering a name associated with a face after 25 minutes
- remembering to ask for an item and where it was hidden, again after 25 minutes
- remembering to question the examiner after 20 minutes
- recognising 10 pictures
- recognising five faces
- orientation
- immediate and delayed recall of a story and a route.

There are four parallel forms, allowing change in patients' performance on the test to be monitored, unconfounded by the patient remembering stimuli from previous testing. The Rivermead Behavioural Memory Test samples a range of memory functions. It is a useful tool both for clinical screening and monitoring change. Normative data are available from 137 normal control subjects aged between 16 and 75 years.

Clinical observations of memory dysfunction

A patient with memory dysfunction may fail to remember many kinds of information. Perhaps the most common demonstration in therapy is a failure to carry over techniques from a previous session, or to apply techniques to everyday life that have been rehearsed in therapy. However, a patient with a dense amnesic syndrome can exhibit far more extensive and disabling memory dysfunction. For example, if a therapist leaves an amnesic patient for a few minutes to answer a telephone, the amnesic patient may well be bewildered when the therapist returns and ask who the therapist is. In the few minutes the therapist spent answering the telephone, all recall of the therapist, the therapy session and the location has vanished.

Discrepancies in different types of memory function can be observed. For example, a patient may have difficulty remembering words and other verbal material, but remain competent at remembering pictures and other visual material. This can be elucidated by discrepancies on the verbal and visual sections of the RMT (Warrington 1984), if a neuropsychological assessment is available. Otherwise, a simple test of telling the patient his appointment time (a verbal strategy) for one session and then showing him a picture of a clock set at the time of his appointment (a visual strategy) for the next session and observing the patient's attendance, might well indicate which memory system is the most efficient.

Apart from a general memory dysfunction for either verbal information or visual information, memory for certain types of verbal and visual information can be selectively impaired. For example, although a patient may be able to perceive an object efficiently (i.e. her visual perceptual processes are intact), she may not be able to remember any knowledge about the object, for example its purpose. In the pure form, this impairment is termed visual agnosia. This syndrome can have devastating results in everyday life, because patients may not be able to recognise a door handle or a toothbrush. In therapy, they may not be able to recognise a wheelchair brake and it will be hard for them to plan their movements in relation to objects, if they are uncertain how to operate or manipulate them.

Similarly, aspects of visual memory can be affected in isolation. Some patients can have a particular difficulty in recognising faces, a syndrome termed prosopagnosia. Others may have a selective impairment in remembering routes within the hospital or around their home locality, which is termed topographical memory dysfunction. Patients who cannot find their way around are clearly seriously disadvantaged when trying to improve their mobility.

As well as different types of memory being selectively impaired, different ways of remembering can be affected to varying degrees. For example, the RMT (Warrington 1984) requires patients to recognise words or faces that they have just seen and is thus a test of recognition memory. The test stimuli act as a prompt or a cue to help the patient remember. Patients remember far more words in this recognition format than they would if they were asked to recite all the words that they had just been shown, that is to recall the words without cue or prompt. For patients with memory dysfunction, the difference between their ability to recall information unaided and their ability to remember information aided by a cue or a prompt can be very great.

As well as recall and recognition memory procedures, another format is paired-associate memory. Pairs of words are shown to the patient; then the first word of each pair is shown and the patient is required to produce the second word that was its associate in the previously seen pair. The association can be strong (e.g. tea–cup) or so weak as to be simply that they were two unrelated words that had been previously seen together (e.g. gate–carpet). The importance of this format is its apparent link to everyday memory function (Wilson et al 1985).

When assessing a patient's ability to remember information in therapy, it is important to be alert to how much prompting and cueing the patient is receiving. A patient may be able to recite perfectly the procedures for transferring safely from a wheelchair to a bed, in response to a series of questions, but that procedure assessed his prompted verbal memory function. The memory function required to perform transfers safely at home is recall performance memory, which could be assessed by observing the patient perform unprompted.

Treatment strategies for patients with memory dysfunction

A detailed account of neuropsychological treatments of memory dysfunction can be found in Wilson & Moffat (1984) and Wilson (1987). The first step to devising treatment strategies to overcome memory dysfunction in therapy is to assess the nature and extent of the patient's difficulties. If verbal memory function appears to be generally more efficient than visual memory function, then a written protocol for transferring from a wheelchair to a bath could be devised. It should be tested by observing the patient transferring when following the written protocol. If any further prompts or explanation are required from the therapist, then these should be added as amendments to the protocol or extra steps. Once the patient has demonstrated step 1 – independent transfers using the protocol (which includes remembering to use the protocol) – then it may be possible for her to learn the protocol by heart and recite it aloud to guide her transfers; this is step 2. Step 3 would be for the patient to rehearse the protocol silently during the transfer. Even if a patient's general intellectual function means that she can never move beyond using the written protocol, she has still achieved independence in that task.

Conversely, if visual memory function appears to be generally more efficient than verbal memory function, then pictures and other visual material may be used to good effect. The pictured information can be used explicitly, for example a set of drawings to prompt each item in a home exercise programme. Or it may be implicit, for example encouraging a patient to visualise striking images that link his therapist to the day of the week when he must attend for his outpatient treatment. The use of visual imagery is extensively reported by Wilson (1987).

The first general principle is, therefore, to identify and utilise competent areas of memory function.

The second principle is to reduce the memory load for the patient at any one time. A task is broken down into components, each of which is sufficiently small for the patient to grasp immediately. Each component is practised extensively, as a single movement with many repetitions. This increases the chances of the component being learnt in the long term. Sometimes this is termed 'overlearning', which indicates the large number of repetitions of a single component that may be required to consolidate the learning, before proceeding to the next component. This breaking down of an activity into separate, smaller components does not fit comfortably with the idea of educating a patient to perform normal movements. However, some patients' memory deficits may be so severe that practising an activity as a whole will never register sufficiently for adequate carry-over and, if they are to make essential functional gains, then the task may need to be broken down into component actions ('chunking') with separate practice of each activity component.

The third principle is 'errorless learning', a technique whereby the patient is taught to perform correctly from the start and not left to arrive at a correct solution by trial, error and feedback. As in the chunking approach described above, errorless learning goes some way against the grain of conventional therapy wisdom, which usually advocates observing the patient and giving feedback concerning the good and bad aspects of the patient's movement. For example, allowing a patient under close supervision to position a splint wrongly, then removing it and replacing it correctly with an explanation. In most therapy situations it clearly makes sense to discover where a patient is going wrong so that effort and expertise can be targeted efficiently.

However, for patients with severe memory dysfunction, there is evidence that once they have tried an incorrect manoeuvre, it is very difficult for their compromised memory systems to erase the incorrect manoeuvre from their plan of that activity. An incorrect manoeuvre can include an omission. For example, patients transferring for the first time from a wheelchair to a bed may move their hands straight from the wheels, which they were turning, to the bed, omitting to put on the wheelchair brakes. Their learnt manoeuvre is to move their hands from the wheels to the bed. It would be very hard for patients with severe memory problems to then 'unlearn' that manoeuvre and insert the 'brakes on' manoeuvre into their recorded plan of the activity. Errorless learning is probably most useful for patients with very severe memory dysfunction. Some detailed experiments which demonstrate how errorless learning benefits amnesic patients are described by Wilson et al (1994).

ATTENTION

Neurological tests of attention

In some ways the most fundamental cognitive faculty, attention underpins all other cognitive activities. If patients can not concentrate, they can not employ any other cognitive function effectively, however efficient their other cognitive processes may be. Attention must be directed and sustained if more (apparently) sophisticated cognitive systems are to be brought to bear on either external information or internal processing. Perhaps the best-known and most widely used clinical test of attention is the Digit Span subtest of the WAIS-R (Wechsler 1981; discussed above under the heading 'Neuropsychological tests of general intellectual impairment'). The repetition of random digit strings will be compromised if the patient has an attentional deficit. It appears that repetition of lists of unrelated items can be achieved with very little additional processing of the items. For most patients, it is a relatively pure test of attention. Sometimes Digit Span is mistakenly thought of as a general memory test. Because it does not necessarily involve the registration and remembering processes of memory (see p. 45), it is best thought of as a test of attention.

A test of attention which illustrates this emphasis on concentration and relatively low demands on other processing is the Paced Auditory Serial Addition Task (Gronwall 1977).

The patient listens to single digits spoken aloud on an audio tape. There are various rates of presentation, for example one digit every second or one digit every 4 seconds. The patient's task is to add together the last two digits he or she has heard. For example, the number 1 might come first, followed by 4. The correct response from the patient is 5. Then the patient hears the next number in the series on the tape, which is 7. The last two numbers the patient has heard are now 4 and 7 and the correct response is 11. Clearly, the arithmetic demands are small, just the addition of pairs of single digits. However, the attentional demands are very exacting, requiring the patient to remain alert to the two digits which constitute the last pair heard whilst performing the simple serial additions correctly.

Robertson et al (1994) have developed the Test of Everyday Attention (TEA), which samples selective attention (the ability to filter out unnecessary information), sustained attention and attention switching. The tasks utilise both visual and auditory stimuli, for example searching a telephone directory for specified symbols and counting tones from an audio tape. There are three parallel versions. The TEA allows three types of attention to be assessed separately and any change in attention skills to be monitored.

Clinical observations of attentional deficits

In therapy, the most common and disruptive attentional deficit will probably be distractibility, that is a failure to ignore irrelevant stimuli. This occurs when the selective function of attention is compromised. Think for a moment of all the detail and activity in a hospital ward or treatment gym (if this is not immediately clear, just imagine how long it would take to make a detailed drawing of the scene and activity and then write out a record of all speech and other sounds occurring in the room, from an audio tape left running during the therapy session). All humans filter out vast amounts of information in their immediate environment so that the stimuli they process are of manageable quantity and appropriate type. The distractible patient, however, may not be able to exclude the conversation that another therapist is having with a patient on the next mat. It may intrude into his processing and prevent him fully comprehending your comments and suggestions.

Pointers towards poor selective attention are that patients may fail to respond appropriately, or at all, in conversation. They may look away, towards another conversation or a sudden activity in another part of the room, when you would expect them to be maintaining eye contact with you as you speak. A detailed qualitative and quantitative account of attentional problems experienced by patients following head injury is given by Gronwall (1977).

Sustained attention deficits will manifest themselves as poor concentration. After a brief, successful period at the start of a therapy session, things will rapidly go downhill. Movements which were performed efficiently at the start become inconsistent or even impossible. A law of diminishing returns has clearly set into the session. Another stumbling block in therapy can be the patient's inability to switch attention. For example, a patient working hard to preserve her midline whilst practising indoor mobility may topple over as she opens a door, because she had been concentrating on her midline to the exclusion of the balance requirements of opening doors.

Treatment strategies for patients with attentional deficits

Studies of treatment for attentional deficits have tended to use computers for training and evaluation and for research purposes, and the tasks have been abstract (for example Gray et al 1992). However, one home-based programme to improve attention in reading, has been described (Wilson & Robertson 1992). Broadly, there are two possible approaches which are likely to reduce the effect of a patient's selective attention deficits on therapy. The first way is to change the therapeutic environment. A quiet, single treatment room is probably an unobtainable ideal in most hospital settings but can often be easily achieved in a patient's home. It may be

best to speak only when you have the patient's eye contact and discontinue when it is broken. Talking patients through a task may help to keep them focused. The second way to minimise the effects of selective attention deficits is for the patients to implement strategies themselves. These can range from imagery guided techniques to verbal commentaries, which can either be spoken aloud or rehearsed internally.

Difficulties in sustaining attention are usually best tackled by simple pacing techniques. Rest periods can be scheduled during a therapy session to allow patients to refocus their concentration, or a number of short sessions may be spaced throughout the day. Switching attention can be facilitated by verbal prompts or commentaries from either the therapist or patient.

LANGUAGE FUNCTION

Neuropsychological tests of language

A detailed historical introduction to the assessment of language dysfunction is given by Howard & Hatfield (1987). A widely used clinical test of naming is the Graded Naming Test (GNT; McKenna & Warrington 1983). It consists of 30 black and white line drawings. The objects depicted range from those which everyone in the normal sample could name ('kangaroo') to rare items that only a small percentage of the normal sample were able to name. It is the less-frequently used words which are most vulnerable to neurological disease. It is often necessary to test patients to the limits of their naming vocabulary in order to discount or demonstrate a naming difficulty. The graded difficulty of the test allows a level of performance to be recorded at any point across the normal range. Thus even mild naming difficulties can be identified. The test is standardised on 100 subjects, mainly inpatients with extracerebral disease.

The Graded Naming Test is a useful diagnostic screening tool; however, sometimes a more detailed assessment of language dysfunction is required. The Psycholinguistic Assessments of Language Processing in Aphasia (PALPA; Kay et al 1992) is based on theoretical models of language function. It comprises 60 tests of different aspects of language such as writing, grammar, speech and comprehension. Tests can be selected according to the pattern of language difficulty a particular patient experiences.

Clinical observation of language dysfunction

Any aspect of a patient's language processing can be affected by neurological disease. Patients may have difficulty in pronouncing words correctly or in finding the right words to say. They may have difficulty in understanding spoken or written words. They may be unable to spell. Patients will sometimes attribute difficulties in reading and writing to peripheral or physical problems, such as failing eyesight or stiff fingers. The terminology is not clear cut for the acquired language disorders. Generally, in all cases where the difficulties are attributed to disease or damage of the cerebral cortex and result in an acquired deficit:

- difficulties with speaking or the spoken word are termed 'aphasias'
- difficulties with reading are termed 'dyslexias'
- difficulties with writing are termed 'dysgraphias'.

In therapy, the patients' difficulties in conversation are likely to be the most problematic. If patients can only partially understand what is being said to them, then they may find it hard either to appreciate the reasons for particular exercises or to grasp what changes and modifications of movement are being required of them. If patients can not express themselves clearly and fluently, then their perceptions and sensations may be hard for the therapist to appreciate fully. Discussion of the home situation will also be limited.

Treatment strategies for patients with language dysfunction

Clearly, the aim of any strategy employed with a patient with acquired language deficits is to optimise communication. A review of specialised aphasia therapy can be found in Howard & Hatfield (1987). If patients have serious speech problems, they may be able to write information that you need to know. If comprehension problems are known or suspected, then using everyday words in short sentences with pauses at the end may help. It may also be the case that the patient's reading comprehension is less affected. If no verbal input is satisfactory, however modified, then pictures and drawings may be helpful. If it can be managed, a set of photographs of the patient moving correctly can be a good compromise.

It is a concern that the use of simple words and pictures may lead the patient to feel patronised. Every effort should be made to avoid this. It is a natural reaction to raise the volume of speech if a patient fails to understand first time, but it is important to keep the voice even toned when repeating or explaining information. Sometimes it helps to frame the simple words and short sentences appropriately if the clinician thinks of him- or herself as speaking to a healthy foreign adult whose knowledge of English is limited. In this way, the tone and style remain appropriate to an adult, whilst the complexity of the language is reduced. Similarly, any stationery, such as folders used to organise written information or pictures, should be as businesslike as possible.

VISUAL PERCEPTION

Neuropsychological tests of visual perception

Neurological disease and damage can result in the disruption of any aspect of visual processing. In rare cases, single aspects such as colour or acuity may be selectively compromised. The breakdown of these early visual processes has been studied in detail by Warrington (1986). Sometimes basic visual information such as colour and form may be processed well, but the integration of these components into an object that can be recognised may be weak. A model of how objects are seen as integrated wholes was devised by Marr (1982).

The Visual Object and Space Perception Battery (VOSP; Warrington & James 1991) includes four tests which are widely used in the clinical evaluation of visual perception. They have been designed to place minimal reliance on other cognitive skills, for example by only requiring simple responses from the patient. The tasks are:

- to identify single, black capital letters, whose form has been degraded by a random scatter of small white squares
- to identify rotated silhouettes of animals and household objects, which thus have an atypical outline
- to select which of four black shapes represents the rotated silhouette of an everyday object
- to identify two objects, which are each presented as a series of rotated silhouettes which become progressively more typical (and thus easier to identify).

The standardisation samples comprise at least 150 subjects.

Clinical observations of visual perceptual deficits

Weak visual perceptual skills can result in quite subtle problems in therapy, which may not be immediately apparent to either the patient or the clinician. It is likely that the patient's interactions with objects will be clumsy and ill-judged. Overlapping objects may pose special difficulties, because the full outline of each object is not in direct sight and therefore only partial visual information on each object is available, which can pose too great a challenge to weakened object perception processes. In general, such patients will exhibit difficulty in making sense of the world around them.

Treatment strategies for patients with visual perceptual deficits

Patients are likely to be helped by objects and equipment being presented in a typical view. For example, they could be advised to approach a door or wheelchair head-on and position themselves straight in front while they take stock of their immediate environment. Once they have processed the visual information correctly, they can then proceed to move more accurately and safely.

SPATIAL PROCESSING
Neuropsychological tests of spatial processing

For people to move and act successfully, they must make a myriad of spatial judgements. They must know where every part of their body is and they must know where every part of their immediate environment is. Any action requires sophisticated computations to determine the precise movement which will, for example, bring a foot to a ball, a hand to a cup, a head to a pillow. Some spatial judgements are very broad, for example taking to the back streets to avoid a traffic jam and managing to drive in the right direction. Other spatial judgements are very fine, for example threading a needle.

The VOSP (Warrington & James 1991) includes four tests which are widely used in the clinical evaluation of spatial perception. They require no manual manipulation of test material by the patient and are therefore free of any effects of praxic difficulties. The tasks are:

- to count random scatters of dots
- to decide which of two dots is exactly centred in its square
- to identify the position of a dot in a square by selecting a number in the identical position in a second square
- to calculate how many cubes would be required to build a pile of cubes, represented in a two-dimensional line drawing.

The standardisation samples comprise at least 150 subjects.

The VOSP provides a stringent, diagnostic screen of the spatial localisation of small visual stimuli. More complex deficits of spatial processing can result in a disregard of parts of space, which is termed a 'neglect'. The Behavioural Inattention Test (BIT; Wilson et al 1987) evaluates a patient's performance on both conventional, table-top tests of neglect and tests of neglect in everyday life. The conventional tests include line bisection, figure and shape copying and cancelling specified shapes presented among distracter shapes. The everyday tests include telephone dialling, telling the time and address copying. The BIT gives a wide-ranging assessment of the patient's spatial neglect. It is based on a control sample of 50.

Clinical observations of patients with spatial impairments

A good review of spatial perception and processing can be found in De Renzi (1982). Patients with spatial processing deficits will often move inappropriately; for example, they may be seen to fumble as they reach for the brake on a wheelchair. If distance judgement is poor, transfers may be unsafe and wheelchair mobility may be inefficient. The transfers are compromised because positioning the wheelchair correctly alongside the bed, for example, and moving the body an appropriate distance, may require a great deal of effort and checking in order to overcome poor distance judgement. Where mid-air corrections are required that place heavy demands on balance, patients may tend to overshoot or undershoot when transferring. Wheelchair mobility may bring special problems when doors have to be negotiated. To propel a wheelchair through a doorway requires fairly precise spatial awareness and calculation.

A unilateral neglect results in patients disregarding up to half of their body or disregarding up to half of the space that surrounds them. This syndrome can occur independently of hemiparesis. An example of the result of a patient with unilateral neglect attempting to copy a symmetrical stack of blocks is given in Figure 3.2. A recent overview of clinical and research findings in unilateral neglect is given in Robertson & Marshall (1993). In clinical settings, patients may be observed to knock into the left side of door frames, because they have failed to allow enough space for the left side of their body to pass through the door frame. They may

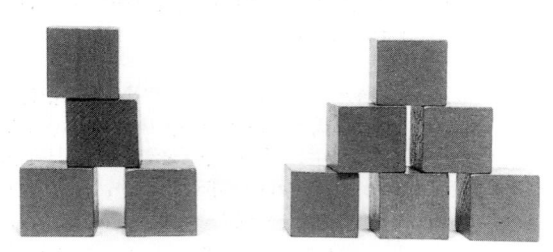

Figure 3.2 The result of a patient with unilateral neglect attempting to copy a symmetrical stack of blocks.

arrive for therapy with the left side of their body undressed, because they have failed to put their left arm into the left sleeve of a garment. Male patients may have neglected to shave the left half of their face. In therapy, the neglected part of the body may be ignored, allowed to slump and the hand and arm may even be left to dangle and risk injury. Patients usually have no insight into the nature or even presence of their difficulty.

Sometimes it can be difficult to determine whether a patient is disabled by a unilateral neglect syndrome or a disturbance of midline perception; for example, a patient who regularly bangs his left arm into the door frame as he walks through the door. The difference can be identified if a minimal contact is maintained with the patient as he walks through a doorway. The minimal contact involves using fingers or hands to keep the patient in an upright stance, but not to influence his walking direction in any way. If he negotiates the door successfully when walking in an upright position, then it is unlikely that a unilateral neglect is the impairment underlying the contact with the door frame. A patient with unilateral neglect would probably neglect his left side, or the left side of space, whatever the angle of his body. If, therefore, the patient bangs into the left side of the door frame even when his body is correctly positioned, it suggests that unilateral neglect is a good candidate to explain his poor negotiation of doorways (because his midline problem has been corrected).

Treatment strategies for patients with spatial impairments

Sometimes making patients aware of the pattern of their difficulties and advising them to take their time and check during activities when spatial judgements are crucial will be enough to overcome the problem. A patient's awareness of her own body positioning may be good, in which case she can usefully employ techniques where she positions a hand or foot as a guide before transferring her weight. As well as being used as a spatial marker, a hand or foot can also be used as a ruler. A wheelchair's distance from a bed can be habitually checked by placing a hand in between, to see if it just touches the bed on one side and the wheelchair on the other. Another approach is to identify a target for the patient through a doorway, for example a picture hung on the wall opposite the doorway, and establishing that if the patient looks at the picture and aims for it as she wheels herself through a doorway, then she will pass centrally through the door frame. An example of a patient using spatial cues is given in Figure 3.3.

There have been some recent interesting developments in techniques for treating patients with unilateral neglect. Robertson et al (1992) used a combination of two techniques when treating three patients with severe left neglect. First, the patients were trained to use their left arm as a spatial marker by positioning it at the

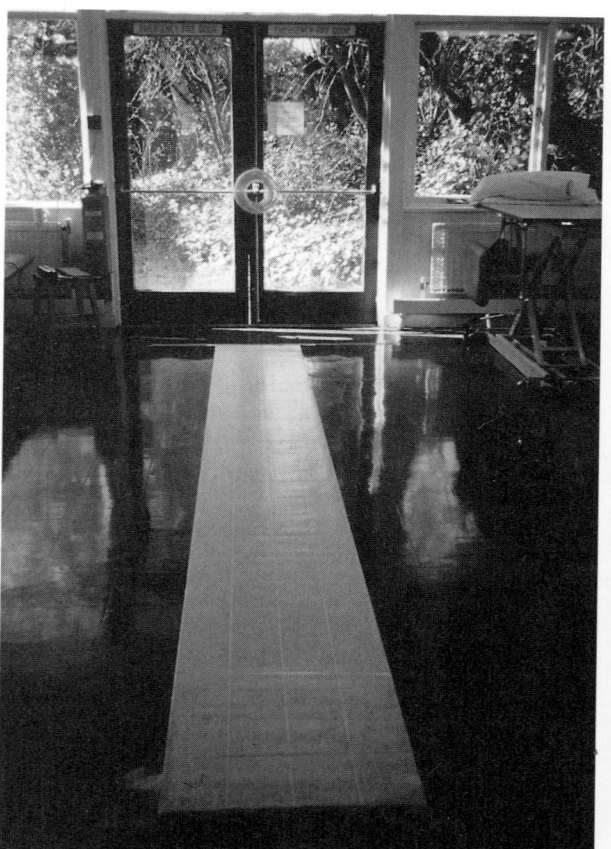
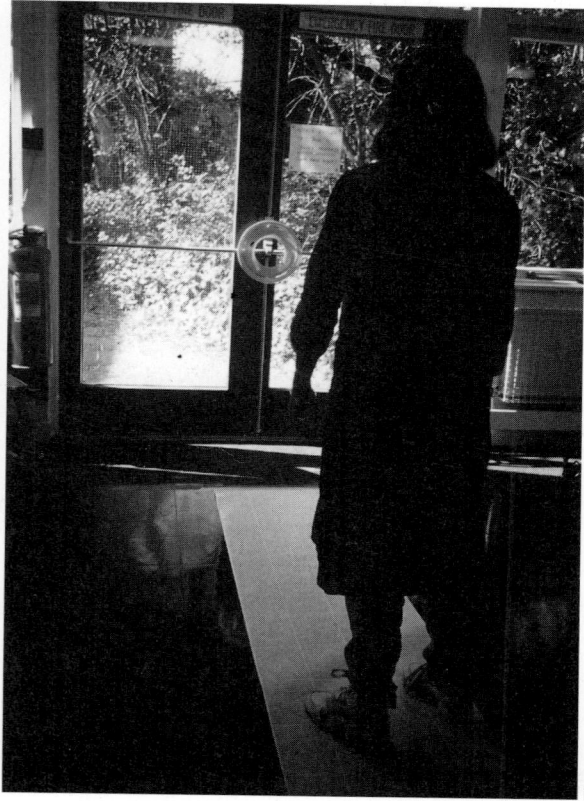

Figure 3.3 The use of salient spatial cues to assist a patient with severe spatial dysfunction to walk in a straight line: (A) the equipment, a length of linoleum to highlight a straight path to the door and a bright plastic disc as the target; (B) the patient using the equipment to walk in a straight line.

left border of any activity. They were also trained to look at it frequently. Secondly, they moved the affected limb. One patient was only told to activate the affected limb. All three patients demonstrated improvements in either table-top neglect tasks or everyday mobility. It appears that by 'activating' the neglected side with simple, repetitive activity, the patient is 'alerted' to the previously neglected hemispace.

Both of these approaches can be adopted, but they require a great deal of prompting and monitoring whilst patients are trained to position and monitor their left hand and then activate it during walking. Clenching and unclenching the left hand is the activation usually employed, but any kind of congenial, sustainable movement would probably suffice. There can be some problems with patient acceptance and compliance because, typically, insight is low and patients may be unwilling to embark on a lengthy retraining programme if they cannot comprehend the need for it.

EXECUTIVE FUNCTIONS
Neuropsychological tests of executive function

The executive functions are the least well understood of the cognitive skills and the tests available to the clinician are generally less robust and reliable than those that test more focal skills. In part this may be because the executive functions are higher order, perhaps supervisory systems that tend to work through other systems, and thus are hard to test precisely and exclusively. Another feature which makes them test-shy is that they tend to become apparent in complicated tasks with many features, which are not easy to package in a cardboard box or rehearse in a clinic setting.

The best-known test of executive function was devised by Milner (1963). It consists of four key cards, which are placed in a row before the patient (Fig. 3.4). A large pack of cards with abstract shapes in various numbers and colours is given to the patient. The patient places a card from the pack with one of the four key cards, in

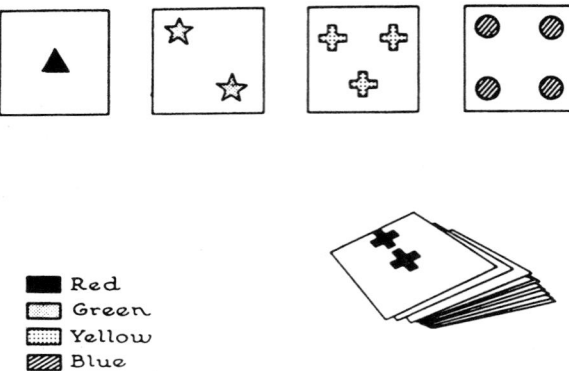

Red
Green
Yellow
Blue

Figure 3.4 The Wisconsin Card Sorting Test. (Reproduced from Milner 1963.)

an attempt to determine a sorting rule. The tester says whether the placed card is right or wrong and the procedure is repeated until the patient demonstrates 10 consistently correct sorts. At this point, the sorting rule is changed. There are three rules which are applied through two cycles.

Clinical observation of dysexecutive syndrome

An overview of research in this area can be found in Perecman (1987). Patients with dysexecutive syndrome can often present as lethargic and poorly motivated. They may be passive. They will often be weak at planning and organisation. Initiation will be especially problematic. They can also be impulsive and disinhibited, the manifestation of which can range from over-jocularity, to over-familiarity, to extreme cases, where the speech can include much swearing and obscenity. Apart from affecting conversation, impulsivity can be observed during activity, when patients who are physically able to walk compromise the safety of their mobility by walking too fast. Similarly, impulsivity in transfers can also compromise safety in patients who have the basic physical ability to transfer easily.

It can be hard for these patients to generate alternative strategies if one movement or action is discovered to be wrong. For example, patients attempting to steer through a doorway can be seen to drive into the frame, hitting the left side of the frame with their left wheelchair footplate. They then reverse and repeat exactly the same trajectory that caused the previous crash. This can be repeated several times. The problem is that they cannot initiate a change of direction, so that their new wheelchair trajectory will take them through the centre of the doorway without incident. They cannot use the feedback of their left footplate crashing into the door frame to make an appropriate modification to their behaviour. Instead, they repeat the identical move that led to the crash.

Sometimes there is clear evidence of poor problem solving at a more complex level. It may be hard for such patients to appreciate the nature and extent of their disease and disability, in which case their application in therapy is likely to be sporadic at best. They will often fail to grasp the implications of threats to their well-being. They may appear unconcerned about their disability. They will probably not be able to think things through and, in conversation, give the impression of not having an understanding of anything beyond the immediate and the obvious.

Treatment strategies for patients with dysexecutive syndrome

A treatment regime of helping brain-injured patients with problem-solving disorders is described by Yves von Cramon & Matthes von Cramon (1992). A combination of individual and group therapy was utilised, taking about 5 hours each week for 5 weeks. Exercises aim to improve selective encoding and comparison, selective combination, idea generation and action planning. Clearly, problem solving cannot be tackled extensively as part of a physiotherapy session, but clear, concrete accounts of the implications of various courses of action and adoption of movement pattern can aid understanding and help patients to overcome their difficulty in grasping the importance of the therapy. It is probably best to start from the premise that nothing is obvious to the patient.

Apathy and poor organisation can sometimes be helped by adding structure. Calendars, diaries and charts of exercises to be performed may help. Prompting and monitoring may be necessary. If there are possible hazards or other problems at home in relation to movement, it is probably best to consider them explicitly and discuss appropriate courses of action in clear, concrete terms. The patients may be unable to realise them for themselves.

For impulsivity in movement, a verbal commentary by the therapist, or patient, which may be internalised eventually, can help. This can range from a simple counting protocol to pace movement to a safely slow pace, to a list of movements and checks to be made during a specific manoeuvre. If initiation of, for example, pressure care is a problem, an electronic beeper may be sufficient prompt to turn in bed.

If disinhibition in conversation and behaviour is a problem in therapy, then a strict behavioural approach may help. This would require that all inappropriate acts and comments are ignored and all appropriate attempts to communicate are reinforced by immediate responses. If this is not enough, then feedback about unacceptable behaviour may be necessary. A consistent approach is essential. It is unfair to patients to smile at a risqué compliment and then later turn your back on them when they tell a crude joke.

INSIGHT
Neuropsychological testing of insight

In essence, insight is determined by the comparison of two things: the first is the patient's view and the second is the clinician's. Usually, if they coincide, the patient's insight is deemed to be good. If they do not, a problem has been identified. Any formal test of insight would thus require two scales and, as insight can apply to any aspect of cognitive function (or physical disability), a multitude of scales would be required. It would be a major undertaking to develop a clinically useful test of insight. Some researchers have attempted to quantify patients' insight, by comparing the patients' ratings of themselves with their scores on formal tests of particular cognitive skills.

McMillan (1984) developed the Subjective Memory Questionnaire (SMQ), which asks patients a number of questions about their everyday memory function, and includes collected comparison data from healthy subjects. Patients with severe head injury and their relatives completed the SMQ and both groups reported the head-injured patients' everyday function to be weaker than a matched control group (Schwartz & McMillan 1989). It appeared that both the patients with severe head injuries and their relatives had some appreciation of the patients' memory dysfunction.

In contrast, patients with MS appear to have less awareness of their memory difficulties in everyday life. Langdon & Thompson (1994) compared the reports of patients with advanced MS and their carers' reports on the SMQ, with the patients' scores on formal tests of memory function (examples of these have been described in the memory section of this chapter). Both patients with advanced MS and their carers reported the patients' general level of everyday memory function to be similar to that of previously reported control groups. The patients' reports were unrelated to formal tests of memory function. However, the patients' reports were related to the patients' level of emotional distress. In contrast, the carers' reports of the patients' everyday memory function were related to the patients' formal memory test performance. However, the carers' reports were not influenced by the patients' emotional distress. It seems that the carers' were able to be more objective, in some sense. The patients were communicating something important when they reported everyday memory dysfunction, probably that their coping skills were not up to the task of managing their day.

Clinical observation of insight

It is arguably the case, that a patient's view of the situation is the most important cognitive factor in his or her recovery or rehabilitation potential. If patients do not think that they have a problem, they are unlikely to attend for therapy. If they do not think the clinician will be able to benefit them significantly, they are unlikely to attend for therapy. If they cannot see the possibility of a worthwhile improvement in their life, they are unlikely to attend for therapy. Patients with weak insight may present as difficult and non-compliant. They may appear unconcerned or off-hand to the clinician. They may be distressed and irritated by attempts at therapeutic intervention. A detailed consideration of difficulties with insight after head injury can be found in Prigatano (1991).

Treatment strategies for patients with poor insight

For some patients, careful discussion and negotiation will enable them to appreciate the need for therapy, and often in these conversations an everyday, low-key tone can be effective. Also the emphasis on the routine nature of the intervention can help to reassure and recruit patients. However, poor insight can be very entrenched and it may be that the patient will never explicitly agree with the therapist concerning the need, efficacy or outcome of treatment. It may still be possible, however, to engage the patient in therapy on a contractual basis. For example, progress in therapy might facilitate an earlier discharge from an inpatient ward. Although it can be hard for clinicians to endure patients constantly decrying the effectiveness of their work, the ultimate goal is the patients' physical progress, not their commendation of the clinician. Sometimes a meeting with a patient in which his or her view is explicitly acknowledged to differ from that of the clinician can be helpful, if some common ground can be found as a result to form the basis of the patient's participation in therapy.

EMOTIONAL DISTRESS

Neuropsychological tests of emotional distress

If patients experience depression, or anxiety, or any affective disturbance, their view of themselves and the world is affected. This shift in outlook and judgement forms the basis of a widely used test of depression, the Beck Inventory of Depression (BID; Beck et al 1979). It consists of 21 sets of four statements, each relating to some aspect of daily life or self-view. The first is a normal response (e.g. 'I do not feel sad') and the statements progress to a very depressed level (e.g. 'I am so sad or unhappy that I can't stand it'). Patients must select one statement from each group of four, which best describes how they have been feeling over the past week. Each statement has a numerical score and these are added together to give a degree of depression, which may fall within the normal or clinical ranges.

Another example of a widely used test of affective disturbance is the State–Trait Anxiety Inventory (STAI; Spielberger 1983). This test examines both immediate, or state, anxiety and background, or trait, anxiety. Items include 'I feel calm', 'I feel nervous'. Patients rate their degree of agreement with 20 statements for each scale.

Clinical observations of emotional distress

Gainotti (1993) has written a good review of work relating to emotional distress following head injury, and many of his observations have a wider application to other neurological conditions. Depressed patients may be tearful. They may be lethargic and find it hard to motivate themselves. They will typically be very negative, constantly producing reasons why there is no reason for therapy, no reason for progress and no reason for hope. They will discount the positive and predict the future negatively. They will present a poor view of themselves and their own effectiveness. They will tend to catastrophise, that is predict disastrous consequences from small setbacks.

Anxiety is usually very apparent. Patients will appear tense and worried. They may voice their worries freely, be over-concerned for their safety, perhaps be seen to delay discharge; certain sticking points may emerge that relate to previous

bad experiences (for example a fall down stairs). In general, if physical progress is not in line with physical ability, then it might be worth considering whether some emotional factor is blocking the patient's advance.

The relation of patients' emotional status to their physical progress is not well understood. The interplay between emotional adjustment and physical disability is especially difficult to determine in an unpredictable condition of varying course, such as MS. Some group studies have examined the relation between emotional distress and the disease process of MS (see Knight 1992, Ch. 5, for a review). The fine detail and temporal dynamics of this relation can only be properly appreciated at the single case level.

A 16-year-old girl experienced her second MS relapse in 8 months. She had suddenly lost a great deal of physical function and had become dependent on a wheelchair for mobility. In July 1994, she was admitted to an inpatient neuro-rehabilitation unit. On admission, the girl was clearly distressed by her current situation and the possibility of permanent physical disability. She had planned to commence a 2-year course of study at her local sixth form college in September. However, on admission she was adamant that she would not attend the college using a wheelchair, or any other aid to mobility. She maintained this view throughout her 7-week stay on the unit.

Assessments were made of the girl's emotional status at approximately fortnightly intervals. The measures used were the BDI (Beck et al 1979), the STAI (Spielberger 1983) and the Spielberger State–Trait Anger Inventory (STAXI; Spielberger 1988). She was also asked to rate how uncomfortable she thought that she would feel in each of 15 everyday situations, on a scale ranging from 0, which represented 'not at all uncomfortable', to 100, which represented 'the most uncomfortable I've ever been'. During her admission, she progressed from using a wheelchair, to a rollator, to walking with two sticks by the time of her discharge. The details of her scores are given in Table 3.2.

Although her score on the BDI never reached the clinically depressed range, there were more

Table 3.2 Changes in measures of emotion and social discomfort across a 7-week neurohabilitation programme

	15.07.94		27.07.94		09.08.94		16.08.94		25.08.94	
Mobility	Wheelchair		Wheelchair		Wheelchair		Rollator		Two sticks	
Depression BDI (not depressed <10)	9		4		2		0		1	
Anxiety STAI										
State (immediate) %	97		45		42		17		3	
Trait (background) %	72		31		10		6		0	
Anger STAXI										
State (immediate) %	81		68		56		56		56	
Trait (background) %	50		10		5		0		2	
Social discomfort	A	F	A	F	A	F	A	F	A	F
Park	61	83	2	14	0	2	0	0	0	2
Supermarket	55	81	2	17	2	2	0	0	0	0
Bus stop	62	82	2	12	0	0	0	0	0	0
Fast food	46	78	1	4	1	1	0	0	0	0
Disco	86	87	—	24	4	5	0	0	0	0
Coffee shop	50	83	—	15	1	1	0	0	0	0
Cinema	50	86	4	—	1	3	0	0	0	0
Home	19	26	1	—	0	0	0	0	0	0
Hospital	20	22	2	4	0	0	0	0	0	0
Cosmetic shop	62	80	2	14	0	2	0	0	0	0
College	83	87	—	54	7	8	0	0	0	0
Corner shop	84	84	3	5	0	0	0	0	0	0
Party	69	94	17	30	2	7	0	0	0	0
Theatre	78	87	2	25	0	3	0	0	0	0
Restaurant	41	93	3	22	0	7	0	0	0	0

A = alone; F = with friends; — = not assessed

negative thoughts reported at the start of the admission, when she scored 9, than by discharge, when she scored 1. In contrast, an abnormal level of anxiety was reported on admission, but this, along with trait anxiety and trait anger, had reduced to very low levels by the time of her discharge. Although state anger also reduced over the same period, a significant level was still being recorded at discharge. Her ratings of predicted discomfort in the everyday situations also reduced, ahead of a full physical recovery. It appears that her anticipation of a full physical recovery led her to predict levels of discomfort in line with physical independence from mobility aids, before her physical progress had reached that point. It is interesting to note that her predicted level of discomfort in situations with her friends, does not reduce as quickly as her discomfort ratings of her being in situations alone. The ratings for the 27th July show this discrepancy. This is probably reflecting her anxieties about her friends' attitudes towards her.

Clearly, the relation between physical progress, fears about disability and emotion is complex. Emotional responses to neurological disease cannot be directly predicted by level of physical disability. They have their own rhythm and rationale, which can only be brought to light by careful discussion and observation.

Treatment strategies for emotionally distressed patients

A significant level of emotional distress will probably require specialist help and certainly any expressions of suicidal intent or other self-harm should be brought to the attention of a psychologist or psychiatrist. But a large number of patients with some degree of emotional distress can be helped through a therapy programme and neither need nor want a consultation with a specialist in abnormal behaviour or mental illness. The basis of formulating a therapy programme is to assess what is the nature of the patients' distress. Are they tense and nervous about their illness or recovery? Then the programme probably needs to take account of their anxiety. Are there problems at home that are overwhelming them? Then they probably need a counselling referral. Are they very negative and pessimistic about everything and everyone? Then the programme needs to be formulated to reduce their negativity.

If patients are very anxious about their illness or recovery, then it may help to arrange a consultation with a member of the medical staff to provide them with information. Some anxieties are not so easily allayed and in most cases it is not a good idea to spend large amounts of therapy time discussing the anxieties. Try to arrange for patients to have specific counselling sessions and agree with them to concentrate on physiotherapy when they are with you. In most instances, an anxious patient is likely to proceed slowly and a paced approach is often most productive, where small agreed increases in physical activity that are well within the patient's capabilities are made each day. Slow, steady progress is the aim and set-backs should be avoided wherever possible.

If the anxiety relates to a past incident, for example a recent fall on stairs resulting in a patient being loath to try stairs again, despite an obvious physical capability, then a brief discussion of the previous event, which includes how the future experience differs (supervision, physical recovery, more effective movement) may help. Sometimes it may be necessary to talk through the feared event. In the current example, discuss what would happen if the patient did fall on the stairs (minimal contact assistance would be maintained, she would not be allowed to injure or hurt herself). It is a characteristic of emotional judgements that the facts often do not speak for themselves. Facts which are apparently obvious may not have gained full acceptance in the patients' mind and may thus fail to influence their perception of risk. By discussing their specific fear, and even what would happen if there was a repeat of the feared event during therapy, patients mentally rehearse the feared event and perceive a happier outcome than they would have imagined without the discussion.

Patients may only feel able to tackle a few stairs at first, but they may be an important learning experience for them – that they can walk up three stairs without falling. Feedback and reassurance will be required constantly, with special emphasis on the safe completion of each activity.

Reassurance and discussion may not be as effective with depressed patients who are very negative. If they are told that everything is all right, they may well be alienated or irritated, because their established view of the world is likely to be bleak and hopeless. For an introduction to psychological techniques used to treat depression, see Beck et al (1979). One approach that is often successful in this situation is a very tight focus of conversation and action towards the specific functional gains identified for the therapy session in progress.

Any negative statements that relate directly to therapy, therapeutic outcome or attendance at therapy should be challenged. Once again a neutral, low-key tone is probably best. Rather than being drawn into an argument about whose view is right, it is best to rely on concrete evidence. If possible, try things out with the patient to demonstrate benefits. Failing that, draw on evidence of previous cases, especially previous cases who started out from the same negative stance. It may be necessary to explicitly acknowledge that patients can see no possible benefit, in which case compliance in therapy can be promoted to patients on the basis that they can not be harmed by the process, or that it might help to take their minds off things. By attending and working in therapy they are at least giving themselves a chance of progress. Once they are involved in therapy, a diary or chart recording their progress in concrete terms can be helpful, in providing evidence for the benefits of the treatment programme.

CONCLUSIONS
Neuropsychological tests

Only a handful of neuropsychological tests have been introduced in this chapter. They have been used to give a brief impression of the kinds of tools that tease out the aspects of a patient's cognitive and emotional skills that have been affected by neurological disease. They are a useful starting point in the design of a treatment programme, but their relation to a patient's physical recovery or rehabilitation needs to be carefully examined. Most patients with cortical involvement of their disease will have widespread cognitive and emotional difficulties. The most striking features of a psychological assessment may not be the most salient in treatment. For any treatment programme, the interaction between all current impairments must be considered and the most appropriate way to achieve necessary functional gains identified.

Clinical observation

There is no substitute for observing a patient's physical activity, if the aim is to understand the nature of their difficulties. It is necessary to monitor constantly for the effects of cognitive and emotional dysfunction. A patient's neurological status can change, affecting the pattern of cognitive impairment. Emotional status can change for a whole host of reasons, many independent of the disease process. Patients who first come to therapy with a high level of physical disability may not demonstrate any cognitive deficits. For example, a patient recovering from a severe head injury, may learn to turn in bed without difficulty. Turning in bed makes relatively low cognitive demands on the patient, in that little precision, timing or spatial calculation is required. However, as the patient's recovery progresses and his physical activity progresses to more complex tasks such as

transfers, the confounding effects of cognitive dysfunction may become obvious.

Treatment strategies

Some patients may have suffered sensory or motor deficits that are relatively peripheral and in addition there is a possibility of cognitive dysfunction. In these cases it may be hard to clarify the pattern of impairment that is causing an observed movement problem. One approach is to try either the most likely or the simplest treatment strategy. If this is sufficiently effective, then there is no need to consider the other option in therapy. If the trial has very disappointing results, it may be best to try a strategy designed to help the other impairment and abandon the first approach. A careful trial of alternative treatment strategies, although initially cumbersome, can eventually be the most efficient intervention, because it avoids spending time on ineffective or inappropriate interventions later. However, many patients suffer from a mixture of peripheral and central impairments. For them, a combined approach may be necessary.

Textbooks can be disappointing, in that they invariably fail to describe the particular constellation of impairment and disability that one's patients demonstrate. But in fairness to textbooks, the neurological patients for whom a 'prêt-à-porter' treatment package can unhesitatingly be adopted are few. It is the absorbing challenge of neurology, to fuse the variety of observed clinical features into a platform on which to build an effective treatment programme. It was the aim of this chapter to help you to add a few planks to that platform.

REFERENCES

Beck A T, Rush A J, Shaw B F, Emery G 1979 Cognitive therapy of depression. Guilford, New York
De Renzi E 1982 Disorders of space exploration and cognition. John Wiley, Chichester
Ellis A W, Young A W 1988 Human cognitive neuropsychology. Lawrence Erlbaum, Hove
Gainotti G 1993 Emotional and psychosocial problems after brain injury. Neuropsychological Rehabilitation 3: 259–277

Gray J M, Robertson I H, Pentland B, Anderson S 1992 Microcomputer-based attentional retraining after brain damage: a randomised group controlled trial. Neuropsychological Rehabilitation 2: 97–115
Gronwall D M A 1977 Paced auditory serial addition task: a measure of recovery from concussion. Perceptual and Motor Skills 44: 367–373
Holden U, Woods R 1995 Positive approaches to dementia care. Churchill Livingstone, Edinburgh

Howard D, Hatfield F M 1987 Aphasia therapy: historical and contemporary issues. Lawrence Erlbaum, Hove

Kapur N 1988 Memory disorders in clinical practice. Butterworths, London

Kay J, Lesser R, Coltheart M 1992 Psycholinguistic assessments of language processing in aphasia. Lawrence Erlbaum, Hove

Kline P 1993 The handbook of psychological testing. Routledge, London

Knight R G 1992 The neuropsychology of degenerative brain disease. Lawrence Erlbaum, Hillsdale

Langdon D W, Thompson A J 1994 Relationship of objective and self-report measures of memory in multiple sclerosis. Journal of Neurology 241: S150

Langdon D W, Warrington E K 1995 The VESPAR: a verbal and spatial reasoning test. Lawrence Erlbaum, Hove

McCarthy R A, Warrington E K 1990 Cognitive neuro-psychology: a clinical introduction. Academic Press, San Diego

McKenna P, Warrington E K 1983 Graded naming test. NFER, Windsor

McMillan T M 1984 Investigation of everyday memory in normal subjects using the subjective memory questionnaire (SMQ). Cortex 20: 333–347

Marr D 1982 Vision. Freeman, San Francisco

Milner B 1963 Effects of different lesions on card sorting. Archives of Neurology 9: 91

Nelson H E, McKenna P 1975 The use of current reading ability in the assessment of dementia. British Journal of Social and Clinical Psychology 14: 259–267

Nelson H E, O'Connell A 1978 Dementia: the estimation of premorbid intelligence levels using the new adult reading test. Cortex 14: 234–244

Nelson H E, Willison J 1992 Restandardisation of the NART against the WAIS-R. NFER, Windsor

Obrzut 1986 Child neuropsychology. Academic, San Diego

Perecman E (ed) 1987 The frontal lobes revisited. IRBN, New York

Prigatano G P 1991 Awareness of deficit after brain injury. Oxford University Press, New York

Robertson I H, Marshall J C 1993 Unilateral neglect: clinical and experimental studies. Lawrence Erlbaum, Hove

Robertson I H, North N, Geggie C 1992 Spatio-motor cueing in unilateral neglect: three single case studies of its therapeutic effects. Journal of Neurology, Neurosurgery and Psychiatry 55: 799–805

Robertson I H, Ward T, Ridgeway V, Nimmo-Smith I 1994 The test of everyday attention. Thames Valley, Bury St Edmunds

Schwartz A F, McMillan T M 1989 Assessment of everyday memory after severe head injury. Cortex 25: 665–671

Spielberger C D 1983 Manual for the state–trait anxiety inventory. Consulting Psychologists, Palo Alto

Spielberger C D 1988 The state–trait anger expression inventory. Psychological Assessment Resources, Odessa

Warrington E K 1984 Recognition memory test. NFER, Windsor

Warrington E K 1986 Visual deficits associated with occipital lobe lesions in man. Experimental Brain Research Supplementum 11: 247–261

Warrington E K, James M 1991 The visual object and space perception battery. Thames Valley, Bury St Edmunds

Wechsler D 1981 Manual for the Wechsler adult intelligence–revised. Psychological Corporation, New York

Wilson B A 1987 Rehabilitation of memory. Guilford, New York

Wilson B A, Moffat N (eds) 1984 Clinical management of memory problems. Croom Helm, London

Wilson C, Robertson I H 1992 A home-based invention for attentional slips during reading following a head injury: a single case study. Neuropsychological Rehabilitation 2: 193–205

Wilson B, Cockburn J, Baddeley A 1985 The Rivermead behavioural memory test. Thames Valley, Bury St Edmunds

Wilson B A, Cockburn J, Halligan P 1987 The behavioural inattention test. Thames Valley Test Company, Bury St Edmunds

Wilson B A, Baddeley A, Evans J, Shiel A 1994 Errorless learning in the rehabilitation of memory impaired people. Neuropsychological Rehabilitation 4: 307–326

Yves von Cramon D, Matthes von Cramon G 1992 Reflection on the treatment of brain-injured patients suffering from problem-solving disorders. Neuropsychological Rehabilitation 2: 207–229

CHAPTER CONTENTS

Introduction   63

Spasticity   64
   Aims of physiotherapy intervention   65
   Specific pathological activity associated with
      patients with spasticity   66

Rigidity   71
   Clinical presentation of parkinsonism   72

Dystonia   74
   Clinical presentation   75
   Treatment   75

Chorea and athetosis   76
   Clinical presentation   77
   Problems associated with communication and
      eating   78
   Problems arising with posture and movement   78

Ataxia   80
   Sensory ataxia   80
   Vestibular ataxia   80
   Cerebellar ataxia   80
   Clinical presentation   82

Summary   83

References   84

4

Abnormal tone and movement as a result of neurological impairment: considerations for treatment

Susan Edwards

INTRODUCTION

Tone is the resistance offered by muscles to continuous stretch, such as that produced by passive flexion or extension of a joint (Brooks 1986). The two mechanisms which contribute to this resistance are the inherent viscoelastic properties of the muscle itself and the tension set up in the muscle by reflex contraction caused by muscle stretch (Rothwell 1994).

Neurological damage is often manifested by diverse physical disability. In some conditions, the presence of abnormal tone dominates the picture. The differing types of abnormal tone are determined by the site and extent of the lesion. At the present time there is no evidence to suggest that physiotherapy can influence the disease processes or pathology of, for example, muscular dystrophy or head injury. However, environmental factors, such as correct positioning and movements to maintain and, where necessary, regain muscle and joint range, are essential in ensuring the optimal level of function for each individual.

The purpose of rehabilitation is to enable the patient to experience as normal a lifestyle as is possible and to minimise the effects of abnormal tone in terms of function. Management and, where appropriate, prevention of abnormal compensatory measures adopted by patients in an attempt to cope with their change in physical status are the remit of all staff involved in this process.

Investigations such as computerised tomography, magnetic resonance imaging and positron emission tomography have revolutionised diagnosis in neurological medicine. Prior to the introduction of this new technology, the site and extent of the lesion was mainly determined by the clinical signs and symptoms. In a sense, the focus of physiotherapy is still at the analytical age where treatment is determined by the clinical presentation and effects of, for example, abnormal tone, sensory impairment, perceptual problems and weakness. It is based on the hypothesis that by providing a more normal, functional environment, therapy can influence outcome. The exact cause and extent of the damage is of secondary importance to the clinical picture of the distribution and severity of the abnormal tone. Even with sophisticated monitoring, exact physical disabilities cannot be predicted from the type and extent of the lesion.

SPASTICITY

This is a disorder of spinal proprioceptive reflexes, manifested clinically as tendon jerk hyperreflexia and an increase in muscle tone that becomes more apparent the more rapid the stretching movement (Lance 1980). Chronic spasticity is often associated with changes in the biomechanical properties of muscle (Thilmann et al 1991, Hufschmidt & Mauritz 1985).

In hemiplegia, spasticity is characterised by increased tendon jerks, the clasp knife phenomenon and an increase in muscle tone which is greater in the flexors of the arm and the extensor muscles of the leg (Rothwell 1994, Petajan 1990).

Spasticity has been considered to be a positive release phenomenon as a consequence of cerebral or spinal cord damage. This gives rise to the characteristic features of spasticity:

- enhanced stretch reflex
- abnormal posture and mass movement patterns
- inappropriate co-contraction and the inability to fractionate patterns and perform isolated movement of one joint
- exaggeration of exteroceptive reflexes of the limbs producing flexor withdrawal or extensor spasms and the Babinski response (Burke 1988, Musa 1986).

These characteristic features may be evidenced immediately after gross cerebral pathology such as may arise from severe head injury. However, in the majority of cases spasticity does not develop immediately (Dietz 1992). Depending on the extent and rate of onset of CNS damage, cerebral or spinal shock may ensue, the duration of which is variable. Emergence from this state and subsequent development of spasticity is often gradual, occurring over days or weeks. This has led to a consideration of spasticity as a phenomenon of plasticity rather than of release (Brown 1994, Kidd et al 1992).

The development of spasticity will be determined not only by the extent and severity of the supraspinal damage but also by environmental influences and psychosocial factors such as posture, effort and patient motivation (Bach-y-Rita 1990). Plastic adaptation of the CNS in response to the neurological damage is felt to be influenced by such environmental factors. The distribution and severity of spasticity will inevitably influence the musculoskeletal system. Length changes imposed by spastic posturing may lead to biomechanical changes within the muscles (Goldspink & Williams 1990) and a transformation of motor unit type, from type II to type I, has been reported in paretic muscles of patients with established spasticity (Dattola et al 1993). Edstrom (1970) found that atrophy of type II fibres in patients with hemiparesis, paraparesis and parkinsonism appeared to be related to the reduction of muscular power and the increase in tone. Therefore, it is impossible to consider the supraspinal damage which leads to abnormal tone and changes in muscle property as separate entities in the management of patients with spasticity (Nash et al 1989).

The intrinsic stiffness of the muscle is one contributor to muscle tone and, given that muscle normally exhibits spring-like behaviour, it is possible that an increase in the intrinsic mechanical stiffness of the muscle is responsible for spastic hypertonia (Brown 1994). This stiffness could be mediated by permanent structural changes in the mechanical properties of muscle or connective tissues, or be variable in character (Katz & Rymer 1989, Carey & Burghardt 1993).

The contribution of these factors to the clinical impression of tone in spasticity is very much a matter of controversy (Rothwell 1994, Dietz 1992, Thilmann et al 1991).

Spasticity will create an imbalance of muscular activity (Knutsson & Richards 1979). In some conditions such as stroke, the pattern of spasticity is often seen as being predominantly in the anti-gravity musculature (Brown 1994). The majority of patients following a cerebrovascular accident demonstrate flexor spasticity in the upper limbs and extensor spasticity in the lower limbs. The severity and distribution of this abnormal tone will be determined both by the site and extent of the lesion and from plastic changes in spinal circuits to compensate for the removal of descending inputs (Burke 1988).

Historical perspective

It is interesting to note that reference to the stroke patient in the literature of some 30 years ago (Smith 1963) describes a somewhat stereotyped picture. Not only is reference made to the patterns of spasticity affecting the anti-gravity musculature, but the reported clinical observation indicates a fairly stereotyped outcome.

Management and treatment of stroke at that time was based on the concept that damage to the CNS was irreparable. Recovery of the affected side was therefore not a consideration. The patients were supplied with a long or short leg caliper to control the affected leg and/or foot, a sling to support the upper limb and a tripod or quadripod stick to provide a means of support. Specific physiotherapy intervention was in many instances directed towards maximising the use of the non-affected side to compensate for the impaired function of the other. No attempt was made to facilitate recovery by means of influencing the spasticity (Partridge et al 1993).

As a result of this approach, patients adopted a stereotyped response which reflected the environment that they were forced to contend with. Effort increases spasticity. The calipers provided at this time were made of metal irons, often extending the length of the leg, and inserting into the shoe. A strap was often incorporated into the design in an attempt to maintain the foot in a neutral position. Special shoes were recommended to ensure an adequate point of fixation for the caliper. The net result was that of a rigid, unadaptable limb and additional weight with which the patient had to cope. Patients supplied with such a caliper would inevitably have to use excessive effort and compensate by hitching the leg forwards in order to step through. This action demands greater activity from, in particular, latissimus dorsi with a resultant shortening of the trunk side flexors. The insertion of latissimus dorsi at the humerus produces medial rotation of the upper limb and compounds the flexor synergy. Each time the patient attempts to hitch the leg forwards, the trunk side flexors and the upper limb, through the action of latissimus dorsi, demonstrate an increase in the spastic flexor activity. A recognised phenomenon at the time was that the severity of spasticity would often increase over a period of time in spite of the stroke itself being recognised as a non-progressive condition.

This analysis provides an illustration of neuroplasticity. Damage to the CNS will determine the initial state in terms of physical and cognitive impairment. Recovery will be dependent upon not only the neurophysiological changes but also the environment in which the patient has to function (Held 1993). Without intervention, patients will develop strategies to compensate for their disability. Whilst some of these may be beneficial, others such as those described above, will cause further impairment of function.

Aims of physiotherapy intervention

Spasticity creates a situation whereby movement is affected and accomplished only with increased effort. Patients attempt to perform the functional skills which are prerequisites of daily living, but unless they have the appropriate background of postural tone and normal active and passive properties of muscle, these movements will be performed in an abnormal way. The effort required to attempt the movement further reinforces the sensation of requiring greater exertion to succeed and the prevailing spasticity is exacerbated.

Physiotherapy intervention aims to provide an improved environment in all aspects of the patient's daily life with a background of tone that allows selective movement. The stroke population of the 1990s is made up of a very different group of individuals in comparison to the stereotyped picture of previous decades. The hypothesis is that by directing treatment at each patient's specific problems in relation to the extent and severity of impaired tone and potential changes in the mechanical properties of muscle, the outcome will be more positive. Only by inhibiting spasticity and facilitating more normal movement on an improved background of postural tone, can the relearning of selective movement occur. Analysis of these individual problems can only be successful if the therapist has a good understanding of basic movement components.

It is essential that physiotherapy treatment is seen to have a functional goal. While in many instances it is necessary to work for component parts of movement patterns, the patient must appreciate that the outcome of this improved activity will have functional significance, otherwise motivation and cooperation will be diminished (Carr & Shepherd 1987, Ada et al 1990).

Specific pathological activity associated with patients with spasticity

Positive support reaction

The positive support reaction was first described by Magnus (1926 as cited by Bobath 1990) as a process by which the movable limb changes into a stiff pillar. It is a static response of the lower limb evoked by a stimulus of pressure on the ball of the foot. It affects agonists and antagonists simultaneously, producing a rigidly extended limb and a subsequent inability to balance with normal alignment of the trunk and pelvis. Bobath (1990) describes a dual stimulus:

- a proprioceptive stimulus evoked by stretch of the intrinsic muscles of the foot, and
- an exteroceptive stimulus evoked by the contact of the pads of the foot with the ground.

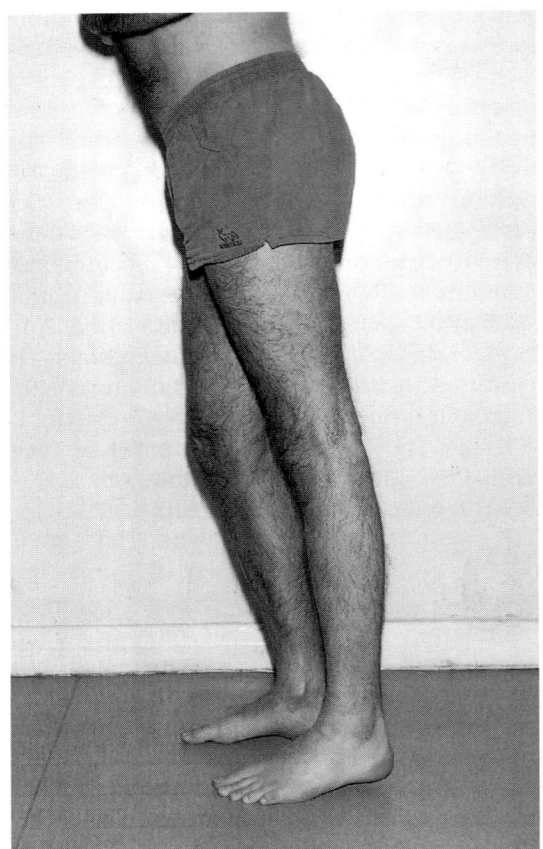

Figure 4.1 Positive support reaction.

The positive support reaction is considered to be of distal origin arising from hypersensitivity which leads to the inability of the foot to adapt and accept the base of support (Fig. 4.1). Compensatory strategies arise proximally in an attempt to maintain balance. This reaction is associated with extensor spasticity in the first instance, although a modification of this response, whereby flexion may dominate, has been observed in clinical practice.

The term 'positive support reaction' would appear to be one used predominantly by physiotherapists. There is little in the literature to clarify this terminology. Rothwell (1994) describes the pressure sensors (mechanoreceptors) in the sole of the foot being used for balance and the importance of mechanoreceptors in the control of movement. The integration of afferent information from these receptors may be impaired following cerebral or spinal cord damage which may give rise to the response described above.

Schomburg (1990) commented that pressure on the plantar skin of the foot leads to what he terms to be an 'extensor thrust', and that activation of the pressure receptors activates the toe extensors without activation of the ankle, knee or hip extensors and without any reciprocal inhibition to the antagonistic toe flexor muscles.

A stereotyped co-activation of muscles during the stance phase of gait was observed in a study of the different types of disturbed motor control in hemiplegic gait (Knutsson & Richards 1979). Dietz (1992) described the spastic gait pattern as being characterised by an inability to increase locomotion speed or to adapt to irregularities in ground conditions, in addition to difficulties in lifting the foot during the swing phase of gait. Thilmann et al (1991) commented that, while at the elbow spastic muscle hypertonia is always associated with velocity-dependent electromyographic activity, this is clearly not the case at the ankle, where a significant contribution to raised tone arises from changes in the passive properties of the ankle.

Ablation of the anterior lobe of the cerebellum has been found to produce deficits in the reflex and proprioceptive control of muscle tone which include increased extensor muscle tone with positive supporting reflexes and tactile supporting reactions (Thompson & Day 1993).

These comments and descriptions may relate to the positive support reaction but with the exception of Thompson & Day (1993), who do not clarify what is meant by 'positive support reflex', no mention is made of this term.

Clinical features. Plantar flexor spasticity is a primary and obvious feature of this reaction and is frequently associated with inversion of the foot due to spasticity of tibialis posterior and the toe flexors. Secondary involvement includes shortening of the intrinsic foot musculature due to the inability to transfer weight across the full surface of the foot and loss of range in the plantar fascia. The posterior crural muscle group

may become shortened due to the inability to attain a plantigrade position during the stance phase of walking, further exacerbating the inability to transfer weight.

A consequence of this reaction is that of compensatory flexion of the trunk in an attempt to maintain balance. The pelvis is retracted as the weight is displaced backwards by the pressure from the ball of the foot against the supporting surface, the patient being unable to transfer the weight over the full support and thus achieve extension at the hip.

Although the knee is maintained in a position of extension this is not achieved on the basis of appropriate quadriceps activity and it is not uncommon to observe wasting of this muscle group. In many instances the knee becomes hyperextended as a result of the inability to attain normal alignment of the pelvis over the foot, impaired reciprocal innervation between the hamstrings and quadriceps muscle groups and shortening of gastrocnemius.

The flexed, retracted position of the hip and pelvis may lead to shortening of the hip flexors, adductors and medial rotators, producing a mechanical obstruction to correct alignment of the hip during stance phase.

The pressure exerted by the foot pushing into extension prevents release of the knee. Attempts by the patient to move the foot away from the floor, result in compensatory strategies being adopted similar to those described in patients contending with a long leg caliper. The predominant extensor spasticity of the lower limb mimics the effect of the caliper. The spasticity of the upper limb is influenced by the amount of effort required to enable the patient to step forwards with the affected leg, primarily through the action of latissimus dorsi. This pathological response, of increased spasticity in the upper limb being determined by the effort necessary to accomplish a step forwards, is an example of what is referred to as an associated reaction (see p. 71).

The positive support reaction will also affect the ability to stand up from sitting and sit down from standing. The resistance from the spastic plantar flexors prevents the transference of weight forwards over the foot as the individual prepares to stand. The leg becomes stiff in extension and the patient is pushed back into the chair. The situation is reversed when attempting to sit down. The leg is unable to release into flexion and the patient falls back into the chair. Patients with hemiplegia will tend to stand up and sit down predominantly on their unaffected leg to minimise the effect.

More recently, a flexor component of the positive support reaction has been observed. As the patient attempts to bring the leg forwards there is a noted increase in flexor activity as a consequence of hypersensitivity of flexor muscle spindles to stretch. In this situation the sensitivity of the foot remains the primary problem but the mechanics in terms of weight-bearing are altered. The foot is maintained in a position of inversion and the ball of the foot does not make contact with the ground, leading to adaptive shortening of affected muscle groups. Weight is taken on the lateral border of the foot with an almost instant withdrawal into flexion as an attempt is made to step through.

Treatment of the positive support reaction must be directed towards mobilisation of the foot, the posterior crural muscle group and the Achilles tendon in the first instance, in an attempt to desensitise against both the intrinsic and extrinsic stimuli (Lynch & Grisogono 1991). Therapists are often advised not to stimulate the ball of the foot but in this instance appropriate handling and facilitation of transference of weight over the foot are important to reduce the effects of this reaction.

Patients with neurological impairment may demonstrate this response in a more stereotyped and consistent pattern. A minimal stimulus, not necessarily noxious, for example removing the bedclothes from a patient following spinal cord injury may be enough to elicit this response. The response in the lower limbs is that of flexion, abduction and lateral rotation at the hip, flexion at the knee and inversion of the foot in conjunction with dorsiflexion or plantar flexion of the ankle. This is illustrated in Figure 4.2.

The problem is often exacerbated by shortening of the dominant muscle groups, particularly the hip and knee flexors which may lead to subsequent shortening of the erector spinae. This response may be stimulated by stretch of these muscles which prevents the patient from standing up effectively (Lynch & Grisogono 1991) and from placing the foot on the floor.

In clinical practice this response may be seen in patients with severe neurological damage such as may occur following head injury or complete spinal cord transection (Brown 1994). It may also be observed in patients with neurological impairment following painful trauma such as a fracture of the neck of femur. Pressure sores, or other painful stimuli of the foot in particular, may also give rise to a flexor response (Schomburg 1990).

Removal of the noxious stimulus and/or management of the primary trauma are of immediate concern in treating the manifestations of this response. The short-term influence of

Flexor withdrawal response of the leg

Flexor withdrawal is a response which occurs in normal subjects and is well illustrated by withdrawal of the hand from a hot stove, or the foot when stepping on a drawing pin. It is associated with the crossed extensor reflex (Magnus 1926 as cited by Bobath 1990, Schomburg 1990, Edwards 1991). The withdrawal response is determined by the direction of the noxious stimulus and therefore may not necessarily be into flexion (Rothwell 1994).

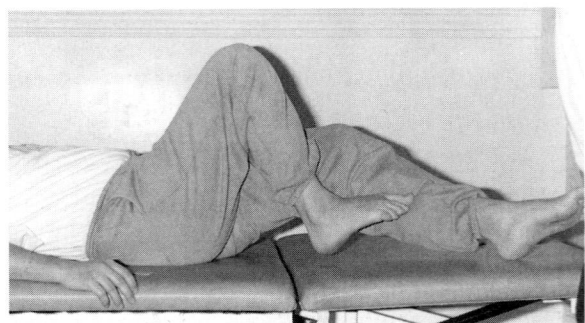

Figure 4.2 Flexor withdrawal.

such a stimulus may prove to be readily reversible, whereas prolonged exposure, particularly to pain, will have more residual effects, such as the establishment of contractures.

Treatment by physiotherapy will be determined by the extent and severity of structural changes which may have occurred. Attempts to stand a patient on a leg which is mechanically shortened due to contracture will further aggravate the situation, not least by imposing an additional painful stimulus. It is essential to first regain the required range of movement at the hip and pelvis, thereby allowing the leg to be released sufficiently to attain its normal length. 'Normal' standing can only be achieved on the basis of mechanical and structural equality of the pelvis and lower limbs. In the absence of equality, compensation, particularly at the trunk and pelvis is inevitable. Mobilisation of shortened muscles and soft tissues may cause some discomfort, but it is important to distinguish between pain resulting from muscle stretch and joint pain which may occur through forcing a malaligned joint. As a general rule, any intervention should be pain-free, it being impossible to inhibit pathological or, indeed, normal protective muscle spasm in the presence of pain.

Davies (1985) advocates the use of a back slab to maintain the leg in extension and thereby facilitate weight-bearing. This procedure may be of benefit in the early stages of counteracting increasing flexor activity of the leg but should be used with caution in patients with more long-standing problems, particularly where there is loss of range. Attempts to force the leg into a back slab may cause pain and thereby nullify any positive effects.

Grasp reflex

The grasp reflex is a normal phenomenon in human infants which disappears within a few months of birth. In the adult it is always pathological.

Rothwell (1994) describes three different types of pathological grasp reflex:

- The classical grasp reflex of neurology, which consists of involuntary prehension elicited by a tactile stimulus to the palm.
- A traction response which usually accompanies the classical grasp reflex. This is a heightened stretch reflex of the finger flexor muscles, such that attempts to remove an object from the hand by extending the flexor tendons results in an increased force of grip.
- The instinctive grasp reflex. This is an involuntary closing of the hand elicited by tactile stimulation on any part of the hand or fingers, not restricted to the palm. The hand is first oriented towards the object so as to bring it into the palm. This stimulus then secondarily elicits a tactile grasp reflex to close the fingers on the object.

The type of grasp reflex more commonly seen by physiotherapists is a combination of the classical and traction response. As described above, the stimulus for initiating this response is to the hand and fingers, particularly the palm. Desensitisation of this reflex must therefore incorporate mobilisation and appropriate tactile stimulation to the hand within the patient's tolerance. This must involve all personnel involved in the management of such patients, not least the patients themselves and their carers. Movements of the hand should also include an appropriate response from the whole of the upper limb and, wherever possible, produce a functional outcome.

The use of splinting to prevent contracture in the presence of a severe grasp reflex remains a controversial issue and is discussed in Chapter 8.

Extensor response

This response may be observed following severe head injury and in people with multiple sclerosis or athetoid cerebral palsy. It is initiated and perpetuated by the contact between the back of the head and the supporting surface and is exacerbated in extensor positions such as supine lying. Extreme cases will include extension of all four limbs with arching of the spine. Patients described as displaying the 'out of line' or 'pusher' syndrome (Davies 1985) will often demonstrate an extensor thrust of the head and upper trunk but in conjunction with flexor spasticity of the affected lower leg.

There are differing degrees of severity, but it is important to recognise the influence of positions of extension and the susceptibility to a stimulus, such as the head support of a wheelchair, in triggering this response. It may be an extensor thrust which is responsible for preventing the patient from accepting the support of a chair with the result that he is constantly pushing himself out. If this is the case, it is important to desensitise this response rather than merely attempting to restrain the patient in the chair.

The extensor response is indicative of gross cerebral pathology, and it may be questioned whether any physiotherapeutic intervention can have an effect on outcome. It is difficult to prevent the development of contractures if the patient is constantly held in this extreme position of extension. Physiotherapy is based on the principle that changes in the environment will influence potential for change in the CNS. Modification of the extended position to introduce an element of flexion will create a temporary release from what can only be assumed to be a painful maintenance of spastic extension. This may be achieved by the use of the gymnastic ball whereby the patient is mobilised into flexion over an adaptable as opposed to a rigid surface (Fig. 4.3).

The patient may also be facilitated into standing, preferably with a therapist in front to support the knees and another behind to provide a mobile support in an attempt to prevent stimulation of the thrust into extension. A tilt table is often used for this purpose and in some instances this may be the only practicable way of the patient attaining the standing position. Difficulties may arise using this method as the table provides a rigid support against which the patient can push and, at the same time, minimises the opportunity of mobilising the patient while upright against gravity (see Ch. 5).

The extensor response is invariably accompanied by plantar flexor spasticity. Treatment as

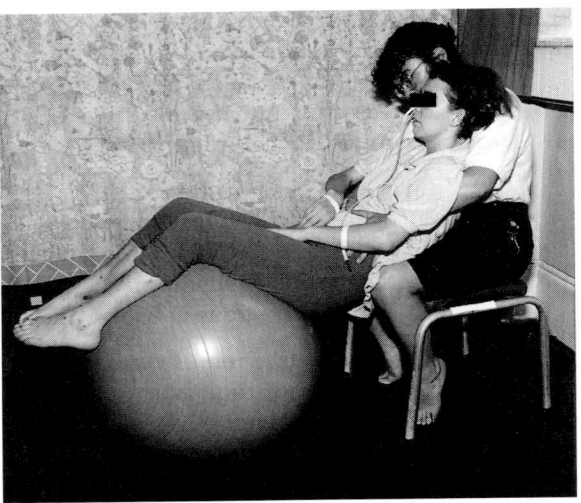

Figure 4.3 Mobilisation of extensor response over ball.

advocated above may have some influence on this particular aspect of management. Unfortunately, contracture of the posterior crural muscles groups is a well-documented complication of extensor spasticity (Yarkony & Sahgal 1987, Booth et al 1983, Kent et al 1990). Application of below-knee inhibitory casts as a prophylactic measure has been recommended as a means of preventing or minimising this disabling complication (Conine et al 1990, Moseley 1993) and is discussed in Chapter 8.

Associated reactions

Associated reactions are pathological movements which are indicative of the potential for development of spasticity or an accentuation of the prevailing spastic synergy. They appear as stereotyped abnormal patterns of movement which are accentuated by effort (Bobath 1990). They may be described as the observable feature of spasticity in that the movement of the limb is directly related to the prevailing tone and the amount of effort that is required to initiate or sustain movement (Dvir & Panturin 1993). These reactions may occur throughout the body but are most apparent in the more distal parts such as the arm and hand and the leg and foot. They may be initiated, not only as a result of attempted movement, but also at the preparatory stage of movement. Attempts to communicate by patients with dysphasia or cognitive problems may also produce this response.

Bobath (1985) makes a clear distinction between associated reactions, which are always pathological, and associated movements, which are normally coordinated movements occurring as a result of reinforcement of movements initiated and performed with effort, such as when learning a new skill. However, Carr & Shepherd (1980) refer to associated movements in the context of both normal and pathological response to concentrated or effortful movement, and Brunnstrom (1970) uses this term to describe involuntary limb movement.

An example of associated reactions has been described previously in relation to compensation for the positive support reaction. They may also be found in a patient following stroke where there is excessive tone at the pelvis and in the lower limb which necessitates increased effort in taking the leg forwards during the swing phase of gait. This increased effort is reflected in an increase of tonus throughout the affected side, producing, in many instances, a stereotyped response of flexor spasticity of the arm and side flexion of the trunk. This pathological response is indicative of the severity of the spasticity.

Dvir & Panturin (1993) found that improvement in effort-related associated reactions mirrored a decrease in tone, and in a study by Cornall (1991) associated reactions were used to assess the effects on spasticity when self-propelling a wheelchair. However, as they are variable depending on the effort involved, they may not be the most appropriate means of measuring spasticity (Haas 1994).

Sustained associated reactions may give rise to a deteriorating level of function in that movement, for example of the arm into flexion, may lead to a gradual loss of range and ultimately contracture (Dvir & Panturin 1993). It must be appreciated that the associated reactions themselves are not the primary problem in this cycle of events. Movement requiring excessive effort as a result of spasticity will invariably produce this pathological response. Unless the true cause is identified, for example instability of the pelvis, and addressed in treatment, inhibition of the associated reactions will have no functional carry-over. Facilitation of more functional movement and advice and explanation to the patient of the cause and effect of this response will go some way to minimising this secondary complication. Both the patient and the physiotherapist may use the associated reactions as a means of monitoring performance. Any activity resulting in marked associated reactions is indicative that it is beyond the patient's control, and appropriate assistance should be given to reduce the amount of effort required (Davies 1994).

RIGIDITY

Rigidity is clinically defined as increased resistance to stretch and the inability to achieve complete muscle relaxation (Wichmann & DeLong 1993). It is present in all muscle groups and has a uniform quality throughout the range of movement. Tendon jerks are normal (Messina 1990).

Features which are associated with rigidity in patients with Parkinson's disease include akinesia and bradykinesia. Neither is caused by the resulting restraint of active movement since both conditions can be present when rigidity is absent (Gordon 1990).

Akinesia. Akinesia has been defined as an impairment in the initiation of movement or delay in the reaction time. In patients with Parkinson's disease this is most prominent for movements which are internally generated rather than those which occur in response to sensory stimuli (Miller & DeLong 1988, Lee 1989). Other characteristics which have been described as features of akinesia in relation to Parkinson's disease are:

- lack of spontaneous movements
- lack of associated movements, such as arm swinging during walking
- abnormally small amplitude movements, such as very small steps during walking or micrographia

- a tendency for repetitive movements to show a decrease in amplitude and eventually fade out
- difficulty performing two simultaneous movements (Lee 1989).

Bradykinesia. Bradykinesia is a term which should be used exclusively to refer to slowness in the execution of the movement (Lee 1989). It appears as a disorder in voluntary movement in daily life and is considered to be partly responsible for disorders in posture and locomotion (Yanagisawa et al 1989).

Although these different definitions are used, they would appear to be of academic rather than practical value. Marsden (1986) and Hallett (1993) provide a more global definition in referring to akinesia as an inability to move and bradykinesia as slowness of movement. In Parkinson's disease, rigidity is considered to be a positive symptom resulting from release of other brain structures that are normally inhibited by basal ganglia function, whereas akinesia and bradykinesia are the key negative features of loss of normal basal ganglia function (Marsden 1982).

Although the most common neurological disorder which produces the akinetic-rigid syndrome is Parkinson's disease, it may occur in many other pathologies. However, most of the causes of symptomatic parkinsonism involve widespread brain damage in addition to lesions of the basal ganglia. Symptomatic parkinsonism may be seen as the overall picture in diffuse brain disease such as Alzheimer's disease and after severe head injury. Other diseases which cause parkinsonism, such as multiple system atrophy and progressive supranuclear palsy, have more restricted pathology, but even this spreads well beyond the confines of the basal ganglia (Marsden 1984).

Treatment of the disease process and basic research into the primary problem lies in the hands of the medical staff. Physiotherapists must consider the resulting disability in terms of the movement deficit. People with Parkinson's disease support physiotherapy intervention and claim beneficial effects of exercise (Banks & Caird 1989) and yet only about 15% of patients see a physiotherapist or occupational therapist (Pentland 1993).

Normal movement is dependent upon an intact CNS providing for an adaptable and integrated level of tonus. Patients with Parkinson's disease become more flexed as their condition deteriorates (Gordon 1990). Rotation is dependent upon the balanced activity between flexor and extensor muscle groups and, as previously described in Chapter 2, a dominance of either muscle group will impair rotation. The lack of rotation with reduced or loss of arm swing is a notable feature of Parkinson's disease (Pentland 1993, Marsden 1984, Lee 1989).

Clinical presentation of parkinsonism

The delay in initiation of movement in Parkinson's disease is more evident with internally generated or self-initiated movements than with movements occurring in response to sensory stimuli (Lee 1989). Various types of sensory input may partially compensate for akinesia. Brooks (1986) suggests the use of visual, auditory and vestibular cues, such as bouncing a ball, rocking the patient's shoulders back and forth or tilting the patient forwards to facilitate movement. It is well recognised that patients with Parkinson's disease may 'freeze' at a doorway and yet have no problem passing through if a stick, for example, is placed on the floor for them to step over. They may be unable to reach forwards with their arm on command but may be able to pick up a glass.

The inability to perform two simultaneous voluntary motor acts was illustrated by Schwab et al (1954 as cited by Marsden 1982):

A patient with Parkinson's disease seated in a hotel lobby notes an acquaintance entering the door. He starts to rise from the chair, which is motor activity No. 1, a complicated postural action involving balancing the body as it reaches the erect position. After this motor activity has been started and is perhaps 50% completed, the normal pattern would include the extension of the right hand in greeting the acquaintance, a second motor activity not related to the first. The person without Parkinsonism will execute these two motor patterns without difficulty so that they blend into a smooth complex of social behaviour. However, when the Parkinsonian patient starts the second motor act, he finds the first one has ceased. This results in his falling back to his chair in an embarrassing and unceremonious manner. If he again attempts to get out of the chair, the second motor activity of the greeting ceases and the right hand falls away awkwardly. In this struggle to perform successfully these common motor acts the Parkinsonian patient is left in a state of agitated frustration and anger, which leads to an increase in rigidity and tremor.

In the past, the emphasis of physiotherapy treatment was to improve rotation. To that effect, walking sticks were placed in the patient's hands with which the therapist would initiate arm swing. In normal subjects, arm swing, a relatively passive action, occurs as a result of interaction between the pelvis and shoulder girdles on the basis of an extended, upright posture. The ageing process clearly supports this analysis, in that, as the elderly adopt a more flexed posture, the arm swing is reduced (Elble et al 1991).

Patients with parkinsonism may become more flexed both through the CNS pathology and the ageing process. Attempts to superimpose arm swing as described above, on the basis of this predominantly flexed posture, will inevitably be doomed to failure. Analysis of the primary movement disorder will identify the lack of extension as a significant factor. Although the increased tone is equally distributed on passive manipulation of the joints, the evidence of increasing flexion is evident (Fig. 4.4). Patients with Parkinson's disease may well benefit from early intervention by physiotherapy in terms of introducing an exercise programme to reduce the insidious onset of flexion. Awareness on the part of the patient of this expected progression of the disease in terms of the impairment of movement and an appropriate home exercise programme to maintain extension may go some way to maintaining function.

The administration of dopamine derivatives often has a dramatic effect for patients with parkinsonism and in many cases determines the functional options (Marsden 1986). In severe cases, it may be that physiotherapy will only be possible after administration of these drugs. In

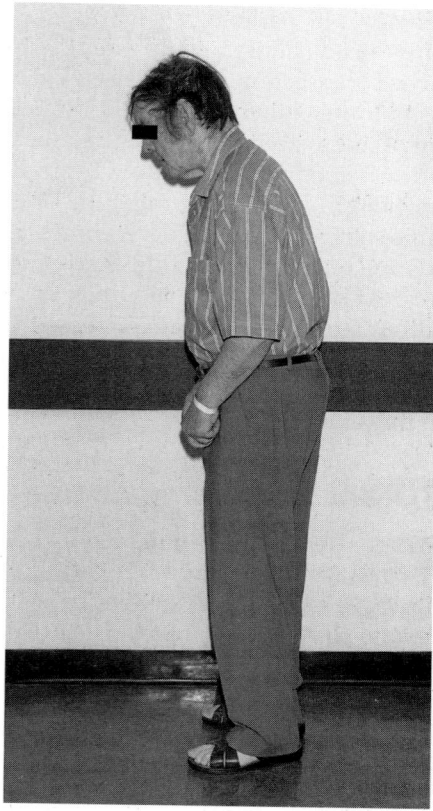

Figure 4.4 Parkinson's posture.

providing the experience of more normal movement and the maintenance of an upright posture, physiotherapy as an adjunct to medication is appropriate and beneficial in the management of this patient group. Equally, advice and management of specific problems which arise in the more disabled population, such as the inability to turn over in bed, will be of tremendous benefit to patients and their assistants. They will direct therapy intervention in that it is they who identify the problem and it is the remit of the therapist to analyse the causative factors and instigate appropriate treatment to enable a greater degree of function.

Rigidity produces stiffness which is primarily static. Patients with Parkinson's disease demonstrate 'plastic' or 'lead-pipe' rigidity with a dominance of flexion. Rigidity may also result from gross CNS pathology such as may occur following head injury, brain stem infarct or spinal cord transection. The extreme case is that of opisthotonus where the body is held in a position of mass extension resembling the rigidity induced in experimental animals by transection at the midbrain level. With this type of rigidity, sometimes referred to as decerebrate rigidity, the muscles resist lengthening; the resistance is independent of the velocity at which the force is applied but increases as length increases (Gordon 1990). These patients are in great danger of developing contractures as the body is constantly held in this extreme position.

DYSTONIA

Dystonia is a syndrome dominated by sustained muscle contractions frequently causing twisting and repetitive movements, or abnormal postures that may be sustained or intermittent (Fahn et al 1987). The cause of dystonia is not fully understood but it is thought to be caused by a biochemical disturbance within the basal ganglia. It is estimated to be more common than other well-known neurological diseases such as Huntington's disease, motor neurone disease and myasthenia gravis (Marsden & Quinn 1990) and yet many general practitioners consider it to be a rare disorder and are unfamiliar with the signs and symptoms (Dystonia Society 1991). For this reason, many sufferers may have considerable difficulty in being correctly diagnosed. It is only quite recently that dystonia has become a recognised, organic condition as opposed to one which, in some instances, was diagnosed as a psychosomatic or psychiatric ailment. However, Rondot et al (1991) found that no fewer than 61% of 220 patients suggested different events which they held responsible for the onset of spasmodic torticollis, and the authors concluded that 'in the complex of factors leading to spasmodic torticollis, psychological aspects do indeed play a role'.

There are several different types of dystonia which may be idiopathic or secondary to, for example, Wilson's disease, brain injury or tumour. It can affect virtually any area of the

Table 4.1 Common names used to describe dystonia affecting specific parts of the body (Marsden & Quinn 1990)

Name	Muscles contracting involuntarily
Blepharospasm	Orbicularis oculi and neighbouring facial muscles
Oromandibular dystonia	Jaw and mouth
Lingual dystonia	Tongue
Spasmodic dysphonia	Laryngeal, causing cord adduction and a strangulated speech, or cord abduction and whispering dysphonia
Dystonic dysphagia	Pharyngeal
Spasmodic torticollis	Sternocleidomastoid and posterior neck
Writer's cramp and other occupational cramps	Hand, forearm and arm
Axial dystonia	Back and trunk, causing scoliosis, lordosis, kyphosis or tortipelvis
Leg dystonia	Foot, leg and thigh

A combination of blepharospasm and oromandibular and lingual dystonia is known as cranial dystonia, Meige's or Brueghel's syndrome.
A combination of cranial dystonia and torticollis is known as craniocervical dystonia.

body and there are familiar names for dystonia at many different sites (Table 4.1). Dystonia affecting only one part of the body (for example spasmodic torticollis or dystonic writer's cramp) is known as a focal dystonia; if two or more adjacent parts are affected (for example torticollis with dystonic arms) as a segmental dystonia; two or more non-contiguous parts (for example eyes, neck and one leg) as multifocal dystonia; ipsilateral arm and leg as hemidystonia; and a whole body, or most of it including legs, as generalised dystonia.

Most patients with generalised, multifocal or segmental idiopathic dystonia of onset in childhood have an inherited disorder, and it may prove that inheritance plays a much larger part than is appreciated at present in the focal idiopathic dystonias of adult onset (Marsden & Quinn 1990). Trauma is considered to be of significance particularly in situations whereby spasmodic torticollis develops after neck injury and focal dystonias of the hand or foot arise after trauma to the affected part (Markham 1992, Anderson et al 1992, Chan et al 1991, Fletcher et al 1990).

Clinical presentation

Dystonic spasms are characterised by co-contraction of antagonist muscles rather than the more usual reciprocal pattern seen in normal voluntary movement (Rothwell 1994, Hallett 1993). Although there have been no studies reported on change in the biomechanical properties of muscle, Hallett (1993) suggests that such changes are as likely to occur in dystonia as in any other long-standing disease where there have been fixed postures.

The spasms may contort the body into grotesque postures which may severely limit activities of daily living. While this is more apparent in those with generalised dystonia, problems also arise for those with focal dystonia. For example, a person with spasmodic torticollis may be unable to drink from a glass, and one with blepharospasm may be unable to drive.

Dystonia can be present at rest but, in general, is more likely to appear during voluntary activity (Hallett 1993). It exhibits a variability under different conditions such as stress, fatigue and performance of certain motor acts such as walking (Lorentz et al 1991). Dystonia occurs characteristically and, especially in the early course of the disease, on certain actions such as the arm hyperpronating on writing but not when performing other manual tasks (Marsden 1984).

Treatment

Symptomatic treatment, particularly of the focal dystonias, has been revolutionised with the advent of botulinum toxin. Its use has proved so successful that Marsden & Quinn (1990) recommend that every regional neuroscience centre needs to provide this treatment. Botulinum toxin is a potent neurotoxin which produces temporary muscle weakness by presynaptic inhibition of acetylcholine release (Anderson et al 1992). Administration of this drug is by injection to the primarily affected muscles. This is now the treatment of choice for most focal dystonias, particularly blepharospasm (Grandas et al 1988) and spasmodic torticollis (Anderson et al 1992). The effect lasts from 2 to 4 months and then wears off as terminal sprouting restores muscle end-plate neurotransmission (Marsden & Quinn 1990). The injections are therefore repeated, on average, at 3-monthly intervals (Lorentz et al 1991, Anderson et al 1992).

Surgical treatment has been advocated in the past, such as facial nerve sectioning or myectomy for patients with blepharospasm and various procedures for spasmodic torticollis. These include selective peripheral denervation and stereotactic thalotomy (Bertrand et al 1978, 1987). Surgery may still be indicated for some patients who do not respond to botulinum toxin.

There is little documented on physiotherapy for patients with dystonia. Marsden & Quinn (1990) consider that physiotherapy is of great benefit in preventing contractures (although they feel that these are unlikely to occur) but cannot yet teach the brain to deliver normal motor programmes. Passive manual techniques, active cervical exercises and electrical neuromuscular stimulation are recommended for patients with spasmodic torticollis (Rondot et al 1991, Bleton 1994). Bertrand et al (1987) considers physiotherapy to be essential following selective denervation for spasmodic torticollis but no mention is made of modalities utilised. Braces and other forms of restraint are thought to be ineffective (Marsden & Quinn 1990).

Physiotherapy has an important role to play in the overall management of patients with dystonia. People with dystonia are unable to control specific voluntary movements and therefore 'exercises' as such are generally inappropriate and often frustrating for these patients. Although, as previously mentioned, Marsden & Quinn (1990) consider that contractures are unlikely to develop, Hallett (1993) suggests that changes in the mechanical properties of muscle are likely to occur. Lorentz et al (1991) describe muscle shortening and fibrosis in some patients with spasmodic torticollis.

On clinical observation, patients with severe spasmodic torticollis, dystonia of the hands or foot and those with generalised dystonia often have a restricted range of movement within the affected muscle groups. Emphasis on a more passive approach to treatment such as massage and specific mobilisation may be of value in preventing or reducing these structural changes. The constant torsioning effect of a sustained posture can also give rise to pain in the dystonic muscles (Anderson et al 1991, Lorentz et al 1991) and any treatment which gives even temporary relief is of benefit to the patient.

There is little evidence to support the effectiveness of this intervention, although patients report that they derive some relief from massage and specific mobilisation of the affected muscle groups. For example, facial and cranial massage for patients with dystonia affecting the face, and neck and shoulder massage for patients with spasmodic torticollis, may well prove of benefit. To date, there have been no clinical trials to evaluate the efficacy of such intervention.

In many instances, people develop their own strategies to control their movements; those with torticollis may touch the side of the chin, and people with blepharospasm, the lateral border of the eyebrow. As with all people with disability, it is important to recognise that the individuals with the disability are often more knowledgeable about the management of their condition than the majority of medical personnel involved in their care.

Advice with posture and seating for people with generalised dystonia is of paramount importance. The term 'torsion dystonia' is frequently used with these patients. This aptly describes the effect of the dystonic movements pulling the patient into distorted asymmetrical postures. Patients requiring wheelchairs must have a detailed assessment of their particular needs with appropriate adaptations as indicated (see Ch. 7).

Other treatments which have been tried include homeopathy, acupuncture, dietary management, hypnotherapy and relaxation but are considered to be of little long-term benefit (Dystonia Society 1991). Another somewhat bizarre treatment for spasmodic torticollis is advocated by Just Christensen (1991). This is the use of a close-fitting cardboard box to produce an involuntary torsion of the head in the contralateral direction. This sensory stimulus which was found to be effective for two patients is aimed at the afferent component of head control. Supportive psychotherapy is felt to be important for patients with dystonia (Marsden & Quinn 1990).

CHOREA AND ATHETOSIS

Chorea and athetosis are common symptoms of basal ganglia disease or damage and describe involuntary, writhing movements of the body. Chorea usually is applied to movements at proximal or axial joints, while athetosis is used more frequently to describe movements of the distal parts of the limbs (Rothwell 1994). All muscle groups tend to be affected, including those of the eyes and tongue, with the movements moving randomly from one part of the body to another. Writhing of the head and limbs, grimacing and twitching often occur unpredictably. Speech is invariably affected. Hallett (1993) comments that the most appropriate adjective to describe chorea is 'random'. Random muscles throughout the body are affected at random times and make movements of random duration. Chorea occurs at rest, on posture and on movement whether it be fast or slow (Marsden 1984).

It is difficult to distinguish between chorea and athetosis as they display similar characteristics. Athetosis is the term most frequently used to describe this dyskinesia in children with cerebral palsy whereas chorea is used to describe the movement disorder in, for example, Huntington's disease. In most cases there is involvement of both proximal and distal musculature and for the purpose of discussion regarding treatment the two will be considered as one.

The motor plan involves the selection, sequencing and delivery of the correct collection of motor programmes required to achieve the desired motor behaviour. In chorea, the correct attempt to move is made by the patient but its success is disrupted by the abnormal co-contraction of synergists, antagonists and postural fixators, so the details of the motor programme are abnormally specified. Both the initiation and execution of movement are disturbed but function may be achieved, often in a somewhat contorted manner, in spite of the severity of the dyskinesia (Marsden 1984).

Clinical presentation

Bobath (1974) describes three types of abnormal movement associated with the athetoid cerebral palsy patient:

- *Intermittent tonic spasms.* These are predictable in pattern and are due to the influence of the tonic labyrinthine and neck reflexes. The individual may be temporarily fixed in extreme patterns representative of these reflexes. This extreme response is more commonly seen in children, but the influence of these intermittent tonic spasms may persist throughout life.

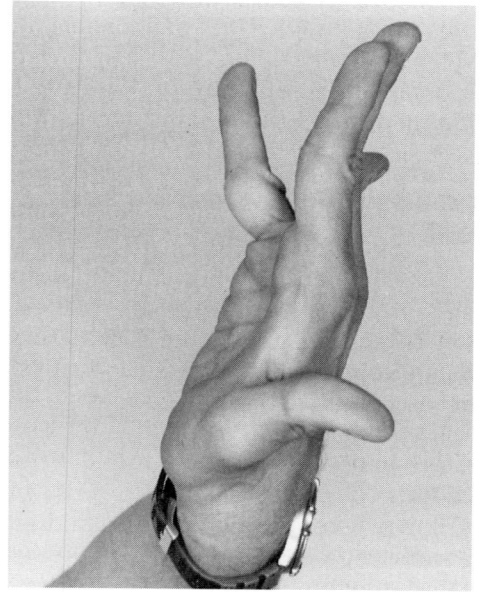

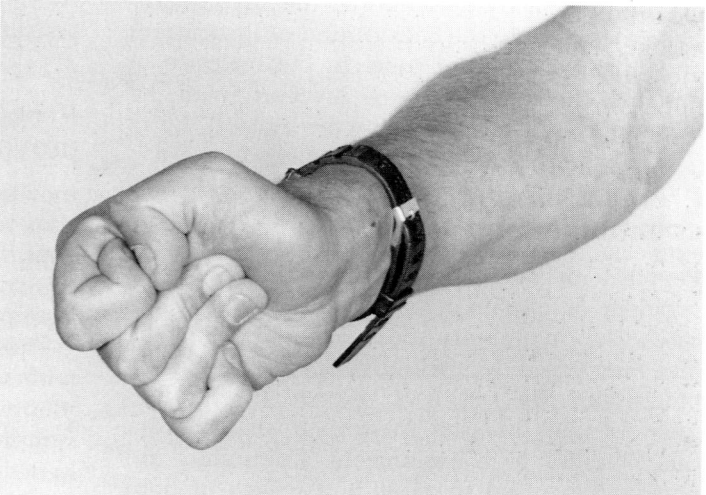

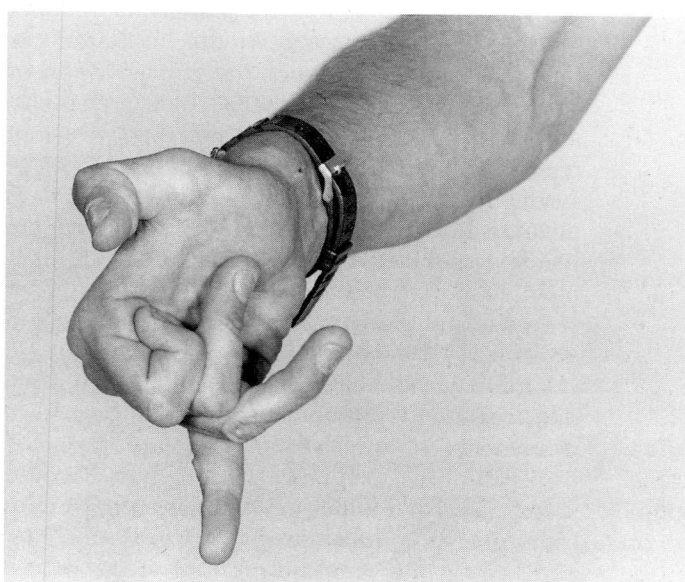

Figure 4.5 Athetoid hands.

- *Mobile spasms.* These are alternating movements, particularly of the limbs and are often rhythmical in nature.
- *Fleeting localised contractions.* These affect muscle groups throughout the body and, if severe, may produce exaggerated postures and movements such as facial grimacing and bizarre movements of the hands and fingers (Fig. 4.5). More localised or weaker contractions may be observed as minor twitches.

The resting tonus is generally low but attempts at volitional activity reinforce the involuntary movement due to the background of insufficient and unstable postural tone. In the majority of patients, the whole body is involved with the upper part more affected than the legs.

Problems associated with communication and eating

People with athetosis often have the additional problem of impaired communication. In some cases, the involuntary movements affecting the face may preclude intelligible speech. The autobiography, *My Left Foot* (Brown 1989), gives great insight into the frustration arising from this inability to communicate. Computers are now widely used to provide a means of both communication and education. Although communication may be considered primarily the remit of the speech therapist, control of posture and respiration are essential prerequisites and will also be addressed by the physiotherapist in collaboration with the speech therapist.

Similarly, eating is a problem both in terms of the uncontrolled tongue movements and the mechanical difficulty of taking the food to the mouth. Very few people with athetosis are overweight, which may be a combination of the eating difficulties and the constant involuntary movement throughout the body. Advice and treatment to address this problem should include:

- Desensitisation of the mouth including the lips, tongue, gums and, where present, the bite reflex. Instruction should be sought from an experienced speech therapist or physiotherapist.

- Supported sitting, with the arms resting forwards supported on a table. This will reduce the tendency to push back into extension as the food approaches the mouth.
- Maintenance of elongation of the cervical spine to facilitate movement of the head towards the food.

Communication and eating difficulties are two of the most distressing aspects of athetosis and, for this reason, treatment techniques or strategies which prove to be of benefit must be constantly reinforced by the patient and/or his assistant.

Problems arising with posture and movement

Inevitably there are many patients with athetosis who will become, or remain, wheelchair dependent. Determining the appropriate chair and adaptations is complex and requires detailed assessment and continual reappraisal.

Those born with athetosis initially present with very low tone and may be referred to as 'floppy children'. Depending on the severity of symptoms, it may take several years for children to develop sufficient tone to maintain themselves upright against gravity. The constant fluctuations of tone throughout the body severely hamper grading of all movement. As the child attempts to stand up from sitting, there is mass extensor activity, the result being that the child 'overshoots' and falls backwards. Facilitation and constant repetition of a more controlled movement of sitting to standing is essential for the child to develop adequate stability. Positioning of the hands together with the arms held forwards may help to break up the mass extensor response and thereby produce more coordinated activity.

People with athetosis who are ambulant often demonstrate a somewhat bizarre gait pattern characterised by marked retraction of the head, trunk and hips. On clinical observation it would seem that the shoulder girdles are retracted with the arms in either flexion or extension depending on the stability afforded at the pelvis.

This stability may be provided by adequate tone in the less severely affected or by mechanical factors, as in the patient with lower tone, who may stabilise the hip in extension by 'hanging' on the iliofemoral ligament.

The swing-through phase differs depending on the fluctuations and degree of increased tone:

- Those people with greater fluctuations in tone tend to initiate a step using a total pattern of flexion to break up the prevailing extensor tone required to maintain them upright against gravity. In this instance the impression is one of utilisation of alternate flexor and extensor synergies, affecting the whole body.
- People with predominantly low tone, using the iliofemoral ligament to provide stability, demonstrate increased extensor activity in the head and trunk in their attempt to step forwards.

Similarly the stance phase differs:

- People with marked fluctuations in tone demonstrate a more rigidly extended leg in the extensor synergy, often with flexion of the hip due to the overall increase in flexion as the opposite leg steps through.
- Those with lower tone use the more mechanical stability of extension of the hip and hyperextension of the knee counteracted by increased extension of the trunk.

Pure athetosis is rare, particularly in the cerebral palsy population. Many athetoids with predominant low tone tend to have some element of ataxia, whereas others with higher and greater fluctuations of tone may also demonstrate spasticity (Fig. 4.6).

People with pure athetosis are unlikely to develop contractures due to the prevailing low tone and constant movements. Those with spasticity are more susceptible to the development of contractures in that there is less variety of movement and the basic tone is higher and in more stereotyped patterns.

People with long-standing athetosis/chorea develop strategies, often unique to each individual, to compensate for their unstable tone and involuntary movement. These strategies are

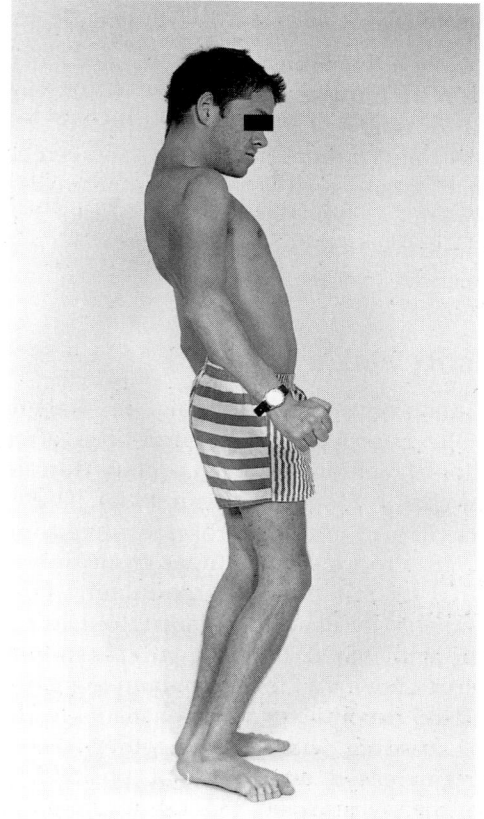

Figure 4.6   Athetoid standing position.

essential for them to function. In most instances, physiotherapy intervention is required for complications arising from the disability, such as pain or contracture, as opposed to treatment of the movement disorder itself. Invariably it is the abnormal movement which causes the problem for which the person seeks treatment, but mutually agreed goals must be established to determine appropriate treatment. For example, many athetoids defy the laws of balance in their means of ambulation, and physiotherapists must recognise that this is successful and functional for them. Attempts to improve their gait pattern, unless this is established to be the cause of the complication, will generally be met with a distinct lack of enthusiasm.

ATAXIA

Ataxia is a general term meaning a decom-position of movement (Holmes 1939). Morgan (1980) describes three main types of ataxia; sensory, labyrinthine (vestibular) and cerebellar. Some diseases such as multiple sclerosis and Friedreich's ataxia demonstrate mixed ataxias, as symptoms may be the result of two or more of the above groups.

Sensory ataxia

This may occur, for example, in diabetic or alcoholic neuropathies or conditions affecting the dorsal columns such as tabes dorsalis or spinal cord tumours (Morgan 1980). These dis-orders disrupt afferent proprioceptive input to the CNS. Proprioceptive input from the legs is essential for initiating and modulating postural adjustments in standing (Mauritz & Dietz 1980, Diener et al 1984b). Patients with sensory ataxia therefore show a wide-based stamping gait with eyes fixed upon the ground for visual feedback. When standing with heels together, there will be an increased amplitude of postural sway when the eyes close. This is Romberg's test (Bannister 1992). These patients are particularly disadvantaged when in the dark.

Vestibular ataxia

This may occur with peripheral vestibular disorders or central disorders which affect the vestibular nuclei and/or their afferent/efferent connections, for example with medullary strokes (Keshner 1994, Dieterich & Brandt 1990).

The vestibular system is involved in initiating and modulating postural reactions and in stabilising the head via the vestibulospinal reflexes. It also helps to sense the body's orientation to the vertical (Horak & Shupert 1994). A patient with vestibular ataxia therefore shows disturbances of equilibrium in standing and sitting. The patient tends to stagger when walking, has a broad base of support and may lean backwards or towards the side of the lesion. Head and trunk motion and subsequently arm motion are often decreased (Borello-France et al 1994). Vestibular ataxia may be accompanied by vertigo, blurred vision and nystagmus due to the vestibular system's role in sensing and perceiving self-motion and in stabilising gaze via the vestibulo-ocular reflex (Horak & Shupert 1994).

Cerebellar ataxia

This results from lesions affecting the cerebellum or its afferent or efferent connections. The cerebellum may be divided into specific functional areas (Thompson & Day 1993). Lesions of the midline structures, the vermis and flocculonodular lobe, produce bilateral symptoms affecting axial parts of the body, which manifest as truncal ataxia and titubation and abnormalities of gait and equilibrium. Dysarthria and nystagmus may also be associated with this pathology. Lesions affecting the hemispheres give rise primarily to ipsilateral limb symptoms (Ghez 1992a).

Symptoms associated with cerebellar ataxia include:

Dysmetria. This refers to inaccuracy in achieving a final end position (hypermetria equals overshoot; hypometria equals under-shoot). This is clearly demonstrated by the patient attempting the finger–nose test. The movement may overshoot or undershoot the target with over-correction resulting in additional movements.

Tremor:

- Kinetic tremor, which is the oscillation that occurs during the course of the movement.
- Intention tremor, which is the increase in tremor towards the end of the movement.
- Postural tremor, which occurs when holding a limb in a given position.
- Titubation, which is tremor affecting the head and upper trunk typically occurring after lesions of the vermis.
- Postural truncal tremor, which affects the legs and lower trunk, is typically seen in anterior cerebellar lobe lesions and often results from chronic alcoholism (Thompson & Day 1993).

Dyssynergia and visuomotor incoordination. Dyssynergia is the incoordination of movement involving multiple joints. The cerebellum is involved in programming, initiation and ongoing control of multi-joint movements towards visual targets (Stein 1986, Haggard et al 1994, Thach et al 1992). The influence of the cerebellum in the initiation of a movement can be seen in the increased reaction time to a given task after cerebellar dysfunction (Diener & Dichgans 1992).

The cerebellum is also vitally important for the control of eye movements and eye–hand coordination (van Donkelaar & Lee 1994, Dichgans 1984). During reaching, coordination of the eye and hand is essential for reaching accuracy (Jeannerod 1988). Abnormalities in multi-joint movements, eye movement and their coordination all occur in cerebellar ataxia and therefore all contribute to the inaccuracy of reaching seen after a cerebellar lesion (van Donkelaar & Lee 1994).

Dysdiadochokinesia. This is the inability to perform rapidly alternating movements such as alternately tapping with palm up and palm down. The rhythm is poor and the force of each tap is variable (Diener & Dichgans 1992, Rothwell 1994).

Posture and gait. Patients with anterior lobe lesions show an increased postural sway in an anteroposterior direction, which is increased with eye closure. Patients with lesions of the vestibulocerebellum (flocculonodular lobe) show an increased postural sway in all directions. The effect of eye closure on postural sway in these patients is minimal (Diener et al 1984a, Mauritz et al 1979). The degree in increase in postural sway with eye closure (Romberg's test) is far greater in patients with sensory ataxia than in those with cerebellar ataxia (Notermans et al 1994).

Experiments on humans and animals have shown that the lateral cerebellar hemisphere not only controls limb movements but also the associated preparatory activity (Massion 1984, Diener et al 1992). The anterior lobe plays a role in modulating more automatic postural adjustments which are thought to arise from the lower centres of brain stem and spinal cord. Patients with anterior lobe damage show hypermetric responses to a sudden unexpected movement which leads to instability (Horak & Diener 1994, Ghez 1992b).

Abnormalities of gait with cerebellar ataxia include difficulty with precise placement of the feet, which are usually too far apart. Dysmetria is common but elevation of the leg is not as exaggerated as in sensory ataxia (Dichgans 1984).

Other symptoms associated with cerebellar dysfunction

Hypotonia. This occurs with acute cerebellar lesions (Holmes 1922) but it is rarely seen in chronic lesions (Gilman 1969, Diener & Dichgans 1992, Rothwell 1994). Physiotherapists often view hypotonia as a symptom of ataxia (Davies 1994, Atkinson 1986). However, although hypotonia is a symptom of cerebellar dysfunction it is not a causative factor of ataxia and usually disappears within a few weeks following acute lesions (Diener & Dichgans 1992).

Weakness and fatigue. Holmes (1922, 1939) describes a generalised non-specific weakness as a feature of cerebellar dysfunction. This occurs more often with extensive and deep lesions and is most apparent in the proximal musculature. It is considered to decrease over months. A recent experimental study has shown that the maximal voluntary contraction of a patient with a chronic cerebellar disorder is similar to that of a normal subject (Mai et al 1988). However, on clinical observation, it would seem that patients with long-term ataxia do show signs of weakness. This may result from their lack of spontaneous normal movement and the adoption of compensatory movement strategies. Frustration may lead to the patient with chronic ataxia becoming increasingly inactive and dependent and, therefore, merely preventing disuse may be helpful (Hardie 1993). Fatigue has also been noted as a common feature of cerebellar dysfunction (Holmes 1922).

Motor learning. It is generally agreed that motor learning is a process which involves the whole nervous system (Eccles 1986). However, some researchers feel the cerebellum to be a major site of motor learning in that it is specialised to combine simple movements into more complex synergies. These synergies or motor patterns are then stored in the cerebellum (Thach et al 1992). This theory remains somewhat controversial (Llinas & Welsh 1993, Bloedel 1994). Patients with cerebellar cortical atrophy have recently been shown to be deficient in learning a conditioned reflex (Topka et al 1993) and more complex motor skills (Sanes et al 1990, Thach et al 1992). This may have implications for the effectiveness of physiotherapy intervention (Hardie 1993).

Clinical presentation

Ataxia is primarily a disorder affecting postural control and the coordination of multi-joint movements (DeSouza 1990). The patient is aware of the movement disorder and adopts compensatory strategies to effect function (Gordon 1990).

Many strategies have been advocated in the treatment of ataxia. These tend to refer to the more cerebellar-type presentation. They include the use of weights (Morgan et al 1975), manual guidance/resistance (DeSouza 1990), rhythmic stabilisations (Gardiner 1976), horse riding (Saywell 1975) and the gymnastic ball (Hasler 1981). Factors which increase the weight of a limb or its resistance to movement, such as the application of weights, decrease tremor (Morgan et al 1975). However, tremor will return after removal of a weight, often greater than before, and can cause fatigue, particularly in patients with multiple sclerosis (DeSouza 1990). The use of weights to reduce truncal ataxia has shown variable results (Lucy & Hayes 1985).

The re-education of proximal control and the performance of goal-directed, multi-joint movements are recommended (DeSouza 1990) rather than strengthening proximally to improve distal control. Patients may require specific mobilisation, particularly of the head, trunk and pelvis following long-term fixation but they must also be given the opportunity to learn their own movement control.

Patients with vestibular ataxia may benefit from a somewhat different approach. The general

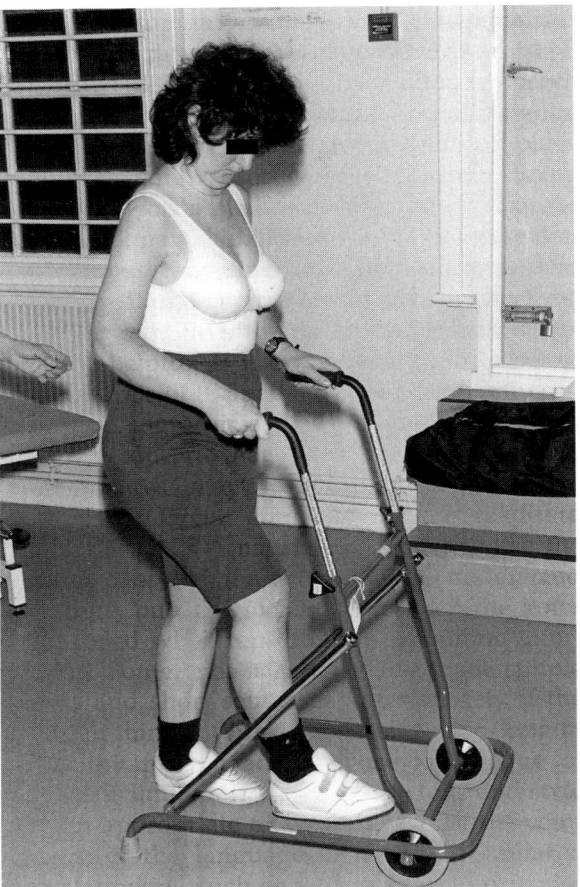

Figure 4.7 Patient with ataxia using a rollator walking frame.

rationale for improving the postural dysfunction and symptoms of vertigo and gaze instability associated with vestibular pathology is that vestibular adaptation is facilitated by stressing the relevant system (Herdman et al 1994). As Brandt et al (1981) state, a therapist should 'expose the patient increasingly to instable body positions in order to facilitate rearrangement and recruitment of control capacities. Stance and gait aids will alleviate only transiently patients' balance problems, but when used continuously, they will worsen the symptoms'. However, in clinical practice it has been observed that use of a rollator walking frame often serves to provide the patient with a means of more independent control. Used selectively, with emphasis on it being an aide to balance as opposed to a point of fixation, patients may use this aid as a means of progression to an independent gait (Fig. 4.7).

Vestibular compensation takes time. With a unilateral disorder there is potential for long-term adaptation in the vestibular system (Zee 1994) and treatment should be aimed at improving remaining vestibular function and not over-reliance on the two remaining sensations, vision and somatosensory (Herdman et al 1994).

With a bilateral vestibular lesion, improvement in ataxia can only occur by substitution of visual and, more importantly, somatosensory cues for the loss of vestibular function. Recovery after a bilateral vestibular lesion takes longer and is more incomplete than after a unilateral lesion. Even so, physical exercise has been demonstrated to affect the rate of recovery (Igarashi et al 1988). A patient with a bilateral lesion may need to be taught compensatory strategies where there is conflict of, or inadequate sensory information from, the two remaining senses. For example, a patient should be taught to turn the lights on prior to getting out of bed (Herdman 1994).

Central lesions also demonstrate more variable recovery as the very areas damaged such as the brain stem, cerebellum and vestibular nuclei are implicated in the process of recovery (Igarashi 1984). This is of particular relevance in the treatment of traumatic head injury where vestibular disorders are thought to occur in 30–65% of patients. Often these patients have associated central deficits which amongst other factors can affect recovery (Shumway-Cook 1994).

Patients with vestibular disorders, in addition to disequilibrium and ataxia, show symptoms of vertigo and often secondary symptoms of poor endurance. This may be due to the imposed inactivity and muscle tension or stiffness, particularly of the head and neck. Progressive exercise such as Cawthorne Cooksey exercise for vertigo can improve these symptoms (Shumway-Cook & Horak 1989, Herdman et al 1994).

Vestibular rehabilitation aimed at the specific areas which affect the individual patient can and does improve functional outcome (Cohen 1994).

Treatment of sensory ataxia follows similar lines to that of vestibular ataxia in the fact that substitution of the remaining senses needs to be encouraged. Although compensation with visual information is required, such as is advocated by Frenkel's exercises (Hollis 1989), the over-reliance on conscious effort with these exercises detracts from the desired automatic response.

The treatment of patients with ataxia requires a balance between the facilitation of improved control and the recognition and acceptance of necessary compensation which is essential for function.

SUMMARY

Physical disability is often characterised by abnormal tone and movement which contribute to the functional deficit. Some of the different types of movement disorders have been described, with emphasis on the clinical presentation and examples of physiotherapy intervention which may prove of benefit.

Although the neurological impairment in many instances is non-progressive, the disability arising from the pathology may increase over time. This deterioration may occur as a result of enforced immobility or dominance of stereotyped movement patterns. Any individual who is restricted to a limited or inappropriate repertoire of movement is in danger of developing structural changes of affected muscle groups, which may further decrease functional capability.

Physiotherapists should have a basic understanding of the pathophysiology of the different types of movement disorder to formulate effective treatment interventions. Many patients, particularly those with severe symptoms, develop compensatory strategies which are appropriate to their functional needs. The physiotherapist must recognise that restoration of 'normal movement' is often an unattainable goal and work with the patient to ensure the optimal functional outcome. In the majority of cases, there should be a balance between re-education of more normal movement patterns and acceptance and promotion of necessary and desirable compensation to attain optimal function.

REFERENCES

Ada L, Canning C, Westwood P 1990 The patient as an active learner. In: Ada L, Canning C (eds) Key issues in neurological physiotherapy: physiotherapy foundations for practice. Butterworth-Heinemann, Oxford

Anderson T J, Rivest J, Stell R, Steiger M J, Cohen H, Thompson P D, Marsden C D 1992 Botulinum toxin treatment of spasmodic torticollis. Journal of the Royal Society of Medicine 85: 524–529

Atkinson H W 1986 Aspects of neuroanatomy and physiology. In: Downie P A (ed) Cash's textbook of neurology for physiotherapists. Faber & Faber, London

Bach-y-Rita P 1990 Brain plasticity as a basis for recovery of function in humans. Neuropsychologia 28(6): 547–554

Banks M A, Caird F I 1989 Physiotherapy benefits patients with Parkinson's disease. Clinical Rehabilitation 3: 11–16

Bannister R 1992 Examination of the limbs and trunk. In: Bannister R (ed) Brain and Bannister's clinical neurology, 7th edn. Oxford University Press, Oxford

Becker W J, Kunesch E, Freund H-J 1990 Co-ordination of a multi-joint movement in normal humans and in patients with cerebellar dysfunction. Canadian Journal of Neurological Sciences 17(3): 264–274

Bertrand C, Molina-Negro P, Martinez S N 1978 Combined stereotactic and peripheral surgical approach for spasmodic torticollis. Applied Neurophysiology 41: 122–133

Bertrand C, Molina-Negro P, Bouvier G, Gorczyca W 1987 Observations and analysis of results in 131 cases of spasmodic torticollis after selective denervation. Applied Neurophysiology 50: 319–323

Bleton J-P 1994 Spasmodic torticollis. Handbook of Rehabilitative Physiotherapy. Editions Frison-Roche, Paris

Bloedel J R 1994 Functional heterogeneity with structural homogeneity: how does the cerebellum operate? In: Cordo P, Harnard S (eds) Movement control. Cambridge University Press, Cambridge

Bobath B 1985 Abnormal postural reflex activity caused by brain lesions, 3rd edn. Heinemann Physiotherapy, London

Bobath B 1990 Adult hemiplegia: evaluation and treatment, 3rd edn. Heinemann Medical Books, London

Bobath K 1974 The motor deficit in patients with cerebral palsy. Clinics in Developmental Medicine. No. 23. Spastics International Medical Publications, William Heinemann Medical Books, London

Booth B, Doyle M, Montgomery J 1983 Serial casting for the management of spasticity in the head-injured adult. Physical Therapy 63(12): 1960–1966

Borello-France D F, Whitney S L, Herdman S J 1994 Assessment of vestibular hypofunction. In: Herdman S J (ed) Vestibular rehabilitation. F A Davis, Philadelphia

Brandt T H 1990 The vertigo syndromes. Springer, London

Brandt T H, Krafczyk S, Malsbenden I 1981 Postural imbalance with head extension: improvement by training as a model for ataxia therapy. Annals of the New York Academy of Sciences 374: 636–649

Brooks V 1986 The neural basis of motor control. Oxford University Press, Oxford

Brown C 1989 My left foot. Mandarin Paperbacks, London

Brown P 1994 Pathophysiology of spasticity. Journal of Neurology, Neurosurgery and Psychiatry 57: 773–777

Brunnstrom S 1970 Movement therapy in hemiplegia. Harper & Row, New York

Burke D 1988 Spasticity as an adaptation to pyramidal tract injury. Advances in Neurology 47: 401–423

Carey J, Burghardt T 1993 Movement dysfunction following central nervous system lesions: a problem of neurologic or muscular impairment? Physical Therapy 73(8): 538–547

Carr J H, Shepherd R B 1980 Physiotherapy in disorders of the brain. Heinemann Medical Books, London

Carr J H, Shepherd R B 1987 A motor relearning programme for stroke, 2nd edn. Heinemann Medical, Oxford

Chan J, Brin M F, Fahn S 1991 Idiopathic cervical dystonia: clinical characteristics. Movement Disorders 6(2): 119–126

Cohen H 1994 Vestibular rehabilitation improves daily life function. American Journal of Occupational Therapy 48(10): 919–925

Conine T, Sullivan T, Mackie T, Goodman M 1990 Effects of serial casting for the prevention of equinus in patients with acute head injury. Archives of Physical Medicine and Rehabilitation 71(5): 310–312

Cornall C 1991 Self propelling wheelchairs: the effect on spasticity in hemiplegic patients. Physiotherapy Theory and Practice 7: 13–21

Dattola R, Girlanda P, Vita G, Santoro M, Tascano A, Venuto C, Baradello A, Messina C 1993 Muscle rearrangement in patients with hemiparesis after stroke: an electrophysiological and morphological study. European Neurology 33: 109–114

Davies P M 1985 Steps to follow: a guide to the treatment of adult hemiplegia. Springer-Verlag, Berlin

Davies P M 1994 Starting again: early rehabilitation after traumatic brain injury or other severe brain lesions. Springer-Verlag, London

DeSouza L 1990 Multiple sclerosis: approaches to management. Chapman & Hall, London

Dichgans J 1984 Clinical significance of cerebellar dysfunction and their topo-diagnostical significance. Human Neurobiology 2: 269–279

Diener H-C, Dichgans J 1992 Pathophysiology of cerebellar ataxia. Movement Disorders 7(2): 95–109

Diener H-C, Dichgans J, Bacher M, Gompf B 1984a Quantification of postural sway in normals and patients with cerebellar diseases. Electroencephalography and Clinical Neurophysiology 57: 134–142

Diener H-C, Dichgans J, Guschlbauer B, Bacher M, Rapp H, Klockgether T 1992 The coordination of posture and voluntary movement in patients with cerebellar dysfunction. Movement Disorders 7(1): 14–22

Diener H-C, Dichgans J, Guschlbauer B, Mau H 1984b The significance of proprioception on postural stabilisation as assessed by ischaemia. Brain Research 296: 103–109

Dieterich M, Brandt T H 1990 Postural imbalance and subjective visual vertical in medullary infarctions. In: Brandt T H, Paulus W, Bles W, Dieterich M, Krafczyk S, Straube A (eds) Disorders of posture and gait. Xth International Symposium of the Society for Posture and Gait Research. Georg Thieme, New York

Dietz V 1992 Human neuronal control of automatic functional movements: interaction between central programs and afferent input. Physiological Reviews 72(1): 33–69

Dvir Z, Panturin E 1993 Measurement of spasticity and associated reactions in stroke patients before and after physiotherapeutic intervention. Clinical Rehabilitation 7: 15–21

Dystonia Society 1991 Dystonia: your questions answered. Porton Products (Leaflet available from the Dystonia Society UK)

Eccles J C 1986 Learning in the motor system. In: Freund H-J, Buttner U, Cohen B, Noth J (eds) Progress in Brain Research. vol. 64: 3–17

Edstrom L 1970 Selective changes in the sizes of red and white muscle fibres in upper motor lesions and parkinsonism. Journal of Neurological Sciences 11: 537–550

Edwards S 1991 The incomplete spinal lesion. In: Bromley I (ed) Tetraplegia and paraplegia: a guide for physiotherapists, 4th edn. Churchill Livingstone, Edinburgh

Elble R J, Sienko Thomas S, Higgins C, Colliver J 1991 Stride-dependent changes in gait of older people. Journal of Neurology 238: 1–5

Fahn S, Marsden C D, Calne D B 1987 Classification and investigation of dystonia. In: Marsden C D, Fahn S (eds) Movement disorders 2. Butterworths, London

Fletcher N A, Harding A E, Marsden C D 1990 The role of trauma in the development of idiopathic torsion dystonia. Journal of Neurology 237 (Suppl. 1): S5

Gardiner M D 1976 The principles of exercise therapy. G Bell, London

Ghez C 1991a The cerebellum. In: Kandel E R, Schwartz J H, Jessell T M (eds) Principles of neural science, 3rd edn. Appleton & Lange, London

Ghez C 1991b Posture. In: Kandel E R, Schwartz J H, Jessell T M (eds) Principles of neural science, 3rd edn. Appleton & Lange, London

Gilman S 1969 The mechanism of cerebellar hypotonia: an experimental study in the monkey. Brain 92: 621–638

Goldspink G, Williams P 1990 Muscle fibre and connective tissue changes associated with use and disuse. In: Ada L, Canning C (eds) Key issues in neurological physiotherapy: physiotherapy foundations for practice. Butterworth-Heinemann, London

Gordon J 1990 Disorders of motor control. In Ada L, Canning C (eds) Key issues in neurological physiotherapy: physiotherapy foundations for practice. Butterworth-Heinemann, London

Grandas F, Elston J, Quinn N, Marsden C D 1988 Blepharospasm: a review of 264 patients. Journal of Neurology, Neurosurgery and Psychiatry 51: 767–772

Haas B 1994 Measuring spasticity: a survey of current practice among health-care professionals. British Journal of Therapy and Rehabilitation 1(2): 90–95

Haggard P, Jenner J, Wing A 1994 Co-ordination of aimed movements in a case of unilateral cerebellar damage. Neuropsychologia 32(7): 827–846

Hallett M 1993 Physiology of basal ganglia disorders: an overview. Canadian Journal of Neurological Sciences 20(3): 177–183

Hardie R 1993 Tremor and ataxia. In: Greenwood R, Barnes M P, McMillan T M, Ward C D (eds) Neurological rehabilitation. Churchill Livingstone, London

Hasler D 1981 Developing a sense of symmetry. Therapy Aug 27: 3

Held J M 1993 Recovery after damage. In: Cohen H (ed) Neuroscience for rehabilitation. J B Lippincott, Philadelphia

Herdman S J 1994 Assessment and management of bilateral vestibular loss. In: Herdman S J (ed) Vestibular rehabilitation. F A Davis, Philadelphia

Herdman S J, Borello-France D F, Whitney S L 1994 Treatment of vestibular hypofunction. In: Herdman S J (Ed) Vestibular rehabilitation. F A Davis, Philadelphia

Hollis M 1989 Special regimes. In: Hollis M (ed) Practical exercise therapy, 3rd edn. Blackwell Scientific Publications, London

Holmes G 1922 On the clinical symptoms of cerebellar disease and their interpretation. Lancet 1: 1177–1182

Holmes G 1939 The cerebellum of man. Brain 62: 1–30

Horak F B, Diener H-C 1994 Cerebellar control of postural scaling and central set in stance. Journal of Neurophysiology 72(2): 479–493

Horak F B, Shupert C L 1994 Role of the vestibular system in postural control. In: Herdman S J (ed) Vestibular rehabilitation. F A Davis, Philadelphia

Hufschmidt A, Mauritz K-H 1985 Chronic transformation of muscle in spasticity: a peripheral contribution to increased muscle tone. Journal of Neurology, Neurosurgery and Psychiatry 48: 676–685

Igarashi M 1984 Vestibular compensation. An overview. Acta Oto-laryngologica (Stockholm) Suppl. 406: 78–82

Igarashi M, Ishikawa K, Ishii M, Yamane H 1988 Physical exercise and balance compensation after total ablation of vestibular organs. Progress in Brain Research 76: 395–401

Jeannerod M 1988 The neural and behavioural organisation of goal-directed movements. Oxford Science Publications, Oxford

Just Christensen J E 1991 New treatment of spasmodic torticollis? Lancet (letter) 338: 573

Katz R T, Rymer W Z 1989 Spastic hypertonia: mechanisms and measurement. Archives of Physical Medicine and Rehabilitation 70: 144–155

Kent H, Hershler C, Conine T, Hershler R 1990 Case control study of lower limb extremity serial casting in adult patients with head injury. Physiotherapy Canada 42(4): 189–191

Keshner E A 1994 Postural abnormalities in vestibular disorders. In: Herdman S J (ed) Vestibular rehabilitation. F A Davis, Philadelphia

Kidd G, Lawes N, Musa I 1992 Understanding neuromuscular plasticity. A basis for clinical rehabilitation. Edward Arnold, London

Knutsson E, Richards C 1979 Different types of disturbed motor control in gait of hemiparetic patients. Brain 102: 405–430

Lance J W 1980 Symposium synopsis. In: Feldman R G, Young R R, Koella W P (eds) Spasticity: disordered motor control year book. Year Book Publishers, Chicago

Lee R G 1989 Pathophysiology of rigidity and akinesia in Parkinson's disease. European Neurology 29 (Suppl. 1): 13–18

Llinas R, Welsh J P 1993 On the cerebellum and motor learning. Current Opinion in Neurobiology 3: 958–965

Lorentz I T, Shanthi Subramaniam S, Yiannikas C 1991 Treatment of idiopathic spasmodic torticollis with botulinum toxin a: a double-blind study on twenty-three patients. Movement Disorders 6(2): 145–150

Lucy S D, Hayes K C 1985 Postural sway profiles: normal subjects and subjects with cerebellar ataxia. Physiotherapy Canada 37(3): 140–148

Lynch M, Grisogono V 1991 Strokes and head injuries. John Murray, London

Mai N, Bolsinger P, Avarello M, Diener H-C, Dichgans J 1988 Control of isometric finger force in patients with cerebellar disease. Brain 111: 973–998

Markham C H 1992 The dystonias. Current Opinion in Neurology and Neurosurgery 5: 301–307

Marsden C D 1982 The mysterious motor function of the basal ganglia: the Robert Wartenburg Lecture. Neurology 32: 514–539

Marsden C D 1984 Motor disorders in basal ganglia disease. Human Neurobiology 2: 245–250

Marsden C D 1986 Movement disorders and the basal ganglia. Trends in Neuroscience October: 512–515

Marsden C D, Quinn N 1990 The dystonias. British Medical Journal 300: 139–144

Massion J 1984 Postural changes accompanying voluntary movements. Normal and pathological aspects. Human Neurobiology 2: 261–267

Mauritz K-H, Dichgans J, Hufschmidt A 1979 Quantitative analysis of stance in late cortical cerebellar atrophy of the anterior lobe and other forms of cerebellar ataxia. Brain 102: 461–482

Mauritz K-H, Dietz V 1980 Characteristics of postural instability induced by ischaemic blocking of leg afferents. Experimental Brain Research 38: 117–119

Messina C 1990 Pathophysiology of muscle tone. Functional Neurology 5(3): 217–223

Miller W, DeLong M R 1988 Parkinsonian symptomatology: an anatomical and physiological analysis. Annals of the New York Academy of Sciences 515: 287–302

Morgan M H 1980 Ataxia: its causes, measurement and management. International Rehabilitation Medicine 2: 126–132

Morgan M H, Langton Hewer R, Cooper R 1975 Application of an objective method of assessing intention tremor: a further study on the use of weights to reduce intention tremor. Journal of Neurology, Neurosurgery and Psychiatry 38: 259–264

Moseley A M 1993 The effect of a regimen of casting and prolonged stretching on passive ankle dorsiflexion in traumatic head-injured adults. Physiotherapy Theory and Practice 9(4): 215–221

Musa I M 1986 The role of afferent input in the reduction of spasticity: an hypothesis. Physiotherapy 72(4): 179–182

Nash J, Neilson P D, O'Dwyer N J 1989 Reducing spasticity to control muscle contracture of children with cerebral palsy. Developmental Medicine and Child Neurology 31(4): 471–480

Notermans N C, van Dijk E W, van der Groaf Y, van Gijh J, Wokke J H J 1994 Measuring ataxia: quantification based on the standard neurological examination. Journal of Neurology, Neurosurgery and Psychiatry 57: 22–26

Partridge C, Cornall C, Lynch M, Greenwood R 1993 Physical therapies. In: Greenwood R, Barnes M, McMillan T, Ward C (eds) Neurological rehabilitation. Churchill Livingstone, London

Pentland B 1993 Parkinsonism and dystonia. In: Greenwood R, Barnes M, McMillan T, Ward C (eds) Neurological rehabilitation. Churchill Livingstone, London

Petajan J H 1990 Spasticity: effects of physical interventions. Journal of Neurological Rehabilitation 4: 219–225

Poewe W, Schelosky L, Kleedorfer B, Heinen F, Wagner M, Deuschl G 1992 Treatment of spasmodic torticollis with local injections of botulinum toxin. Journal of Neurology 239: 21–25

Rogers M W 1991 Motor control problems in Parkinson's disease. In: Lister M (ed) Contemporary management of motor control problems. Foundation for Physical Therapy, Alexandria VA

Rondot P, Marchand M P, Dellatolas G 1991 Spasmodic torticollis–review of 220 patients. Canadian Journal of Neurological Sciences 18: 143–151

Rothwell J 1994 Control of human voluntary movement, 2nd edn. Chapman & Hall, London

Sanes J N, Dimitrov B, Hallett M 1990 Motor learning in patients with cerebellar dysfunction. Brain 113: 103–120

Saywell S Y 1975 Riding and ataxia. Physiotherapy 61(11): 334–335

Schmidt R A 1991 Motor learning and performance: from principles to practice. Human Kinetics Publishers, Leeds

Schomburg E D 1990 Spinal sensorimotor systems and their supraspinal control. Neuroscience Research 7: 265–340

Shumway-Cook A 1994 Vestibular rehabilitation in traumatic brain injury. In: Herdman S J (ed) Vestibular rehabilitation. F A Davis, Philadelphia

Shumway-Cook A, Horak F B 1989 Vestibular rehabilitation: an exercise approach to managing symptoms of vestibular dysfunction. Seminars in Hearing 10(2): 196–209

Smith G 1963 Care of the patient with stroke. Tavistock Publications, London

Stein J F 1986 Role of the cerebellum in the visual guidance of movement. Nature 323: 217–221

Thach W T, Goodkin H P, Keating J G 1992 The cerebellum and the adaptive coordination of movement. Annual Review of Neuroscience 15: 403–442

Thilmann A F, Fellows S J, Ross H F 1991 Biomechanical changes at the ankle after stroke. Journal of Neurology, Neurosurgery and Psychiatry 54: 134–139

Thompson P D, Day B L 1993 The anatomy and physiology of cerebellar disease. Advances in Neurology 61: 15–31

Topka H, Valls-Sole J, Massaquoi S E, Hallett M 1993 Deficit in classical conditioning in patients with cerebellar degeneration. Brain 116: 961–969

Traub M, Rothwell J C, Marsden C D 1980 Anticipatory postural reflexes in Parkinson's disease and other akinetic-rigid syndromes and in cerebellar ataxia. Brain 103: 393–412

van Donkelaar, Lee R G 1994 Interactions between the eye and hand motor systems: disruptions due to cerebellar dysfunction. Journal of Neurophysiology 72(4): 1674–1685

Wichmann T, DeLong M R 1993 Pathophysiology of parkinsonian motor abnormalities. Advances in Neurology 60: 53–61

Yanagisawa N, Fujimoto S, Tamaru F 1989 Bradykinesia in Parkinson's disease: disorders of onset and execution of fast movement. European Neurology 29 (Suppl. 1): 19–28

Yarkony G M, Sahgal V 1987 Contractures: a major complication of craniocerebral trauma. Clinical Orthopaedics and Related Research 219: 93–96

Zee D S 1994 Vestibular adaptation. In: Herdman S J (ed) Vestibular rehabilitation. F A Davis, Philadelphia

CHAPTER CONTENTS

TREATMENT AND MANAGEMENT OF RESPIRATORY DYSFUNCTION 87

Acute brain injury 87
Intracranial pressure, cerebral perfusion pressure and cerebral blood flow 88
Factors affecting the cerebral vasculature 89
The effect of brain injury on the lungs 90

Respiratory muscle impairment 90

Physiotherapy intervention 91

Summary 94

MANAGEMENT OF NEUROLOGICAL DYSFUNCTION 94

Basic principles 94

Positioning 95
Principles of positioning in bed 96
Principles of positioning in sitting 99
Principles of positioning in standing 100

Movements 106
Orofacial movements 106
Shoulder girdle and upper limb 107
The elbow joint 110
The wrist and fingers 110
The lower limb 110
The foot and ankle 111

Summary 111

References 112

5

General principles of treatment

Philippa Carter
Susan Edwards

The purpose of this chapter is to describe principles of treatment which apply to all stages of management of patients with neurological disability. This includes both those with acute onset and those with progressive disorders. The emphasis is on early physiotherapy intervention when patients are usually hospitalised and includes management of respiratory and neurological dysfunction.

Some sections of this chapter are well referenced whereas in others there is no literature to support current practice. The description of physiotherapy management is based on the authors' clinical experience and should not be considered as definitive, proven intervention. It is hoped that many research questions will be raised to substantiate or disprove this treatment approach.

TREATMENT AND MANAGEMENT OF RESPIRATORY DYSFUNCTION

This section concentrates on how the neurological status of a patient may affect the respiratory management rather than on examining the more detailed aspects of respiratory care.

ACUTE BRAIN INJURY

Brain injury can be divided into primary and secondary brain damage. Primary damage is caused at the time of the insult and irreversibly affects the brain tissue. Secondary damage occurs at some time later and results from raised intracranial pressure (ICP) and decreased cerebral perfusion with oxygenated blood secondary to hypotension and hypoxia.

Medical intervention is directed at promoting adequate cerebral blood flow (CBF) and minimising damage arising from secondary complications which have devastating effects on the survival of the patient and the quality of overall outcome (March et al 1990, Snyder 1983). The physiotherapist participates closely in the patient's management, primarily in assessment, maintenance and treatment of respiratory conditions and in patient handling and positioning.

Intracranial pressure, cerebral perfusion pressure and cerebral blood flow

Intracranial pressure (ICP) is described as the pressure exerted by the cerebrospinal fluid (CSF) within the lateral ventricles of the brain (Allan 1989) or as 'the pressure exerted within the skull and meninges by the brain tissue, the CSF and the cerebral blood volume (CBV)' (Andrus 1991). It is measured via a subarachnoid or intraventricular catheter and more recently by intraparenchymal fibreoptic devices.

The normal range of values for intracranial pressure is between 0 and 15 mmHg (Andrus 1991, Garradd & Bullock 1986, Johnson et al 1989, Allan 1989). Intracranial hypertension occurs when the pressure exceeds 15 mmHg, and treatment is required for levels greater than 25 mmHg. A persistently high ICP may be associated with a poor prognosis, and an uncontrollable ICP is often fatal (Tobin 1989).

Intracranial pressure is one of the determinants of the cerebral perfusion pressure (CPP), the other being systemic blood pressure. The CPP is calculated as the difference between the mean arterial pressure (MAP) and the mean intracranial pressure (ICP) (Prasad & Tasker 1990, Lindsay et al 1991). CPP is the pressure at which brain tissue is perfused with blood and is a measure of the adequacy of the cerebral circulation (March et al 1990). For this reason,

great care and consideration must be given to any procedure which may increase the intracranial pressure or lower the blood pressure and consequently decrease the CPP.

The normal range of values for cerebral perfusion pressure is between 60 and 90 mmHg (Andrus 1991, Tobin 1989). When CPP falls below 50 mmHg, cerebral blood flow decreases by about 25%. When it falls below 40 mmHg, cerebral perfusion is severely compromised resulting in reflex vasodilatation of the cerebral vasculature. The increased cerebral blood volume further increases intracranial pressure and ultimately reduces the cerebral blood flow (Ciesla 1989, Tobin 1989).

To understand the relationship between intracranial pressure, cerebral perfusion and cerebral blood flow, it is useful to consider the Monro Kellie doctrine (Andrus 1991). The skull is a rigid compartment filled to capacity with three non-compressible components, brain matter (80%), blood (10%) and CSF (10%). Monro Kellie proposed that the total volume of the intracranial contents must remain constant for intracranial pressure to be maintained at a non-pathological level (Snyder 1983). If one component increases in volume, there is a concomitant decrease in volume of one or both of the remaining components to compensate for the rise and maintain normal ICP and adequate cerebral blood flow. This physiological mechanism is the intracranial pressure–volume response or compliance of the brain. With an expanding intracranial mass, the compensatory mechanisms are:

- displacement of CSF from the cranial to the spinal subarachnoid space
- decreased CSF production
- decreased cerebral blood volume
- decreased extracellular fluid.

Therefore a relatively large change in intracranial volume can occur before there is a subsequent increase in intracranial pressure. This is best demonstrated by the pressure–volume curve in Figure 5.1 (A–B) (Andrus 1991, Snyder 1983, March et al 1990, Lindsay et al 1991).

Under normal conditions, cerebral autoregulation maintains cerebral blood flow (CBF) at a

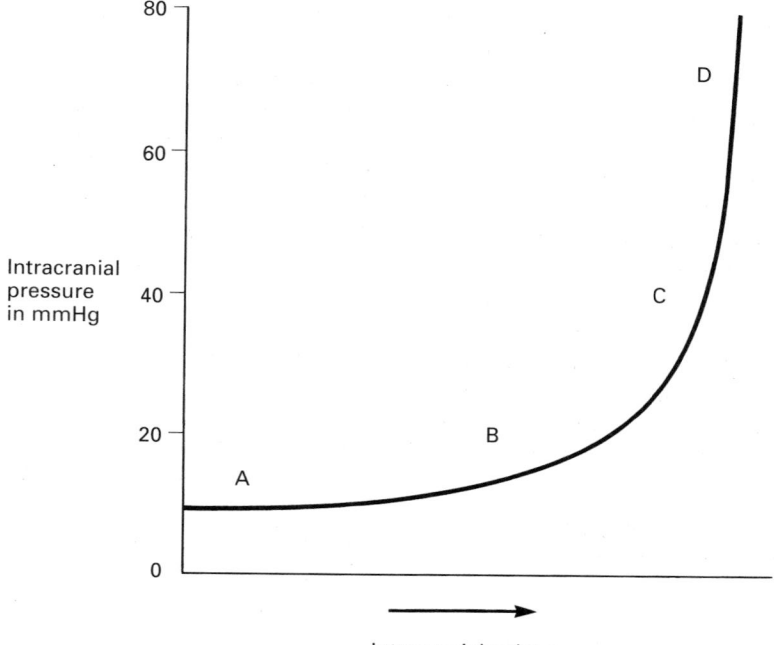

Figure 5.1 Intracranial pressure–volume curve.

level sufficient to meet metabolic demands by regulating the cerebral vascular resistance (CVR) over a range of perfusion pressures (Ellis 1990, Andrus 1991, Johnson et al 1989, Lindsay et al 1991). It has a normal value of 50 ml/100 g per minute, and is calculated as:

$$CBF = \frac{CPP}{CVR} \qquad (CPP = MAP - ICP)$$

The CVR is the pressure across the cerebro-vascular circulation from the arteries to the jugular veins and it may be altered by oedema, vasospasm and pre-existing hypertension (Johnson et al 1989). Cerebral blood flow may be measured clinically using radioactive xenon techniques.

Following head injury, autoregulation and compliance may be severely impaired and therefore when the compensatory mechanisms are exhausted even a small rise in the intracranial volume will result in marked intracranial hypertension (Shapiro 1975) (Fig. 5.1 B–C).

Factors affecting the cerebral vasculature

Cerebral vasodilatation is caused by:

↑ PCO_2
↓ PO_2
↓ extracellular pH
↑ products of metabolism.

The result of cerebral vasodilatation is to increase the cerebral blood volume and hence the intracranial pressure. If systemic blood pressure remains unchanged, this results in a fall in the cerebral perfusion pressure which in turn leads to a reduction in the cerebral blood flow.

As there is a direct relationship between intra-cranial pressure (ICP), cerebral perfusion pressure (CPP) and cerebral blood flow (CBF), physio-therapy intervention may have an effect on this relationship by affecting the ICP, but the positive benefits gained by the treatment often far outweigh the temporary increase in ICP. It is also worthy of note that, although there may be an increase in the ICP, the CPP often remains unchanged because of a corresponding rise in systemic blood pressure (Garradd & Bullock 1986, Parataz & Burns 1993). The decision, whether or not to treat, must be made in conjunction with the medical and nursing staff.

Patients in the acute stage following head injury are often mechanically ventilated. Sedative and paralysing agents are used in the early stages, usually for the first 48–72 hours, and then withdrawn to assess the patient's conscious state (Garradd & Bullock 1986). Patients are often deliberately hyperventilated; hypocapnia causes cerebral vasoconstriction by decreasing the H^+ ion concentration of the blood and CSF.

Hyperventilation can be described as 'ventilation in excess of that required to maintain normal arterial CO_2 levels' (Kerr et al 1993). During hyperventilation the arterial partial pressure of carbon dioxide ($PaCO_2$) is usually kept between 3.8 and 4.2 kPa. Hyperventilation may become ineffective at controlling the intracranial pressure after 36–48 hours as CSF pH returns to normal due to compensatory mechanisms such as the excretion of bicarbonate by the kidneys (compensatory metabolic acidosis) (Tobin 1989, Kerr et al 1993). If the patient is excessively hyperventilated and the $PaCO_2$ falls below 3 kPa, severe vasoconstriction may result in cerebral hypoxia because of a reduction in the cerebral blood flow to below a critical level. Cerebral ischaemia and a further increase in intracranial pressure will then occur. It is therefore vital that regular arterial blood gas (ABG) readings are taken to monitor the $PaCO_2$ levels.

Regular assessment of the patient, recorded ICP, CPP, cardiovascular parameters, ABGs, X-rays, auscultation and Glasgow Coma Scale (GCS) are all vital in determining the appropriateness of physiotherapy intervention. The benefits of treatment must always be carefully balanced against the potential harmful effects.

The effect of brain injury on the lungs

Central nervous system (CNS) damage may impair lung function both directly and indirectly, resulting in respiratory insufficiency leading to hypoxia and hypercapnia.

Direct damage to the chest wall, pleura or lungs may occur and cause, for example, fractures, pneumothorax and contusions (Parataz & Burns 1993, West 1985, Prasad & Tasker 1990, Ellis 1990). At the time of the original trauma, the patient may vomit and aspiration may occur, further compromising the respiratory system.

Indirect respiratory insufficiency may be due to:

- Depressed level of consciousness, which leads to an inability to maintain an adequate airway, with suppressed gag and cough reflexes (Andrus 1991, Warren 1983).
- Altered respiratory patterns as a result of an increase in pressure on the respiratory centre in the brain stem (Prasad & Tasker 1990).
- Reduced lung compliance which may be up to 50% due to changes in the pulmonary surface tension (Beckman et al 1971).
- Neurogenic pulmonary oedema, the occurrence of which is rare and somewhat debatable. Recent studies suggest that it may present acutely or be delayed. It is thought to be due to systemic hypertension, pulmonary venoconstriction, negative and positive inotropic factors and impairment of intrinsic myocardial function. The neurologic pathways responsible for initiating these responses are unknown (Tobin 1989).
- Immobility resulting in reduced tidal volumes leading to small airway closure and patchy areas of microatelectasis (Parataz & Burns 1993, Warren 1983).
- Tonal changes (Thomas & Ellis 1992, Ellis 1990).

RESPIRATORY MUSCLE IMPAIRMENT

Respiratory muscle function may be compromised directly, due to diseases affecting the muscles themselves, such as in patients with muscular dystrophy, or indirectly due to a disorder of the motor pathways of the central and peripheral nervous system. This results in weakness or paralysis of the respiratory muscles as may occur in patients with Guillain–Barré syndrome or following spinal cord injury (Thomas & Ellis 1992, Bromley 1991). In both these cases there is reduced intercostal activity with poor diaphragmatic excursion. This results in reduced expansion of the chest wall and a poor inspiratory effect. Coughing is severely affected due to paresis of the abdominal muscles. Signs of alveolar hypoventilation appear and this may lead to areas of atelectasis and retention of secretions (Thomas & Ellis 1992, Ciesla 1989).

Regular assessment of respiratory function is essential but intracranial pressure monitoring is not indicated. Potential deterioration in the patient's condition should be monitored by measuring and recording the vital capacity (VC) at regular intervals. If the VC falls below 1 litre, assisted ventilation may be indicated.

PHYSIOTHERAPY INTERVENTION

An understanding of intracranial dynamics and the effect of physiotherapy techniques on these is of vital importance to the physiotherapist treating the acutely ill neurological patient in order to accurately assess and treat the patient safely and effectively (Ada et al 1990). The techniques employed are no different from those used for the non-neurological patient with respiratory complications; however, they may need some modification.

Manual hyperinflation

This is a means of providing artificial ventilation in the intubated patient by use of a rebreathing or nonrebreathing (Ambu) bag attached to an oxygen source. If the patient has raised intracranial pressure, an Ambu bag is preferred as this prevents rebreathing and the retention of CO_2.

The aim of manual hyperinflation is to increase lung volume and re-expand areas of atelectatic lung, by utilising and increasing gaseous exchange at alveolar level (Hough 1991, Ada et al 1990).

Manual hyperinflation with a quick release stimulates a cough and is beneficial in mobilising

and assisting the clearance of excess bronchial secretions, especially when 'hands-on' techniques may be inappropriate (Webber & Pryor 1993).

With a large tidal volume being delivered, there is an increase in intrathoracic pressure which in turn leads to a decrease in cerebral venous return and subsequent increase in cerebral blood volume. This results in an increase in intracranial pressure and a decrease in cerebral perfusion pressure (Snyder 1983, Ciesla 1989, Ada et al 1990). If the blood pressure is low, the induced increase in intrathoracic pressure reduces systemic venous return, lowering the cardiac output, which further lowers the systemic blood pressure and compromises the cerebral perfusion pressure (Prasad & Tasker 1990, Webber & Pryor 1993). If the blood pressure is high at rest, then manual hyperinflation can further increase it to what may be critical levels (Ada et al 1990).

Application of manual hyperinflation should be used with caution and kept as brief as possible, as this technique has been shown to increase the intracranial pressure over time (Parataz & Burns 1993, Garradd & Bullock 1986). The instillation of 2–3 ml of normal saline prior to manual hyperinflation may help to loosen tenacious secretions (Webber & Pryor 1993). However, it may elicit a cough, which increases the intracranial pressure. Rapid manual hyperinflation or hyperventilation without the use of an inspiratory hold may be used as a temporary measure in reducing intracranial pressure by 'blowing off' CO_2 and is often used prior to or following suction (Ada et al 1990).

Shaking/vibrations

These techniques consist of intermittent, fine or coarse compressions of the chest wall during expiration and are usually combined with manual hyperinflation in the intubated patient. They augment the expiratory flow and facilitate large and small airway clearance by mobilising and advancing secretions centrally in order for them be suctioned clear (Ciesla 1989, Webber & Pryor 1993). Manual hyperinflation with shaking has been shown to increase the intracranial pressure over time by increasing intrathoracic pressure (Ciesla 1989, Prasad & Tasker 1990) and should therefore be used with caution, but vibrations in isolation have been found to have no effect on intracranial pressure (Parataz & Burns 1993).

Percussion/chest clapping

This technique consists of slow, rhythmical clapping with cupped hands over the affected lung segment. This produces an energy wave transmitted through the chest wall to the airways (Ciesla 1989, Pryor 1992) and is used to mobilise secretions from the bronchial walls (Ada et al 1990). Percussion has been shown to lower intracranial pressure if performed slowly with a single hand action (Garradd & Bullock 1986, Parataz & Burns 1993).

Positioning

Generally, the patient is positioned either supine or with the head elevated to 30 degrees. The head and neck must always be kept in neutral alignment with the trunk. Any deviation may lead to restricted or obstructed cerebral venous return and consequently a rise in the intracranial pressure. This also applies if the hips are flexed beyond 90 degrees (Allan 1989, Andrus 1991, Garradd & Bullock 1986, March et al 1990, Shallit & Umansky 1977).

There is an extremely important relationship between the position of the patient and the ratio of ventilation to perfusion (V̇/Q̇). In the non-ventilated patient, the ventilation and perfusion are greatest in the dependent areas of the lung; for example, in left side-lying, the left lung is better ventilated and perfused than the right. Conversely, in the ventilated patient or in the case of respiratory muscle paralysis, ventilation takes the path of least resistance. Therefore in left side-lying, the right lung is better ventilated, with perfusion still greater in the dependent lung. Turning the patient regularly, if medically stable, is therefore of great value in the management of the respiratory status (Ciesla 1989, West 1985, Hough 1991).

Postural drainage is a method of positioning the patient that enables gravity to drain local areas of the lung. Positions which include a head-down tilt increase the intracranial pressure by impairing cerebral venous return. If indicated, postural drainage positions may have to be modified and it should be performed with extreme caution and close monitoring of intracranial pressure and cerebral perfusion pressure, and only following discussion with the medical staff (Prasad & Tasker 1990, Ada et al 1990).

Suctioning

Suctioning is used to remove secretions from the upper airways. It is a potentially hazardous technique and should be carried out with extreme care and skill (Prasad & Tasker 1990, Garradd & Bullock 1986). In the ventilated, non-sedated patient it can produce reflex coughing and, whilst this may assist with sputum clearance, it also increases the intrathoracic pressure and subsequently the intracranial pressure. Ventilated patients who are paralysed and sedated may also demonstrate a rise in intracranial pressure which is due to direct tracheal stimulation (Ada et al 1990, Garradd & Bullock 1986, Shapiro 1975). Frequently, a bolus dose of sedating agents or painkillers prior to treatment settles the patient and considerably lessens any adverse effects of treatment. However, care must be taken as some sedative agents can lower the blood pressure. The timing of this drug administration is vital if it is to be effective as an adjunct to treatment, and close liaison with all staff concerned is essential.

Hyperoxygenation by use of the ventilator or manually using the bag prior to suctioning has a slightly vasoconstrictive influence on the cerebral arteries, decreasing the cerebral blood volume and lowering the intracranial pressure (Garradd & Bullock 1986, Parataz & Burns 1993, Kerr et al 1993).

The suction pressure should be kept at the lowest possible level which enables effective removal of secretions. High pressure can reduce the functional residual capacity (FRC) and cause aveolar collapse leading to hypoxia. As a general rule, the suction catheter should not exceed half the internal diameter of the endotracheal tube and the procedure should be quick but effective (Young 1984, Kerr et al 1993). In most cases, the rise in intracranial pressure is only temporary and it returns back to its baseline within 30–60 seconds. To avoid or minimise cerebral hypertension particularly in the severely head injured patient, suction should be limited to a maximum of two to three passes in one treatment session. Consecutive suction has a cumulative effect on intracranial pressure and may produce potentially dangerous elevations (Garradd & Bullock 1986, Prasad & Tasker 1990, Kerr et al 1993).

For patients who are self-ventilating, suction is performed through either a nasal-pharyngeal or an oral airway. Nasal suction is contraindicated in patients who have facial or base of skull fractures, rhinorrhoea, or who have undergone transphenoidal surgery. Great care must be taken when orally suctioning a patient who has undergone transoral surgery. In many cases, both the physiotherapist and nursing staff may find it preferable to use a mini-tracheostomy for clearing secretions.

Humidification

Patients with a raised intracranial pressure may have a restricted fluid intake, which can lead to drying of the mucosa, reduced ciliary action, and thickening and retention of secretions. Both ventilated and non-ventilated patients must therefore be adequately humidified at all times, especially if they are on any form of oxygen therapy (Linden 1993, Ada et al 1990).

Positive end expiratory pressure (PEEP)

The effect of PEEP is to maintain the patency of the airways at the end of expiration in the intubated patient (Pryor 1992). PEEP in excess of 7.5 cmH$_2$O may increase the intracranial pressure by increasing the intrathoracic pressure and must therefore be used with caution.

Continuous positive airway pressure (CPAP)/intermittent positive pressure breathing (IPPB)

CPAP is the application of positive airways pressure throughout the respiratory cycle in a patient who is breathing spontaneously. It reduces the work of breathing, improves collateral ventilation and increases the functional residual capacity (FRC) (Hough 1991, Pryor 1992).

IPPB is the maintenance of positive pressure within the airways throughout inspiration with airway pressure returning to atmospheric pressure during expiration (Webber & Pryor 1993). This also reduces the work of breathing and increases the tidal volume (TV). Both these techniques improve ventilation in the patient who is not mechanically ventilated. However, they may increase the intracranial pressure by increasing the intrathoracic pressure.

Assisted coughing

The assisted cough is used for patients with a cough reflex but who lack the intercostal and abdominal force to produce an effective cough. It is best illustrated in the management of patients with cervical or upper thoracic spinal cord lesions. The therapist can replace the function of the paralysed abdominal muscles by creating increased pressure underneath the working diaphragm. The patient takes a large inspiration followed by a forceful expiration during which the chest and upper abdomen is compressed

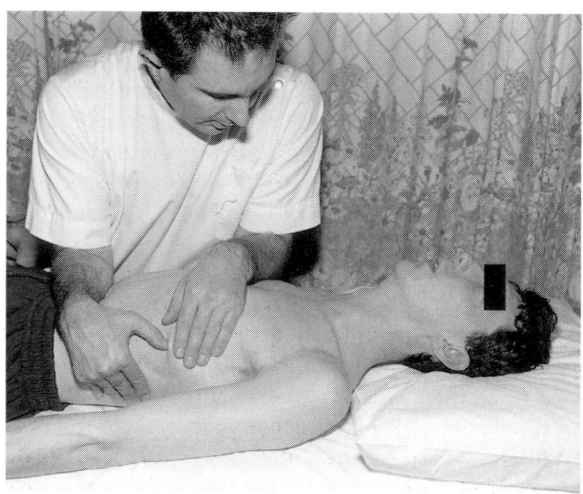

Figure 5.2 Assisted cough/expiration.

upwards and inwards creating a push against the diaphragm (Fig. 5.2) (Bromley 1991, Ward 1993).

SUMMARY

Nowhere is accurate, skilled clinical judgement more important than in the management of the acutely brain-injured patient. Physiotherapists have a vital role to play in the prevention of secondary brain damage which may result from hypoxia arising from respiratory dysfunction.

It is essential that the physiotherapist has an understanding of the relationship between brain and lung function, intracranial dynamics and the potential effects of physiotherapy. This knowledge enables the therapist to plan effective intervention and prevent therapy-induced problems.

MANAGEMENT OF NEUROLOGICAL DYSFUNCTION

BASIC PRINCIPLES

The control of body posture includes the alignment of body segments to each other and to the supporting surface. It requires a fixed, or reference, point around which movement can occur. The choice of position, both for support and for the performance of movement, must be considered in respect of the prevailing abnormal tone, the influence of gravity, the potential structural deformities and the preservation of tissue viability (Pope 1992, Dufosse & Massion 1992).

Movements are regularly performed on patients who are unconscious, paralysed, or who have hypertonus, in order to maintain muscle and joint range. An understanding of normal movement as described in Chapter 2 is essential to ensure that movements are performed correctly. Emphasis should be placed on functional movements, ensuring an appropriate response throughout the whole body rather than movements purely of an isolated part.

Passive joint motion refers to any movement of an articulation that is produced by some external force (Frank et al 1984). By implication,

the term 'passive' indicates that what is done is outside the patient's control and, as such, passive movement must be considered a powerful tool. Patients who are unconscious or who have a flaccid paralysis have no resistance to any force applied, whereas those who are dominated by stereotyped spastic posturing tend to resist movements out of these patterns.

In the clinical setting, the term 'passive' is often inappropriate in that, irrespective of their level of consciousness, patients should be involved in the activity. Verbal instruction should be given as each movement is carried out, to inform patients of the desired response and what is expected of them, and attention given to the degree of proximal mobility and alignment to effect optimal limb movement. It is only in this way that the maintenance of muscle and joint range becomes a dynamic activity rather than a mindless, routine procedure performed on the patient.

It is impossible for the physiotherapist to replicate, for a paralysed patient, the full gamut of functional activity undertaken in everyday life. Normal movement is dependent upon the activation of appropriate agonists and antagonists, with adjustment of synergists and postural fixators (Marsden 1984). Appropriate positioning is of great importance in enabling effective movement with this concurrent response throughout the body. For example, elevation of the arm in the normal subject is influenced by the degree of thoracic excursion which complements this action. If the spine becomes stiff and immobile and is unable to accommodate to the arm movement, this movement will be performed ineffectively and may traumatise the shoulder joint and surrounding structures.

Limitation of range of movement is a common complication in patients with musculoskeletal and neurological conditions (Williams 1990, Pope 1992). Many authors stress the importance of passive movements to prevent this occurrence (Frank et al 1984, Pope 1992, Soryal et al 1992, Daud et al 1993, Davies 1994). However, Davies (1994), while advocating the use of passive movements, emphasises the need for caution, and Silver (1969) and Daud et al (1993) identified a relationship between passive movement and heterotopic bone formation in patients with spinal injury. Patients who are unable to signify pain and discomfort are at particular risk if the limb is taken to the extreme of range by a therapist intent on 'maintaining range of movement'.

The use of passive movement remains controversial. Vigorous, forceful movements carried out in the presence of severe spasticity may cause microtears in muscle which may lead to calcification of the muscle (Ada et al 1990). Movement of a joint where there is inadequate muscular control may also lead to overstretching of tissues around the joint (Frank et al 1984). This is in part due to the lack of reciprocal activity which under normal circumstances provides proximal control and stability. Soryal et al (1992) described three patients with Guillain–Barré syndrome who had 'profound disability and social handicap over 1 to 3 years after acute neurological presentation primarily as a result of reduced joint mobility rather than neurogenic weakness'. This was considered to be the result of either inadequate passive movement or excessive passive movement, in the presence of hypotonia, traumatising the joints and surrounding structures.

When muscle is immobilised in a shortened position there is a reduction in both the muscle fibre length due to a loss of serial sarcomeres and a remodelling of the intramuscular connective tissue, leading to increased muscle stiffness (Goldspink & Williams 1990). Mobilisation of the muscle is therefore essential to minimise these structural changes. Periods of stretch as short as half an hour each day have been found to be effective in preventing loss of sarcomeres and reducing muscle atrophy in neurologically intact mice (Williams 1990). Tardieu et al (1988), in a study of the soleus muscle of children with cerebral palsy, demonstrated that it was necessary for the muscle to remain in a lengthened position for 6 hours to prevent contracture.

Passive movements of the limbs may be performed on patients once or twice a day. This is particularly so for patients in an intensive care setting where passive movements are often carried out as a routine procedure. The time

taken in carrying out these movements varies, but due to other constraints, rarely exceed 1 hour a day in total. If the rest of the time, the patient is dominated by spastic patterns which maintain the muscles in a shortened position, this intervention is unlikely to be effective in the maintenance of muscle and joint range. Other strategies must be developed to produce a more lasting effect in the control of body posture and movement.

Early mobilisation of the patient should be encouraged as and when the medical condition allows. Movements of the limbs while the patient is confined to bed are difficult in terms of facilitating activity within the trunk. Where bed rest is unavoidable, it is essential to maintain adequate movement of the trunk to maintain mobility and to stimulate postural adjustments when moving the limbs.

Of equal importance is the mobility of the nervous system itself and how it adapts to body movement (Hall et al 1993, Maitland 1986, Butler 1991, Shacklock 1995). Mobilisation of the nervous system is used extensively in the assessment and treatment of pain syndromes but it is only quite recently that its importance has been recognised in the treatment of patients with neurological disability (Davies 1994). Patients who are unable to move or who are dominated by spastic stereotyped postures are in as great a danger of developing shortening of neural structures as they are of loss of range of the musculoskeletal system.

Davies (1994) advocates the use of specific tension tests for the maintenance or restoration of adaptive lengthening of the nervous system. Therapists are advised to study the techniques carefully and to practice them on normal subjects prior to using them in the treatment of patients with neurological dysfunction.

POSITIONING

Different postures and positions, and their influence on tone and movement, are discussed in Chapter 2. These should be considered in determining the most appropriate position for treatment of patients with differing types of

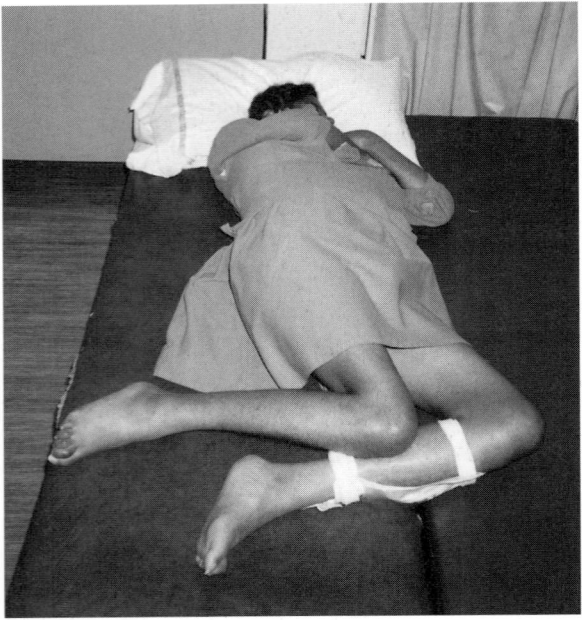

Figure 5.3   Windswept hips.

abnormal tone. However, the optimal position is not always possible due to the patient's medical condition or the presence of contractures, and modification is necessary.

Throughout this section 'acceptance of the base of support' refers to the ability of the patient to adjust appropriately to the contours of the supporting surface.

Positioning in a variety of postures is recommended particularly for patients dominated by severe hypertonus. Many patients with increased tone demonstrate a degree of asymmetry which, without treatment, may lead to contracture within the spastic pattern. An example of this pattern of contracture is illustrated in Figure 5.3.

The pattern includes:

- rotation of the pelvis relative to the thorax
- lateral flexion of the trunk
- 'windswept' lower limbs
- unilateral hip adduction
- abduction of the opposite hip
- bilateral knee flexion (Pope et al 1991).

This pattern of contracture not only precludes sitting and standing but also adversely affects the patient's ability to accept the base of support in supine and side-lying.

Principles of positioning in bed

The patient may be confined to bed, particularly in the early stages, and is therefore only able to experience a limited variety of positions and movement. The positions are generally restricted to those of side-lying, supine, half-lying and occasionally prone. Movements are dependent upon the position and are compromised by limitations imposed by proximal inactivity or inappropriate activity as may result from hypertonus. The positions and movements must not be seen as separate entities; each is dependent on the other to ensure the maintenance of function.

Supine lying

Patients with low tone totally accept the large supportive surface. It is not uncommon to find that, after prolonged periods in bed with reduced muscle tone, the spine adapts to the contours of the support. Supine lying predisposes to the lumbar spine becoming flatter with a posterior tilt of the pelvis and the thoracic spine becomes more extended as the shoulder girdles elevate and fall back into retraction. The feet, unless supported, tend towards plantar flexion with the danger of contracture of the posterior crural muscle group.

Patients with increased extensor tone may be unable to accept the large base of support, pushing back against the resistance offered by the surface and thereby exacerbating the extensor spasticity. The patient with increased flexor tone may be unable to release this tone to accommodate to the base of support. In most instances, either the extensor or flexor tone is compounded by an element of asymmetry, making appropriate placement virtually impossible. Adaptations to spinal and pelvic alignment are determined by the prevailing tone.

Modification of supine lying, by the use of a wedge and/or pillows, may be of value in controlling the alignment of the spine and in

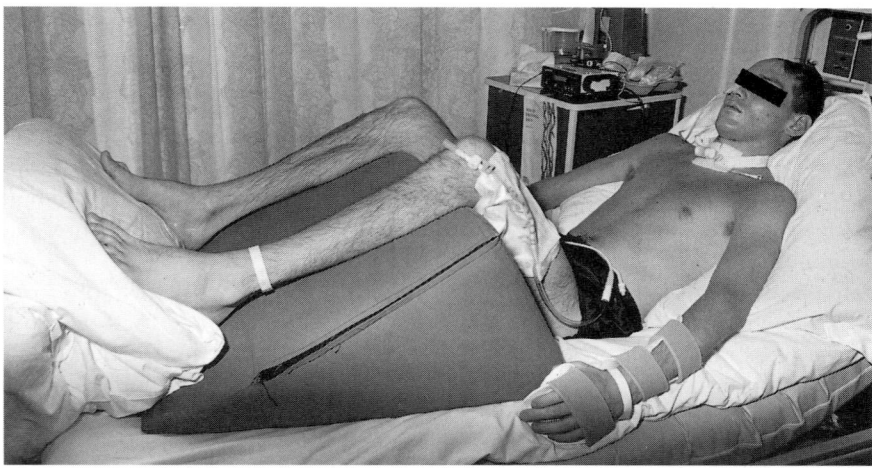

Figure 5.4   Supine lying with wedges.

facilitating acceptance of this position. Wedges may be used to good effect both under the head and shoulders and under the knees (Fig. 5.4). For those with predominant extensor tone, the introduction of flexion provides a point of fixation at the pelvis about which movement from lying can be facilitated. The head is in alignment with the trunk in the sagittal and coronal planes, reducing the tendency for increased extension of the cervical spine and for the shoulder girdles to pull back into retraction. The flexion introduced at the hips and knees breaks up the dominant extensor tone of the legs.

Patients with predominant flexor tone may be unable to release the flexor activity if the supporting surface is flat and fully extended. In cases where the flexor tone is excessive, a larger wedge may be required in the first instance, its size being gradually reduced as the patient becomes able to accommodate to a more extended position. If there is established shortening of the hip flexors, the graduated use of wedges can be effective in regaining range of movement.

Many patients with spasticity present with asymmetrical posture. The use of a T-roll (Fig. 5.5) may be of value in that it promotes more equal loading of tissues and can improve the alignment of body segments (Pope 1992).

Side-lying

This position is often utilised in the management of patients with neurological dysfunction (Bobath 1990, Davies 1994). It introduces opposing influences of tone on the two sides of the body; on the supporting side, one of extension, and on the non-weight-bearing side, one of flexion. The side-lying position is similar for patients with either low tone or increased tone. The patient may be positioned with either the underneath leg extended and the uppermost leg flexed or with both legs flexed. The underneath shoulder is protracted to prevent pressure falling over the acromion process, and the pelvis is rotated

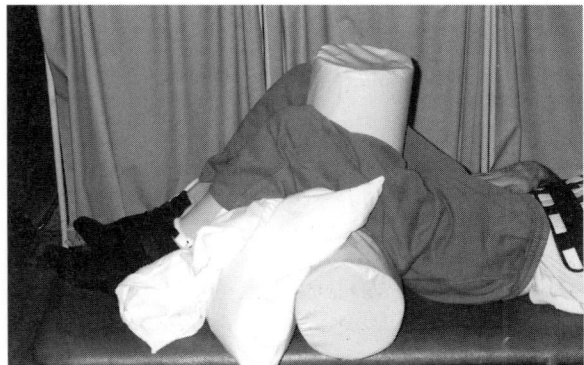

Figure 5.5   Supine lying with T-roll.

slightly towards prone. Pillows are required, one or two in front of the patient to support the arm and encourage maintenance of this position towards prone, and one between the knees to stabilise the pelvis and prevent adduction of the uppermost leg. A pillow behind the patient should not be necessary, providing the pelvis is tilted slightly forwards, unless there is uncontrolled movement.

Asymmetrical posturing of the head and trunk may also be corrected or improved with the use of pillows. For example, pillows are used to maintain the head in alignment in the coronal plane, and positioning of a pillow under the left side, when in left side-lying, may prove effective in maintaining range within the opposing trunk side flexors.

Prone lying

This position is recommended as a means of maintaining or correcting range into extension particularly at the hips and knees (Davies 1994, Pope 1992). However, prone lying should be used with caution in that it may exacerbate flexor tone. Patients with flexor spasticity rarely accommodate to this position without the

additional support of a wedge or pillows in conjunction with specific inhibitory techniques to prepare them. Davies (1994) advocates the use of pillows under the trunk to allow acceptance of the support, gradually reducing them until the patient can lie in full extension. The feet should be positioned over the end of the bed to prevent shortening of the posterior crural muscle group.

For patients with low tone, prone lying may be a useful adjunct to treatment. A wedge or pillows placed under the thorax alters the contour of the spine and enables controlled weight-bearing through the forearms. The protracted position of the arms facilitates flexion at the thoracic spine, thereby overriding the tendency of extension when the patient is positioned in supine. The extended position of the lumbar spine serves to maintain the lumbar lordosis. From this position, normal extensor activity may be recruited in the head and trunk (Fig. 5.6).

Positioning in this way may also be of benefit for patients with extensor spasticity, as the overall influence is one of flexion. For these patients, the emphasis is more on mobilising the shoulders forwards into protraction to counteract the commonly observed retraction. Extensor spasticity

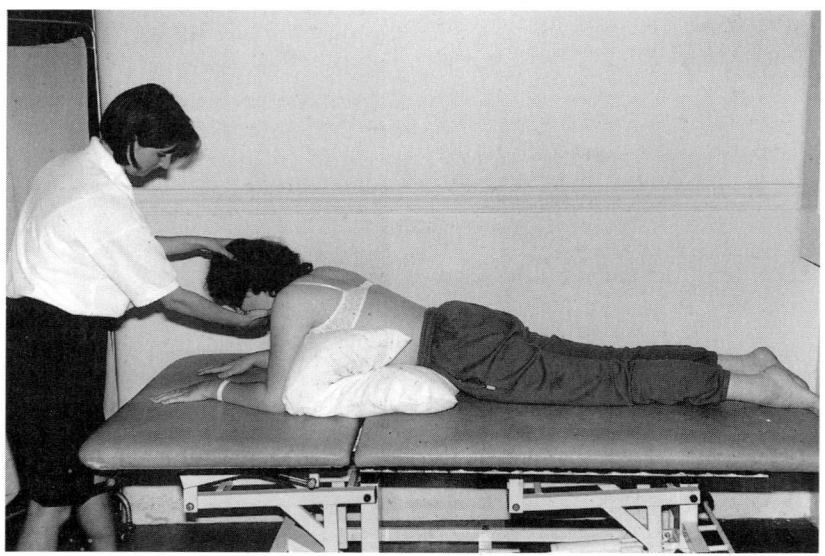

Figure 5.6 Prone lying with forearm support over pillows.

of the cervical spine may also be inhibited when the patient is in prone lying.

Prone lying is rarely used by nursing staff, especially when there are respiratory complications necessitating ventilation. However, Davies (1994) advocates the use of this position as a means of facilitating drainage from the respiratory tract and considers the presence of a tracheostomy not to be a precluding factor. The disadvantage is that there is little stimulation when lying face downwards and, in many instances, the degree of neck rotation required to provide a clear airway may be somewhat restricted.

Summary

Limb movements are compromised if there is reduced spinal mobility and inadequate or inappropriate muscle tone to enable effective proximal adjustments. Where bed rest is unavoidable, it is essential to maintain adequate movement within the trunk to maintain mobility and to stimulate the proximal control associated with limb movements. Although frequently less obvious than contractures affecting the limbs, loss of range and impaired coordination of the trunk musculature has a dramatic effect on function (Davies 1990).

Movement between lying positions and when coming up from lying to sitting should be carried out with care and the patient given time to adjust to the change of position. Turning from side to side or being hurriedly taken into sitting can be a frightening experience particularly if there are perceptual problems and sensory impairment.

Principles of positioning in sitting

The principles for appropriate seating are described in detail in Chapter 7.

Trunk mobilisations

In the treatment of neurological patients, trunk mobilisations refer to movements of the trunk, facilitated by the physiotherapist, which are used to modify abnormal tone and improve alignment. In this context they should not be confused with specific vertebral mobilisations as advocated by manipulative therapists.

Treatment of the patient in sitting provides an opportunity for the physiotherapist to mobilise the trunk and facilitate correct alignment with proximal control and stability. Trunk mobilisation as used in this way is considered by some practitioners to be a somewhat passive form of intervention. However, as with all techniques, it is dependent upon the physiotherapist's skill and expertise to elicit the desired response. Slow, rhythmical movements, providing full support from behind the patient are more effective in reducing tone and increasing mobility. Smaller range movements with less support and intermittent pressure as required to gain a 'holding' response, are more effective in stimulating activity.

Patients with hemiplegia develop compensatory strategies to contend with their asymmetry. Those with low tone may develop excessive activity of the 'unaffected' side as they struggle to support the weight of the flaccid hemiplegic side. It is often the overactivity of the sound side which precludes activity of the affected side. Mobilisation of the trunk is of particular benefit to these patients, as the physiotherapist can facilitate a more appropriate balance of response between the two sides of the body. In this situation, it is the 'unaffected' side which is in danger of becoming shortened.

Hemiplegic patients with spasticity may develop shortening of the trunk side flexors of the affected side. Mobilisation of the trunk is again appropriate but in this instance the emphasis is on reducing tone in the affected side and thereby stimulating more normal activity of the sound side.

This scenario illustrates the holistic effects of neurological impairment. Although hemiplegia is by definition a condition affecting half of the body, the consequences of motor and sensory impairment of one side inevitably affects all aspects of movement.

Use of the gymnastic ball

The ball is made of resilient plastic and comes in

various sizes. In treatment, it is used predominantly in eight directions – forwards, backwards, to each side and diagonally forwards and backwards (Lewis 1989). Klein-Vogelbach (1990) gives detailed reference to specific techniques which may be used to optimise stability and/or mobility. These are active exercises performed by the patient with assistance from the therapist as required. These techniques were originally designed for the treatment of orthopaedic conditions. Hasler (1981) adapted Klein-Vogelbach's method for the treatment of patients with neurological disability and Silva & Luginbuhl (1981) and Edwards (1991) recommended its use in the treatment of patients with incomplete spinal cord injury. The gymnastic ball has also been recommended as a treatment modality for patients with hemiplegia (Davies 1990, Lewis 1989).

The ball is useful:

- to stimulate dynamic co-contraction of the trunk musculature
- to mobilise the trunk and limbs
- in retraining balance reactions and coordination
- in strengthening postural muscles (Hasler 1981).

Patients may be mobilised, sitting on the ball with the physiotherapist supporting from behind. In this way the potential loss of range, especially at the thoracolumbar spine and pelvis may be prevented or minimised. A second person may be required to control the patient's legs to prevent them falling into abduction and lateral rotation (Fig. 5.7). Slow, deliberate movements of the ball both laterally and forwards and backwards can prove most effective in inhibiting tone and maintaining mobility.

Summary. The gymnastic ball may be used to good effect in preserving or regaining range of movement and in stimulating postural adjustments, particularly within the trunk and lower limbs. However, it should be used with caution in that, in some cases, this mobile surface provides insufficient support for the patient to effect the desired response.

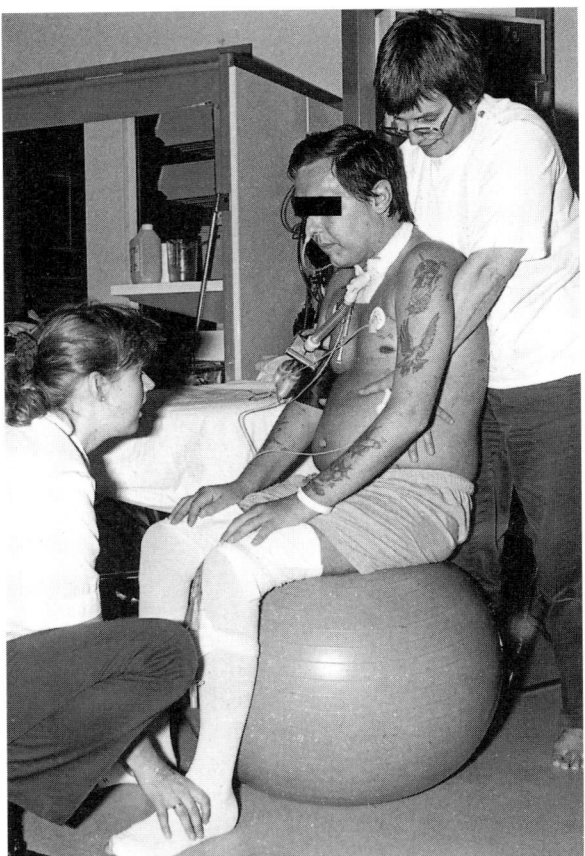

Figure 5.7 Patient on gymnastic ball.

Principles of positioning in standing

Standing is advocated as a means of maintaining joint range and stimulating anti-gravity activity (Ada et al 1990, Pope 1992, Brown 1994). Different types of equipment are recommended to achieve this goal. The selection of the most appropriate aid is dependent upon the size and weight of the patient, the patient's medical status and the assistance available.

Positioning of the feet is of particular concern. Patients with low tone may be placed in standing to maintain the length of soleus and gastrocnemius and thereby prevent development of contractures (Ada et al 1990, Pope 1992). However, loss of range of the posterior crural muscle group is a recognised complication of excessive spasticity

(Yarkony & Sahgal 1987). In this situation, support must be provided under the heel to accommodate this shortening. The effect of this is twofold:

- A foam wedge placed under the heel reduces the stress placed on the shortened structures by increasing the contact area and is therefore more conducive to the patient accepting the support.
- The increased base of support enables more equal weight-bearing through the full surface of the foot. If there is no support under the heel, the pressure is exerted through the metatarsal heads, which may exacerbate the spasticity. The pressure exerted by the patient's own body weight may place unacceptable strain over the medial arch and the plantar fascia, and damage to these structures may ensue.

By using support in this way, the patient may gradually be able to accept a smaller wedge as the range of movement increases. Mobilisation of the plantar flexors while in standing may be effective in maintaining or regaining range of movement.

The tilt table

This is frequently used, particularly in the early stages of treatment. Patients who are unconscious and/or have low tone will require total support to enable them to achieve an upright posture. The tilt table affords this support and is perhaps the most commonly used form of intervention. It is of particular value for patients who are excessively heavy. The patient may be transferred on to the tilt table by means of either a hoist or by sliding them, on a sheet or 'easy-slide', from their hospital bed on to the table. When using the latter technique, attention must be paid to the protection of the skin by ensuring that any rigid points are covered by a towel or other means of padding.

The tilt table, preferably one that is manually operated, is the method of choice where there is cardiovascular and/or autonomic instability with the potential danger of hypotension. In these instances, it is imperative that the patient can be restored to the horizontal position at the first sign of distress. Initially, in many cases, the blood pressure is monitored throughout the procedure to ensure there are no untoward effects. The manually operated table is preferred in that this provides more instant control; the electrically controlled table takes considerably longer to return to the horizontal position and it is not unknown for it to fail.

The tilt table is perhaps the most passive means of taking the patient up into standing. The common characteristics of normal alignment in standing are dependent upon an intact neuromuscular system and have been described in Chapter 2. Where there is abnormal tone caused by neurological impairment, the patient is unable to attain this normal alignment. The use of the tilt table brings the patient up into standing but does little to facilitate the postural adjustments essential for normal standing (Friedli et al 1984).

Patients with predominantly low tone adapt to the gravitational force, supported only by the straps securing them to the table. The pelvis tilts anteriorly with a resultant increase in the lumbar lordosis and consequent flexion of the hips. In this position, the iliopsoas muscle is in a shortened position with the potential for development of hip flexion contractures. The knees tend to hyperextend, with the resultant loss of the plantigrade position at the feet through the relative shortening of gastrocnemius. To prevent the head and shoulders falling forwards and the patient hanging on the trunk strap, the tilt table is frequently positioned a few degrees from the full vertical. The shoulder girdles retract with the head extended precipitating shortening of the extensor muscles of the cervical spine. Clearly, if the therapist is aware of these potential complications, then adjustments can and should be made. Use of the tilt table, purely to attain an upright posture, is of little value to the patient in terms of regaining correct postural control.

The tilt table should be used only as an adjunct to treatment. Where possible the straps should be removed, thereby stimulating the

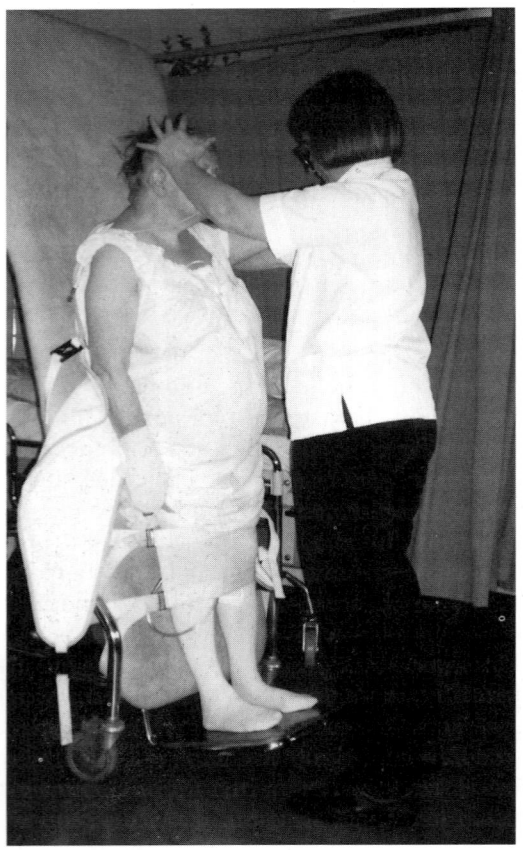

Figure 5.8 Tilt table.

patient's own control. This is of particular relevance to the trunk strap. In the majority of cases this need not be used if the therapist supports the patient from the shoulder girdles with the patient's arms extended over the therapist's shoulders (Fig. 5.8). In this way head and trunk control may be facilitated. A pillow or towel may be used behind the knee to prevent hyperextension, but it must be recognised that this in itself does not address the primary problem, that of the anterior tilt of the pelvis.

The tilt table is not generally recommended for patients with severe extensor spasticity, primarily because it provides an extensor surface against which they may resist, thereby exacerbating their tone. For those with flexor tone the tilt table may be of value in controlling the legs in a more extended position. This positioning

should only be used in conjunction with inhibitory techniques to first reduce the flexor spasticity.

Forcing the legs into extension by means of the knee strap will not only exacerbate the spasticity but may also cause considerable discomfort to the patient. Equally, the attainment of more extension at the knees by these means will inevitably create problems both proximally and distally. Sustained pressure exerted on the knees stretches the iliopsoas, thereby pulling the pelvis into increased anterior tilt with a compensatory lumbar lordosis. There is increased pressure exerted on the posterior aspect of the heels, further increasing the dominant influence of flexion. The use of force to attain improved alignment is ineffective in terms of controlling increased tone or in the prevention of subsequent contractures.

Summary. The tilt table is a valuable tool in enabling the patient to stand. If there is any risk to staff in standing patients by more dynamic means, then the tilt table is the method of choice. Where possible, other means should be considered to ensure correct alignment through concurrent inhibition and/or facilitation to provide for more active and appropriate intervention.

The Oswestry standing frame

Originally developed for standing patients following spinal cord lesions, this frame is widely used, not only in spinal injury units, but also in most general hospitals and certainly in the majority of neuroscience centres in the United Kingdom. The wooden frame affords tremendous stability whilst allowing access for the therapist from behind. Additional trunk supports are available for patients with residual and extensive neurological impairment.

Three sheepskin-covered straps attach behind the ankles, in front of the knees and behind the hips. If correctly applied, these secure the lower limbs in a position of extension and enable the therapist, standing behind the patient, to ensure correct alignment of the pelvis.

Two staff are required to lift the patient from a sitting position, either from the side of the bed

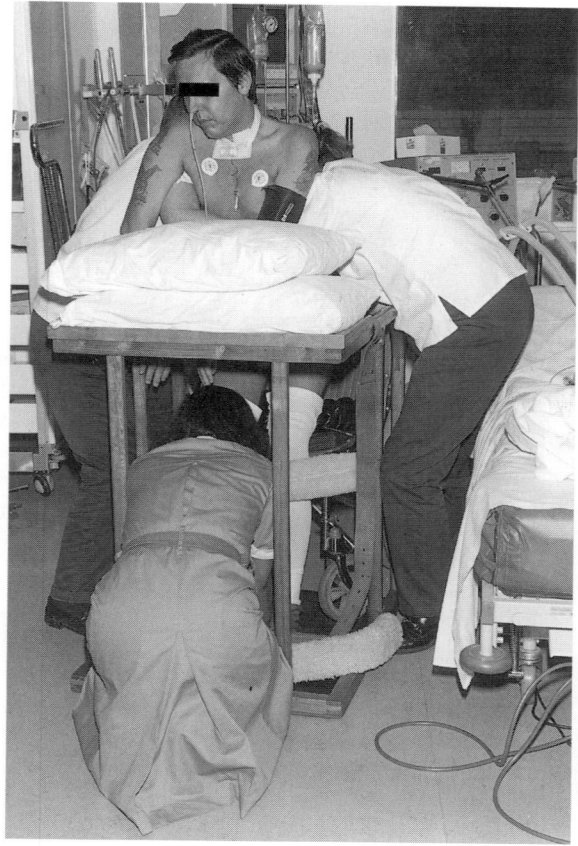
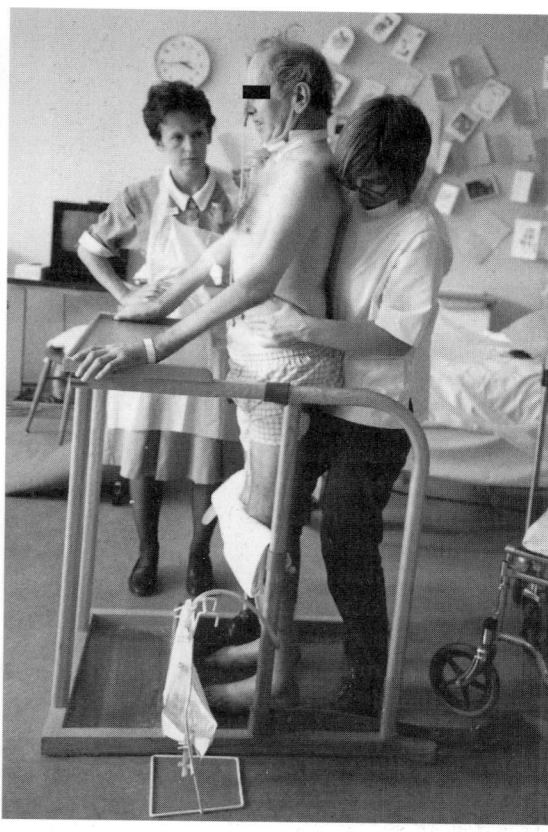

A   B

Figure 5.9   Oswestry standing frame: (A) preparing to stand; (B) upright in frame.

or from a wheelchair (Fig. 5.9). A third person (possibly even a relative) would be required if the patient is intubated or has a tracheostomy and is being ventilated.

In most cases, once the patient has been brought up into standing, only one therapist would be required to maintain the patient upright. A further person may be necessary to support the head and neck and stimulate head control. If the patient is ventilated then this additional person is essential.

The therapist can ensure that the pelvis is in neutral or preferably in a position of slight posterior tilt. This enables full extension at the hips with mechanical lengthening of the ilio-femoral ligament and the iliopsoas muscle. Maintenance of the length of these two struc-tures prevents the compensatory lordosis of the

lumbar spine and extension at the shoulder girdles. This positioning also facilitates abdominal activity.

To achieve this optimal alignment it is import-ant that the straps are correctly applied.

- The hip strap must be taut to prevent the patient 'sitting' on it and thereby producing flexion, adduction and medial rotation at the hips.
- The knee strap must be positioned over the patella tendon, as opposed to over the patella itself, and maintain the knees in extension. A foam wedge or towel may be placed between the knees to prevent valgus.
- The foot strap is attached behind the heels.

The table may be used to advantage by placing the patient's hands over the rim and stimulating extensor activity in the arms. This may also assist in more appropriate alignment of the head and trunk.

The Oswestry frame allows for more dynamic intervention in terms of movement. The hip strap may be removed, with the therapist standing behind and supporting the patient. In this way the therapist can allow the patient to move, in a small range, down towards sitting and facilitate movement back into standing ensuring correct pelvic alignment. The therapist should have a plinth positioned behind her at the correct height to ensure that this activity is safe.

Patients may also be mobilised by use of the table. By gradually taking the patient forwards to rest over pillows or a wedge on the table, the thoracolumbar spine may be mobilised and full extension of the cervical spine obtained. The patient may stand supported in this position to ensure extensibility of the hip extensors, knee flexors and of the neural structures.

Summary. The Oswestry standing frame is designed in such a way as to enable its use for:

- stimulating muscle activity with correct body alignment
- mobilisation of the patient with increased tone to prevent shortening of structures dominated by the increased tone.

It may be considered to provide 'an extra pair of hands' in providing proximal and lower limb stability to allow for functional use of the arms.

Prone standing table

The prone standing table is of particular value for patients with severe extensor tone. Straps over the trunk, hips and feet secure the patient and a table is attached for arm support (Fig. 5.10). The supporting surface is on the flexor aspect, which prevents the patient pushing backwards and exacerbating his extensor tone. At the same time, this positioning may stimulate more normal extensor tone by providing secure and stable proximal support.

The stability afforded to the trunk, pelvis and lower limbs enables more specific intervention for facilitation of, for example, head control or

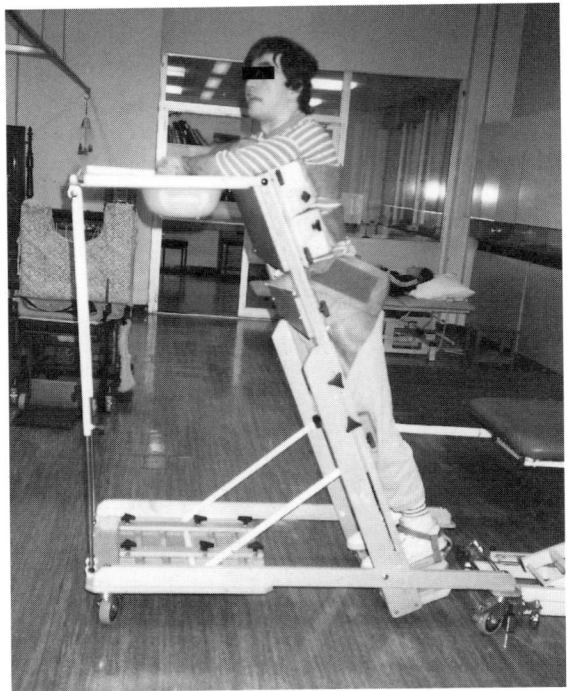

Figure 5.10 Prone standing table.

increased range of movement of the upper limbs.

Standing using two or more therapists

This is a more dynamic intervention in that it provides for instant response and adjustment on the part of the therapist to the patient's changing status. However, standing in this way is more demanding on staff and should only be attempted on patients with whom the therapist feels confident. Therapists new to working with neurological patients should not feel that this method of standing the patient must be used at all costs. In most instances, therapists need time to develop their handling skills, which in turn gives them the confidence to attempt more complex intervention. Many experienced neurological therapists continue to use either the tilt table or a standing frame, and with good reason. The persistent, insidious strain from heavy lifting and supporting patients with severe neurological deficit can have long-term

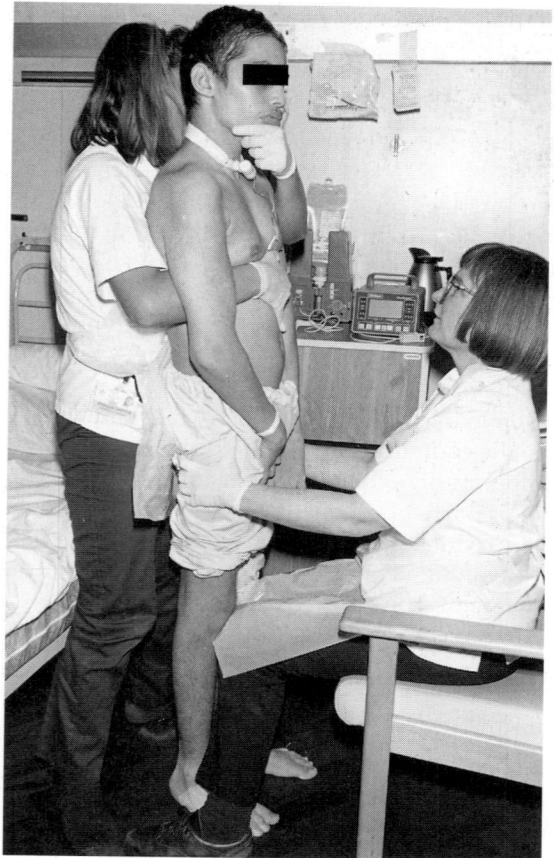

Figure 5.11   Standing, using two physiotherapists.

Standing a patient with increased tone may need to be adapted depending on the severity and distribution of tone with, in some instances, more than two therapists being required.

The advantage of standing the patient in this way is that it enables the therapists to feel and respond to any change in the patient's status. Movements may be facilitated from standing to sitting back on to the therapist behind, and up again into standing.

Transfer of weight from one side of the body to the other, maintaining the correct alignment, provides the sensation of movement between the two sides which is of particular importance for patients with a hemiplegic presentation. Any activity by the patient can be felt immediately. A positive response can be facilitated whereas unwanted activity can be instantly inhibited.

Summary.   Standing patients in this more dynamic way is often of great benefit to the patient. The therapist must be competent and confident to manage this technique. If there is any doubt in the mind of the therapist, or the patient demonstrates any concern, other, less strenuous means should be adopted, utilising equipment aids as indicated.

Use of back slabs

Back slabs, made from either plaster of Paris or glass fibre material, may be used to maintain the legs in an extended position to effect standing. Davies (1994) considers this the method of choice when support is required to stand patients following head injury. They should be made specifically for the individual patient to ensure a correct fit and be securely bandaged in place. (Detailed description is given in Ch. 8.)

The purpose of the slabs is to enable the therapist to work for improved trunk and pelvic control while stabilising the lower limbs. The therapist may choose to stand in front of or behind the patient while stimulating head, trunk and upper limb control, or the patient may stand in the parallel bars to facilitate weight-bearing through the arms (Fig. 5.12). By maintaining a posterior tilt of the pelvis, shortening of the iliopsoas may be prevented.

consequences, particularly in relation to back injuries. Selection of the most appropriate treatment intervention must therefore always consider the therapist as well as the patient.

Standing a patient who is unconscious with no volitional movement requires maximum input from the therapist. The patient should be lifted from the sitting position by a therapist standing in front supporting the knees with the patient resting forwards on the therapists shoulder. The therapist lifts the patient with her hands placed under the ischial tuberosities. A second therapist, standing behind the patient, then brings him into standing and supports the head and trunk. Once the patient is upright the therapist in front of the patient can sit on a chair, maintaining control of the hips, knees and feet (Fig. 5.11).

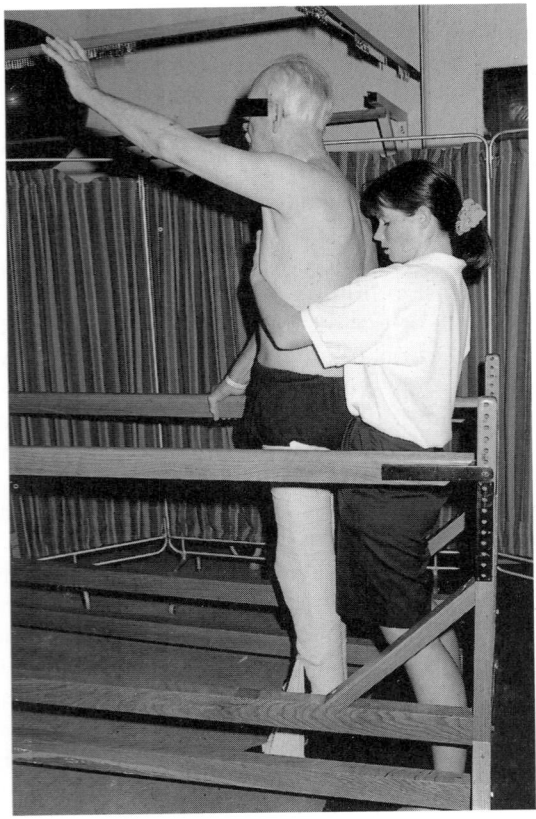

Figure 5.12 Standing with back slabs in parallel bars.

Back slabs may be used to good effect with all unconscious or low toned patients and for those with increased flexor tone. They are rarely appropriate for patients with extensor spasticity.

Patients with flexor spasticity of the legs may have such severe tonus that it is impossible to secure the slabs without the use of excessive force. As previously discussed in relation to the tilt table, inhibitory techniques must first be used to enable the patient to accept this support.

The use of a back slab has been advocated in the early management of stroke patients with lack of midline orientation (Davies 1985). These patients are often referred to as 'pushers' in that they overuse the sound side, pushing themselves off balance to the affected side. The back slab, applied to the affected leg, enables the patient to transfer weight through this limb and thereby regain more body awareness. This should be used with caution if a flexor pattern of spasticity becomes dominant in the lower limb.

The main disadvantage of using this method is that the patient cannot be taken up into standing through sitting. With the legs fixed in extension, the patient has to be helped into standing by the therapist. Once in standing, it is impossible to facilitate release of activity to allow the patient to move towards sitting by coordinating movement between the pelvis, hips, knees and feet. A further disadvantage is that there is little stimulation of the lower limb extensors.

Summary. The use of back slabs allows for specific mobilisation of the trunk on pelvis and the pelvis on extended lower limbs. In this way, it is of particular benefit in preventing the onset of, or reducing, hip flexor contracture. The main disadvantage is that back slabs preclude normal movement from sitting to standing.

MOVEMENTS

In the following section, specific movements of the body are described with identification of problems which may arise as a result of neurological dysfunction.

Orofacial movements

Patients with severe brain damage may demonstrate significant problems relating to impaired control and coordination of facial structures. The mouth is one of the most sensitive areas of the body and yet it is an area which is often neglected in rehabilitation (Davies 1994). There are many aspects which need to be considered in the maintenance of orofacial function. These include:

- The positioning of the head and trunk in that, if the head is held in extension, swallowing becomes difficult if not impossible.
- Many patients have spasticity of the tongue, which may be palpated as a tight ball behind the chin. As with other muscles dominated by spasticity, restricted range of movement results unless passive movement of the tongue is

undertaken by either the physiotherapist or speech therapist.

- Spasticity of the facial muscles may produce grimacing and loss of range of movement of the jaw. In severe cases, the temporo-mandibular joint may sublux.
- A gag, swallowing or bite reflex may be in evidence. These will severely compromise the maintenance of oral hygiene and, where appropriate, feeding. Orofacial therapy is essential to prevent increasing sensitivity to touch of the area within and around the mouth (Davies 1994).

Therapists are often apprehensive about treating facial structures, particularly the mouth, tending to concentrate more on the trunk and limb movements. 'The patient who is unconscious or who's mouth is significantly paralysed, experiences an almost total sensory deprivation interrupted only by certain nursing or medical procedures, sometimes unpleasant ones' (Davies 1994). If something unpleasant is put into the mouth of a normal subject, the response is one of disgust registered by grimacing and possibly spitting the object out. The patient who is unable to respond in this manner may show signs of distress with a general increase in spasticity throughout the body.

Patients respond positively to mobilisation of facial structures, particularly within the mouth and the surrounding area. Orofacial treatment is essential to desensitise these abnormal responses and to enable the patient to receive more appropriate feedback. *Gloves should always be worn when working within the mouth to minimise the risk of cross-infection.*

Examples of techniques which may be used to manage some of the problems listed above include:

- elongation of the cervical spine with extension of the trunk to prevent adaptive shortening of the cervical spine into extension; this is best achieved with the therapist behind the patient, supporting the trunk and holding the chin between the index and middle fingers with the thumb extending to the temporomandibular joint (Fig. 5.13)

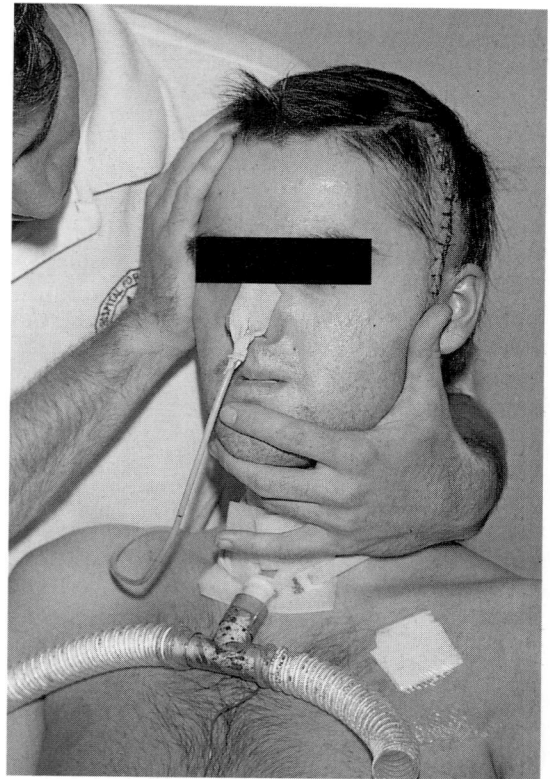

Figure 5.13 Orofacial control.

- maintaining this grip and mobilising the tongue with the middle finger to facilitate swallowing
- taking hold of the tongue using a piece of cotton gauze and gently mobilising to maintain or regain its range of movement
- massage/mobilisation of facial muscles to reduce tone and maintain or restore symmetry
- massage of the gums and the interior aspect of the cheeks after immersing the finger in water, or using a wet piece of gauze.

These techniques and others are described in detail in Davies (1994).

Shoulder girdle and upper limb

The shoulder joint is particularly vulnerable to trauma being the most mobile joint of the body in terms of its anatomical structure. It is dependent upon muscular activity for stability and therefore, when abnormal tone prevails, the mechanics of the joint are compromised (Lippitt & Matsen 1993).

Movements of the upper limb must be carried out with great care and with a detailed knowledge of the shoulder mechanism. The therapist must appreciate the holistic nature of functional activity. Movements of the upper limb cannot be viewed in isolation. Attention must be paid to the position in which the movements are performed, the stability afforded by the supporting surface, the patients' ability to maintain themselves or move against gravity and the ability of the trunk to respond effectively to the imposition of distal movement.

Potential problems affecting the shoulder girdle and upper limb function

The patient with low tone. In sitting or standing, the scapula, with little or no muscular activity to maintain its position of lateral rotation around the chest wall, rotates medially. The inferior angle of the scapula and the medial aspect of its spine are therefore equidistant from the vertebral column (Fig. 5.14). This movement results in a realignment of the position of the glenoid fossa, producing a degree of abduction at the shoulder joint.

In the adducted position, the capsule becomes taut and prevents downward displacement of the humerus (Cailliet 1980). The shoulder is vulnerable in a position of abduction, as the superior portion of the capsule is slack. The 'locking mechanism' is no longer effective, resulting in a subluxation of the glenohumeral joint (Fig. 5.15). This complication will always ensue to a greater or lesser extent in the presence of flaccidity or low tone.

Preventive measures offering support to the upper limb should be employed before irreparable damage occurs. The scapulohumeral rhythm is impaired and therefore movement performed by the therapist at the glenohumeral joint must include adequate excursion of the scapula.

Examples of specific problems which may arise as a result of low tone include:

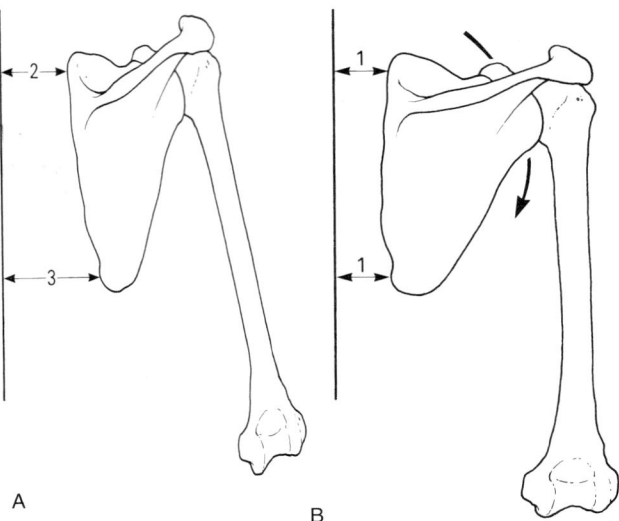

A   B

Figure 5.14 Relationship of the shoulder girdle and vertebral column: (A) normal; (B) abnormal (reproduced from Bromley 1991 with kind permission).

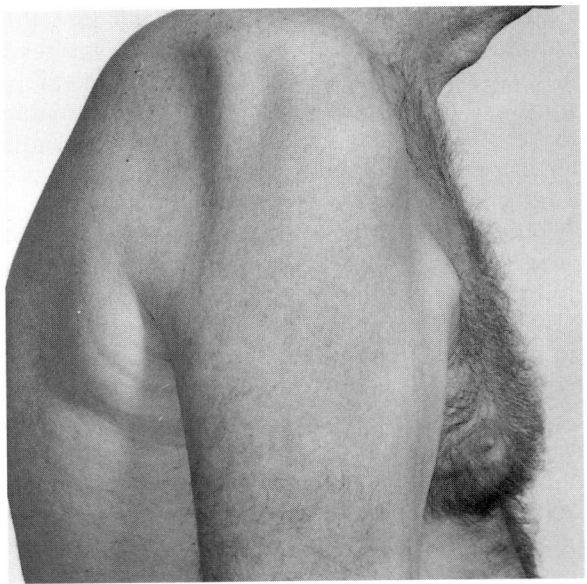

Figure 5.15 Shoulder subluxation.

- hyperactivity of the upper fibres of trapezius in an attempt to support the flail arm
- shortening of the pectorals with reduced range of movement into horizontal abduction

- shortening of latissimus dorsi
- immobility of the scapula
- hypermobility of the scapula should the medial rotators, namely teres major and subscapularis, become shortened.

The patient with increased tone. In patients with spasticity, the most commonly observed posturing of the upper limb is that of retraction of the scapula, adduction and medial rotation of the glenohumeral joint, flexion of the elbow, pronation of the forearm, flexion and ulnar deviation of the wrist, and flexion of the fingers with adduction of the thumb (Rothwell 1994, Bobath 1990).

Spasticity produces a degree of immobility; the dynamic co-contraction and stability afforded by the scapula as described in Chapter 2 being impaired. Reciprocal innervation is compromised; the grading of movement being lost with the static co-contraction of the dominant spastic muscle groups. Selective movement of the upper limb becomes difficult if not impossible with the impaired proximal stability. Shortening of the muscle groups producing the stereotyped posturing may result.

The scapula is pulled closer to the vertebral column by spasticity of the rhomboids. This may be either in a vertical position or with a degree of medial rotation. The angle of the glenoid fossa becomes vertical or possibly even downward facing. This malalignment of the glenohumeral joint produces a degree of relative abduction at the shoulder joint. Spasticity of the pectorals and medial rotators produces an anterior, rotational movement of the humerus, further distorting its position in relation to the glenoid fossa (Irwin-Carruthers & Runnalls 1982).

Movements undertaken by the physiotherapist to maintain range of movement must incorporate inhibition of the prevailing spasticity. Not only is there malalignment of the joint surfaces but also resistance from the spastic muscle groups. Spasticity invariably affects all muscle groups in spite of the predominance of flexion, adduction and medial rotation. Attention must be paid to the position in which the movements are performed. For example, movement of the arm up

into elevation will be more successful with adequate extension of the thoracic spine (Crawford & Jull 1993).

The scapulohumeral rhythm is altered, the extent to which this is disrupted being dependent upon the severity and distribution of spasticity. For example:

- The excursion of the scapula may become limited by the spasticity of its extensive musculature. In this situation, attempted movement of the arm away from the body may traumatise the glenohumeral joint and the surrounding tissues.
- Spasticity of the medial rotators may reduce the range of movement at the glenohumeral joint through shortening of teres major and subscapularis in particular. In this instance, attempted movement of the arm away from

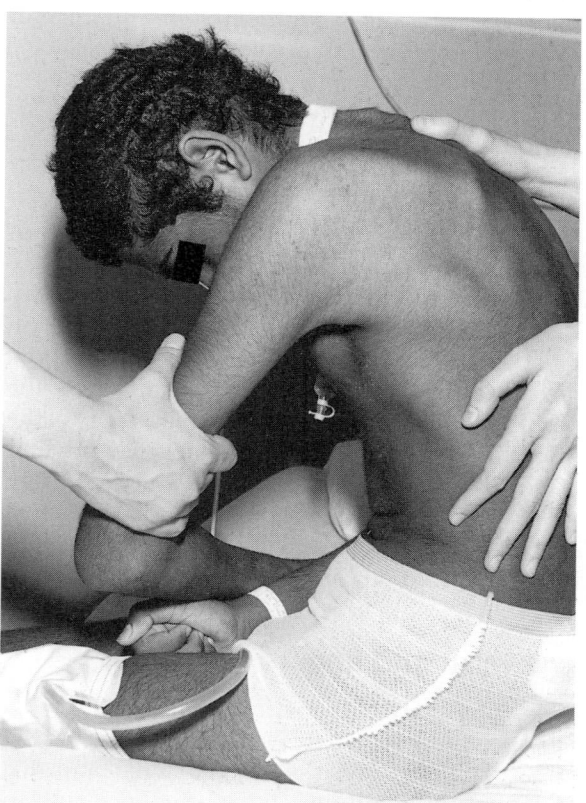

Figure 5.16   Reduced glenohumeral movement resulting in increased excursion of the scapula.

the body produces hypermobility of the scapula to compensate for the immobility at the glenohumeral joint (Fig. 5.16).

Pain may be an additional complication which may develop as a result of the unremitting spastic posturing and/or forcing of range without appropriate inhibition, thereby traumatising the shoulder mechanism.

Prehension is dependent upon the proximal musculature of the shoulder for placing the hand in the correct spatial location to effect function. Neurological impairment affecting the shoulder mechanism will therefore affect the selective use of the hands for function.

The elbow joint

The flexor pattern of spasticity affecting the upper limb may result in shortening of the elbow flexors, most commonly in conjunction with pronation of the forearm. Where spasticity of biceps is dominant, this flexion is seen in conjunction with supination.

Mobilisation/massage of the elbow flexors is of benefit in reducing the flexor tone and improving the malleability of the muscles, thereby facilitating movement into extension. Constant forcing of range against a spastic resistance may be a causative factor in the onset of ossification. Passive movement of the arm into extension must ensure release and elongation of the elbow flexors to prevent excessive strain falling on the periosteum where the muscles insert on to the forearm. Where there is excessive spasticity and extension of the elbow becomes increasingly difficult to maintain, prophylactic or corrective splinting by means of a drop-out cast (see Ch. 8) is the preferred option.

The wrist and fingers

Flexor spasticity of the wrist and finger flexors is most commonly seen with pronation of the forearm, ulnar deviation of the wrist and adduction of the thumb. It is often difficult to prevent shortening of these structures unless splinting is used to maintain a functional

position (see Ch. 8). However, the effects of this intervention must be carefully monitored. Inappropriate splinting may further reinforce spasticity if the patient is unable to accommodate to the support. Depending upon the severity of spasticity, a full cast or a removable splint may be advocated. Where possible, the splint should be able to be taken off to allow for mobilisation of the wrist and fingers as a means of desensitising the grasp response. The family in particular should be instructed in the most appropriate way of mobilising the wrist and hand, the hand being one of the most common points of contact between the patient and his relatives.

Movements of the wrist and fingers can only be effective with a reduction of flexor tone throughout the upper limb. Attempts to straighten the fingers, for example, or radially deviate the wrist, are singularly unsuccessful if the shoulder and elbow are still dominated by flexor spasticity.

Movements of the wrist and hand for patients with cervical cord injuries must be performed with extreme care. For example, a patient with a lesion at the level of the sixth cervical vertebra loses control of the fingers and is dependent upon the wrist extensors to effect function by the use of a tenodesis grip. If the wrist and fingers are passively extended to the extreme of range, the finger flexors may become overstretched and the tenodesis grip thus ineffective. Contracture of the finger flexors is to be avoided but overstretching can have catastrophic functional consequences.

The lower limb

In a normal subject, if the leg is actively lifted on to the chest in supine lying, there is a central stabilising effect. Abdominal and erector spinae activity ensure effective action of the psoas muscle as a hip flexor by stabilising the lumbar spine and controlling the pelvis in a position of posterior tilt. This movement of the pelvis is essential in ensuring effective action of the iliopsoas muscle. As the leg is flexed, the pelvis should be posteriorly tilted and the sacrum

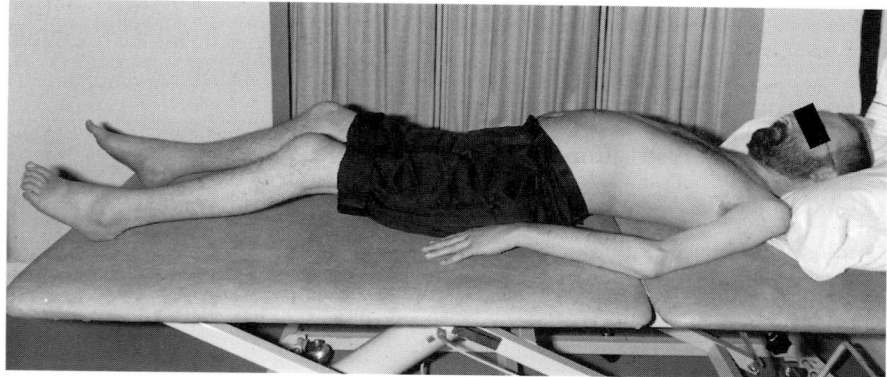

Figure 5.17 Flexion contraction of the hips.

remain in contact with the bed as the leg is extended. In this way, normal range of psoas may be preserved. Patients with long-term immobility invariably lose range in the hip flexors so that in supine, with hips extended, the lumbar lordosis is exaggerated (Pope 1992) (Fig. 5.17).

Hip adduction may accompany either flexor or extensor spasticity. Movements of the leg into abduction must ensure that the movement occurs at the hip joint and does not produce a lateral tilt of the pelvis. In severe cases, ipsilateral shortening of the hip adductors may result in displacement of the hip joint. In this situation, the patient may lose the ability to be positioned in a wheelchair or to stand in a standing frame. Genital hygiene and the management of continence may also be compromised.

The foot and ankle

Movements to maintain muscle and joint range at the foot and ankle is often difficult, more so in patients with spasticity affecting the posterior crural muscle group.

For patients with low tone, maintenance of range of movement at the ankle is not as much of a problem as maintenance of mobility within the foot. The normal activity of the intrinsic foot musculature which occurs, particularly during standing and walking, is hard to replicate. Movements of the metatarsals and maintenance of range at the metatarsophalangeal joints, particularly of the great toe, is essential to enable effective stance and gait. Massage and mobilisation of the calf muscles may also be effective in improving range within these structures.

The effects of force imposed over the forefoot have been described on page 101. In patients with severe spasticity, maintenance of range of movement at the ankle is often best achieved with the use of prophylactic or corrective below-knee casting (see Ch. 8).

SUMMARY

Patients with neurological dysfunction resulting in abnormal posture and movement are at great risk of developing structural deformity. Treatment to control body posture and movement must be initiated at the onset of neurological disease or damage and continued for so long as the danger of secondary complications exists.

Positioning and movement are interdependent on each other. Patients with restricted range of movement of the limbs also often have loss of range within the trunk and around the pelvis and shoulder girdles. Attempts to take the limbs through a full range of movement with impaired range proximally, will almost certainly traumatise the joints and soft tissues. It is therefore essential that the person performing these movements is aware of established limitations in respect of obtainable range. Any forcing of range must be considered detrimental.

REFERENCES

Ada L, Canning C, Paratz J 1990 Care of the unconscious head-injured patient. In: Ada L, Canning C (eds) Key issues in neurological physiotherapy: physiotherapy foundations for practice. Butterworth-Heinemann, Oxford

Allan D 1989 Intracranial pressure monitoring: a study of nursing practice. Journal of Advanced Nursing 14: 127–131

Andrus D 1991 Intracranial pressure: dynamics and nursing management. Journal of Neuroscience Nursing 23(2): 85–91

Beckman D C, Bean J W, Baslock D R 1971 The sympathetic influence on lung compliance and surface forces in head injury. Journal of Applied Physiology 23(2): 223–229

Bobath B 1990 Adult hemiplegia: evaluation and treatment, 3rd edn. Heinemann Medical Books, London

Bromley I 1991 Tetraplegia and paraplegia: a guide for physiotherapists, 4th edn. Churchill Livingstone, Edinburgh

Brown P 1994 Pathophysiology of spasticity. Journal of Neurology, Neurosurgery and Psychiatry 57: 773–777

Buckingham A K 1985 Arterial blood gases. Nursing Life Nov/Dec: 48–51

Butler D S 1991 Mobilisation of the nervous system. Churchill Livingstone, London

Cailliet R 1980 The shoulder in hemiplegia, 5th edn. F A Davis, Philadelphia

Ciesla N 1989 Chest physiotherapy for special patients. In: MacKenzie C F (ed). Chest physiotherapy in the intensive care, 2nd. edn. Williams & Wilkins, London

Crawford H J, Jull G A 1993 The influence of thoracic posture and movement on range of arm elevation. Physiotherapy Theory and Practice 9(3): 143–148

Daud O, Sett P, Burr R G, Silver J R 1993 The relationship of heterotopic ossification to passive movement in paraplegic patients. Disability and Rehabilitation 15(3): 114–118

Davies P M 1985 Steps to follow: a guide to the treatment of adult hemiplegia. Springer-Verlag, Berlin

Davies P M 1990 Right in the middle. Springer-Verlag, Berlin

Davies P M 1994 Starting again. Springer-Verlag, London

Dufosse M, Massion J 1992 Posturo-kinetic interactions: modeling and modes of control. In: Stelmach G E, Requin J (eds) Tutorials in motor behaviour II. Elsevier Science Publishers, London

Edwards S 1991 The incomplete spinal lesion. In: Bromley I (ed) Tetraplegia and paraplegia: a guide for physiotherapists, 4th edn. Churchill Livingstone, Edinburgh

Ellis E 1990 Respiratory function following head injury. In: Ada L, Canning C. (eds) Key issues in neurological physiotherapy: physiotherapy foundations for practice. Butterworth-Heinemann, Oxford

Frank C, Akeson W H, Woo S L-Y, Amiel D, Coutts R D 1984 Physiology and therapeutic value of passive joint motion. Clinical Orthopaedics and Related Research 185: 113–125

Friedli W G, Hallett M, Simon S R 1984 Postural adjustments associated with rapid voluntary arm movements 1. Electromyographic data. Journal of Neurology, Neurosurgery and Psychiatry 47: 611–622

Garradd J, Bullock M 1986 The effect of respiratory therapy on intracranial pressure in ventilated neurosurgical patients. Australian Journal of Physiotherapy 32(2): 107–111

Goldspink G, Williams P 1990 Muscle fibre and connective tissue changes associated with use and disuse. In: Ada L, Canning C (eds) Key issues in neurological physiotherapy: physiotherapy foundations for practice. Butterworth-Heinemann, Oxford

Hall T, Hepburn M, Elvey R L 1993 The effect of lumbosacral posture on a modification of the straight leg raise test. Physiotherapy 79(8): 566–570

Hasler D 1981 Developing a sense of symmetry. Therapy Aug 27: 3

Hough A 1991 Physiotherapy in respiratory care: a problem solving approach. Chapman & Hall, London

Irwin-Carruthers S, Runnalls M J 1980 Painful shoulder in hemiplegia: prevention and treatment. South African Journal of Physiotherapy 36: 18–23

Johnson S M, Omery A, Nikas D 1989 Neurological aspects of critical care, effects of conversation on intracranial pressure in comatosed patients. Heart and Lung 18(1): 56–63

Kerr M E, Rudy E B, Brucia J, Stone K S 1993 Head injured adults: recommendations for endotracheal suctioning. Journal of Neuroscience Nursing 25(2): 86–91

Klein-Vogelbach S 1990 Functional kinetics: observing, analysing and teaching human movement. Springer-Verlag, Berlin

Lewis Y 1989 Use of the gymnastic ball in adult hemiplegia. Physiotherapy 75(7): 421–424

Linden B M 1993 Heat and moisture exchanging bacterial filters. British Journal of Intensive Care September: 330–337

Lindsay K, Bone I, Callander R 1991 Neurology and neurosurgery illustrated, 2nd edn. Churchill Livingstone, London

Lippitt S, Matsen F 1993 Mechanisms of glenohumeral joint stability. Clinical Orthopaedics and Related Research 291: 20–28

Lynch M, Grisogono V 1991 Strokes and head injuries. John Murray, London

Maitland G D 1986 Vertebral manipulation, 5th edn. Butterworths, London

March K, Mitchell P, Grady S, Winn R 1990 Effect of backrest position on intracranial and cerebral perfusion pressures. Journal of Neuroscience Nursing 22(6): 375–381

Marsden C D 1984 Motor disorders in basal ganglia disease. Human Neurobiology 2: 245–250

Moseley A M 1993 The effect of a regimen of casting and prolonged stretching on passive ankle dorsiflexion in traumatic head-injured adults. Physiotherapy Theory and Practice 9(4): 215–221

Parataz J, Burns Y 1993 The effect of respiratory physiotherapy on intracranial pressure, mean arterial pressure, cerebral perfusion pressure and end tidal carbon dioxide in ventilated neurosurgical patients. Physiotherapy Theory and Practice 9: 3–11

Pope P M 1992 Management of the physical condition in patients with chronic and severe neurological pathologies. Physiotherapy 78(12): 896–903

Pope P M, Bowes C E, Tudor M, Andrews B 1991 Surgery combined with continued post-operative stretching and management for knee flexion contractures in cases of multiple sclerosis. A report of six cases. Clinical Rehabilitation 5: 15–23

Prasad A, Tasker R 1990 Guidelines for the physiotherapy management of critically ill children with acutely raised intracranial pressure. Physiotherapy 76(4): 248–250

Pryor J 1992 Mucociliary clearance. In: Ellis E, Alison J (eds) Key issues in cardiopulmonary physiotherapy. Physiotherapy Foundations for Practice. Butterworth-Heinemann, Oxford

Rothwell J C 1994 Control of human voluntary movement, 2nd edn. Chapman & Hall, London

Shacklock M 1995 Neurodynamics. Physiotherapy 81(1): 9–16

Shallit M N, Umansky F 1977 Effects of routine bedside procedures on intracranial pressure. Israeli Journal of Medical Science 13(9): 881–886

Shapiro H 1975 Intracranial hypertension: therapeutic and anaesthetic considerations. Anaesthesiology 43(4): 445–466

Silva A, Luginbuhl M 1981 Balancing act treatment. Therapy Aug 27: 3

Silver J R. 1969 Heterotopic ossification: a clinical study of its possible relationship to trauma. Paraplegia 7: 220–230

Soryal I, Sinclair E, Hornby J, Pentland B 1992 Impaired joint mobility in Guillain–Barré syndrome: a primary or a secondary phenomenon? Journal of Neurology, Neurosurgery and Psychiatry 55: 1014–1017

Snyder M 1983 Relation of nursing activities to increases in intracranial pressure. Journal of Advanced Nursing 8: 273–279

Tardieu C, Lespargot A, Tabary C, Bret M D 1988 For how long must the soleus muscle be stretched each day to prevent contracture? Developmental Medicine and Child Neurology 30: 3–10

Thomas A, Ellis E 1992 Ventilatory dysfunction. In: Ellis E, Alison J (eds) Key issues in cardiopulmonary physiotherapy: physiotherapy foundation for practice. Butterworth-Heinemann, Oxford

Tobin M J 1989 Essentials of critical care medicine. Churchill Livingstone, London

Ward T 1993 Spinal injuries. In: Webber B A, Pryor J A (eds) Physiotherapy in respiratory and cardiac problems. Churchill Livingstone, London

Warren J B 1983 Pulmonary complications associated with severe head injury. Journal of Neuroscience Nursing 15(4): 194–200

Webber B A, Pryor J A 1993 Physiotherapy in respiratory and cardiac problems. Churchill Livingstone, London

West J B 1985 Respiratory physiology: the essentials. Williams & Wilkins, Baltimore

Williams P E 1990 Use of intermittent stretch in the prevention of serial sarcomere loss in immobilised muscle. Annals of Rheumatic Diseases 49: 316–317

Yarkony G M, Sahgal V 1987 Contractures: a major complication of craniocerebral trauma. Clinical Orthopaedics and Related Research 219: 93–96

Young C 1984 Recommended guidelines for suction. Physiotherapy 10(3): 106–108

CHAPTER CONTENTS

Introduction   115

Patient with a right hemiplegia following surgery
   for posterior fossa exploration and removal of
   clivus meningioma   116

Patient with an incomplete spinal lesion at the
   T12–L2 level   121

Patient following head injury   123

Patient with multiple sclerosis   129

Discussion   133

References   133

6

Case histories

Susan Edwards

INTRODUCTION

Rehabilitation is a problem-solving and educational process aimed at reducing the disability and handicap experienced by someone as a result of a disease, always within the limitations imposed by available resources and by the underlying disease (Wade 1992).

The definition from the Oxford Paperback Dictionary is 'to restore to a good condition or for a new purpose'. This is most apt in describing the process of neurological rehabilitation where the aim is to maximise and maintain the residual capability. For this reason rehabilitation must be viewed along a continuum, from the preventive, early-stage management to the on-going, continuing care of patients with chronic, residual disability.

Patients with different and varied pathologies require neurological rehabilitation. The patient, in most instances, is medically stable and able to participate in a rigorous programme of treatment. This is undertaken by all members of the multidisciplinary team and includes physiotherapists, occupational therapists, speech therapists, the nursing and medical staff and, in many cases, the social worker and clinical psychologist. It is therefore impossible to view neurological rehabilitation in professional isolation. Physiotherapy is but a part of the whole and unless the different members of the team complement one another's interventions, patients are unlikely to achieve their optimal level of recovery.

Most importantly, the patient must be involved in the planning of treatment, and in the setting of goals and objectives. This has been shown to increase the motivation and compliance of patients facing what is often an extensive course of rehabilitation (Kaye 1991). The long-term goal may be that the patient will walk independently, but it is important to provide stepping stones along the way, in the form of short-term goals, to enable the patient to realise that, perhaps only small, but substantial progress is being made. Family and friends must also be involved in the treatment programme. This is especially important in the rehabilitation of patients with cognitive deficit. These patients may not be able to comply actively with treatment and it is often through the more constant input of the carers that positive changes can be implemented.

Many rehabilitation centres have been established to cater for the needs of people with neurological disability. Inevitably these units are more able to provide the full gamut of multi-disciplinary intervention and in so doing cater more effectively for the needs of the patients. However, it must be appreciated that not all patients who would benefit from neurological rehabilitation are successful in obtaining a place in such a unit. Many people with neurological disability continue to be treated in general hospitals where the emphasis is more on illness than on the promotion of independence. In this environment it is even more important to co-ordinate the professional/patient/carer intervention and, where appropriate, to enable the person with the disability to have responsibility for its management.

A problem-solving approach is of value in:

- the analysis of the prevailing symptoms
- the prevention of unwanted and unnecessary compensations
- promotion of useful, necessary compensatory strategies to attain the optimal level of function.

The majority of patients with neurological disability demonstrate a complex and varied picture which is potentially changeable depending on the existing pathology and the environment in which they function. For example, a patient with an incomplete lesion of the spinal cord, in many instances, demonstrates an imbalance of muscle activity. If the less-affected muscle groups are allowed to dominate in the attainment of function, these muscles will become even stronger at the expense of potential recovery of the weaker muscle groups (Edwards 1991). Even if the muscle strength were to remain unaltered throughout the course of rehabilitation, the patient must be made aware of the danger of contracture and given advice as to the maintenance of range of movement. Recovery of weakened muscle groups is even more difficult if joint and muscle range is compromised.

The following case histories describe the rehabilitative process which may be instigated for patients with neurological disability.

PATIENT WITH A RIGHT HEMIPLEGIA FOLLOWING SURGERY FOR POSTERIOR FOSSA EXPLORATION AND REMOVAL OF CLIVUS MENINGIOMA

This patient presented with a dense right hemiplegia following his surgery. Physiotherapy commenced immediately post-surgery, his problems being identified as including:

1. inability to communicate
2. dysphagia
3. impairment of respiratory function
4. dense right hemiplegia
5. severe sensory impairment of the right side
6. lack of midline orientation with neglect of the right side
7. overactivity of the left side constantly pushing him over to his right.
8. difficulty in sustaining an appropriate sitting posture due to the overactivity of his left side
9. inability to accept weight on his right side making positioning in bed extremely difficult
10. lack of bladder and bowel control.

This patient illustrates the need for multi-disciplinary treatment, each member of the team being made aware of the others' roles and supporting recommended intervention. During the early stages of rehabilitation, while receiving treatment in the acute environment, the patient was totally dependent upon others for all his functional needs. All problems were immediately addressed.

1. A personalised communication booklet with pictures was issued by the speech therapist to provide a means of communication. The patient was unable to speak but was able to recognise pictures.

2 and 3. The speech therapist and physiotherapist worked together to facilitate swallowing and maintain and restore his respiratory function.

4–9. Treatment intervention for the paralysis of his right side, the sensory impairment and the overactivity of his left side were managed primarily by the physiotherapist, the nursing staff and the occupational therapist. The main problem for the patient was his fear of accepting weight on the right side, which no longer provided appropriate sensory input. Basic management such as turning the patient from side to side in bed, transfers from bed to chair and positioning in a wheelchair was particularly difficult for patient and staff alike. All movements had to be carried out with great care to allow the patient time to accommodate to and accept the change of position.

10. The lack of bladder and bowel control was primarily due to his movement impairment and communication difficulties and was initially managed by means of an indwelling catheter and regular toileting. This problem was of relatively short duration. Once the patient was able to communicate and was able to be moved more readily, the situation was largely resolved. While the catheter was in situ, a leg bag attached to the lower leg, under his trousers, was used whenever the patient was out of bed.

The patient was transferred to a rehabilitation unit 4 weeks after the surgery.

Following a joint assessment involving the patient and all relevant staff, which included the nurse, physiotherapist, occupational therapist and speech therapist, the short- and long-term goals were agreed. The problems listed as numbers 4 to 9 on the original list were considered to be a true reflection of the patient's condition, although improvements could be identified.

Problem 1. His inability to communicate had resolved although his speech remained dysarthric.

Problem 2. Dysphagia remained a problem but had improved in that he was now able to take a soft diet with supervision.

Problem 3. Respiratory dysfunction had resolved.

Problem 10. The lack of bladder and bowel control had resolved.

Physiotherapy intervention was largely directed towards improving the coordination of activity between the two sides of the body. The sensory impairment continued to give rise to severe difficulties in terms of movement, in particular the patient's ability to respond to being moved and handled.

The long-term goal was that the patient would return home independent from a wheelchair in all activities of daily living, he would be able to take a few steps within his own home, with close supervision, and he would have intelligible speech to his family. The timescale for this achievement was 4 months.

The short-term goals were identified as enabling the patient:

1. to accept the right side-lying position and to be positioned in bed on alternate sides with the assistance of one person.
2. to be moved from lying to sitting and from sitting to lying over both sides with the assistance of one person.
3. to be transferred between the bed and wheelchair to either right or left side using a sliding board.
4. to maintain a symmetrical position in the wheelchair.

The timescale for the attainment of these goals was 3 weeks.

These goals were specifically aimed at improving the patient's sensory awareness and restoring his midline orientation. All members of the multidisciplinary team were involved in these activities, each one being aware of the necessity to constantly reinforce the agreed means of achieving these goals.

1. Turning from side to side was reinforced in the physiotherapy treatment area by slowly facilitating the patient on to his right side. Movements of the left side were encouraged while the patient maintained the right side-lying position (Fig. 6.1). This activity stimulated an active response of the right side through his dependency on the weight-bearing side for balance.

2. Movements from lying into sitting and from sitting into lying over the right and left sides were performed with support and facilitation at the right shoulder. This enabled the patient to move his body away from the right upper limb thereby preventing potential problems of shortening of the pectorals and medial rotators. These movements were performed slowly to allow the patient time to respond appropriately. This was of particular relevance in ensuring weight transfer over the right buttock while stimulating activity of the right trunk side flexors. The patient's tendency was to stabilise himself by overuse of the left trunk side flexors, which in turn inhibited recovery of the right side of his trunk. At each stage of the movement, integrated activity between the two sides of the body was facilitated. The patient was also assisted to lie down and sit up over his left side, thereby actively using this side rather than merely pushing.

3. Transfer from the bed to chair and from chair to bed was carried out using a sliding board. This was agreed to be the preferred option in that attempts by the patient to transfer himself without this support required excessive effort. This transmitted itself into overactivity of the left side pushing him across and beyond the right side. Use of the sliding board in the early stages enabled staff to move the patient fairly passively, thereby preventing the excessive use of the left side. In this way the patient accommodated to being moved prior to actively participating in the transfer. Transfers were carried out to both left and right sides.

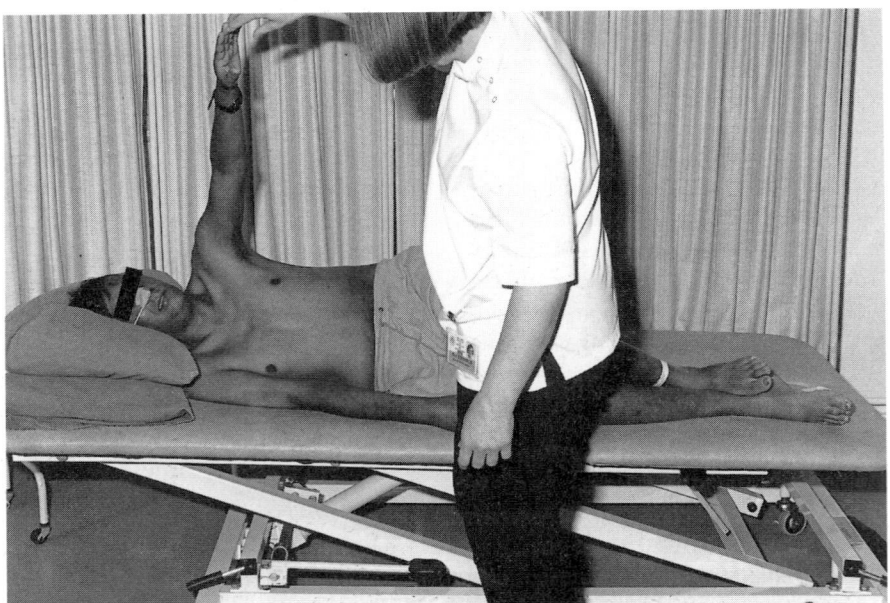

Figure 6.1 Lying on right side.

4. Positioning in the wheelchair ensured that the patient was symmetrical and had appropriate support within the chair. The arms rested forwards on a fitted tray attached to the wheelchair. A Jay cushion was provided, which gave a basis of stability whilst ensuring adequate pressure control. A foam wedge was placed at the back of the chair to provide appropriate support and to counteract sagging. The tray was felt to be essential to support the arms and thereby control subluxation of the right glenohumeral joint, and to improve the patient's awareness of the right upper limb. The tray further encouraged the patient to lean forwards in the chair, thus inhibiting the tendency to push backwards. An electric wheelchair was provided after 2 weeks in the unit to allow increased independence (Fig. 6.2).

All members of the multidisciplinary team ensured each of these goals; all functional requirements at this time were carried out in the way described. Activities such as eating, dressing and toileting complemented this approach.

In physiotherapy, the patient was facilitated into standing and supported in this position by means of a vari-table. This gave the patient a feeling of security and allowed the therapist to work independently with the patient upright against gravity. Without the vari-table, another person was required to stabilise the right knee. The patient was taken up into standing with the therapist standing immediately behind, providing

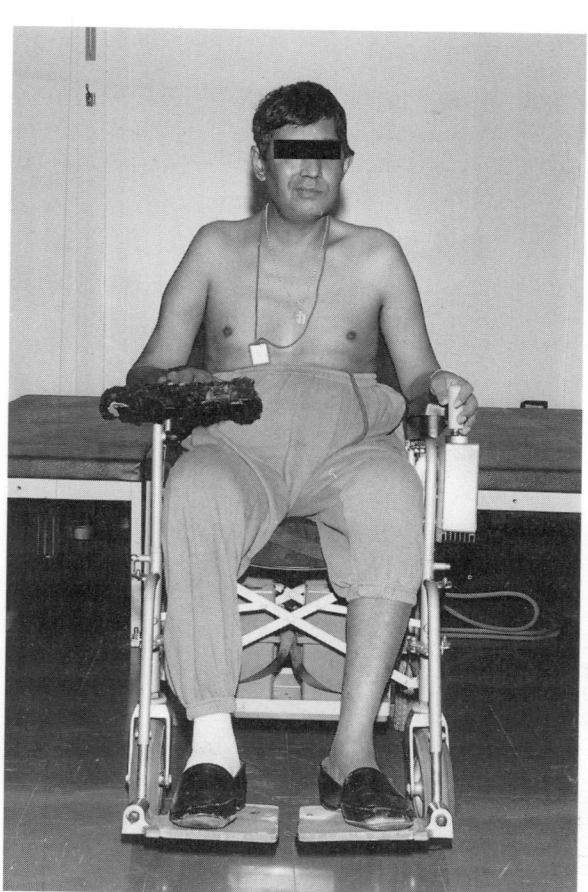

Figure 6.2 Sitting in electric chair.

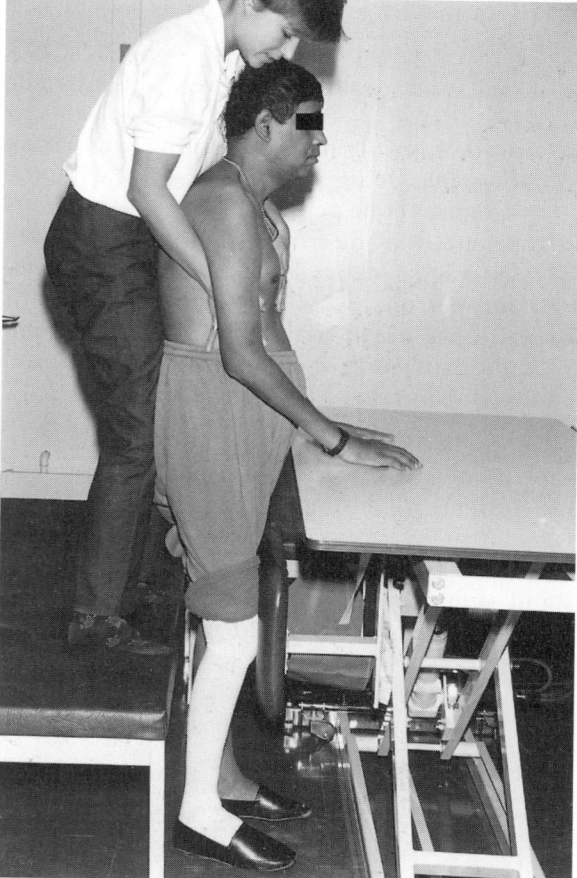

Figure 6.3 Standing using vari-table.

direction and full support (Fig. 6.3). The knee pad maintained the knees in extension enabling the therapist to work for activity in the trunk with improved midline orientation.

This activity was not used purely for the patient to attain standing but also to facilitate movement to and from standing and sitting. Static positioning in standing, tended to make the patient fix, overusing the left side in an attempt to attain stability. Slow, repetitive movements such as letting go into sitting back on to the therapist from the standing position, were used as means to prevent the development of unnecessary fixation.

This additional intervention further helped to restore the patient's midline orientation and sensory awareness, thereby assisting in the achievement of the agreed short-term goals.

Within the 3-week timescale, the patient was able to be:

- turned and could lie securely on alternate sides
- moved from lying into sitting and from sitting into lying over both sides with the assistance of one person
- transferred to and from bed to chair over both sides using a sliding board with the assistance of one person
- positioned appropriately in a wheelchair and could manoeuvre independently by means of electric controls.

Throughout the rehabilitation process new short-term goals were set in conjunction with the patient, to indicate progress. These goals, were in many cases specific to one profession, such as a physiotherapy goal of being able to stand symmetrically using the vari-table. Each new short-term goal would be discussed with the team on a weekly basis to ensure continuity and consistency of care.

Summary

This patient returned home after a 4-month period of rehabilitation. He was able to walk with a stick within the home but required a wheelchair for outdoor use. There was no significant recovery in the right upper limb. In spite of this, the limb was involved in many functional activities; for example, when eating, the arm was positioned forwards on the table and, when dressing, the arm was brought forwards when putting on or taking off clothing. In standing, the patient had sufficient awareness to recognise changes in tonus which depended primarily on the degree of effort used and his ability to transfer weight confidently over the right side. He was generally able to release unwanted activity by ensuring he had adequate weight over his right side. This control enabled him to have a free arm as opposed to one which, with uncontrolled spasticity, may have adversely affected his walking by impairing balance.

A major factor in the outcome was that the patient regained his awareness of the right side in spite of there being little objective change on

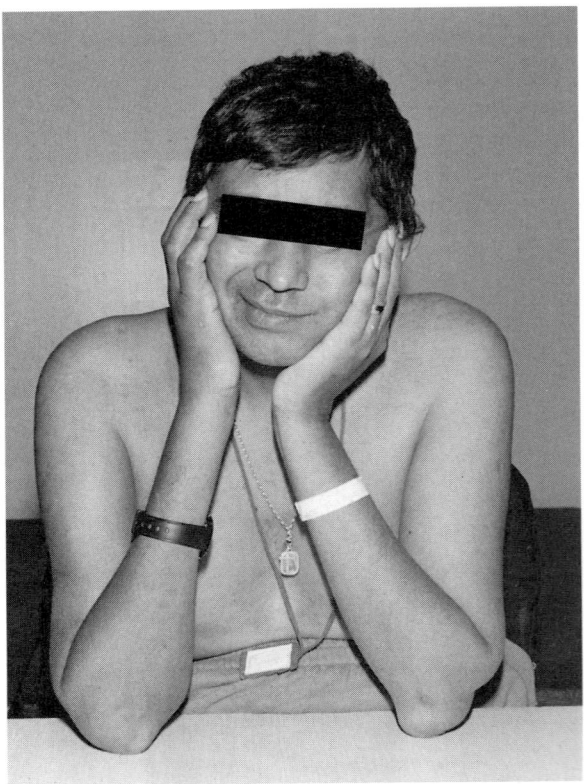

Figure 6.4 Hands on face to increase sensory awareness of the right side.

testing of sensory modalities. Sensory impairment is recognised as a limiting factor in neurological recovery. The treatment of this patient is an example of what may be achieved with consistency of approach by all members of the team including his wife and family and constant reinforcement of the involvement of the right side in all functional activities, an example of which is illustrated in Figure 6.4.

PATIENT WITH AN INCOMPLETE SPINAL LESION AT THE T12–L2 LEVEL

This patient was admitted to hospital for embolisation of a spinal arteriovenous malformation (AVM) at the T12–L2 level. The impairment was one of marked sensory loss, bladder dysfunction and severe muscle weakness affecting all muscle groups innervated from below L2. Following the embolisation, muscle charting using the Oxford Scale was documented weekly for a period of 2 months. After this time, measurement of muscle strength was reduced to fortnightly and, within a further 2 months, to monthly. The initial reading and a further one taken 6 months post-embolisation show little change in terms of the strength of individual muscles.

Specific problems identified

1. Severe weakness of the gluteal muscles. Active extension of the hips was not possible.
2. Attempts to stand without full leg support resulted in flexion of the hips, hyperextension of the knees, lateral rotation of the legs and inversion of the feet. Correct alignment in standing could only be controlled by the physiotherapist ensuring that extension of the hips was maintained.
3. Danger of contracture of the iliopsoas muscle and the foot invertors and plantar flexors.
4. Overactivity of the upper body as a result of wheelchair dependency.
5. Lack of bladder control necessitating self-catheterisation three times daily.
6. Sensory impairment below the knees.

Goal setting

Realistic goals were agreed with the patient, which were a compromise between his determination to achieve an independent gait and the therapist's perspective that this may only be realised, if at all, following a period of gait re-education using long leg calipers. The key to this compromise was the detailed anatomical description of the affected muscle groups and the potential complications, specifically in terms of loss of joint and muscle range, which may have resulted from overuse of the less severely affected muscle groups, particularly the hip flexors.

Treatment plan

1. Active assisted exercises to facilitate recovery of the affected muscle groups, most notably gluteus medius and maximus and the hamstrings. This incorporated exercises in prone (Fig. 6.5), supine and side-lying to stimulate hip extension and knee flexion.

The gymnastic ball was also used to facilitate general activity, particularly at the trunk and pelvis and of the quadriceps and hamstrings.

2. Sitting to standing and the maintenance of standing with assistance as required from the physiotherapist (Fig. 6.6). With correct alignment of the hips, the lateral rotation of the legs, hyperextension of the knees and inversion of the feet could be controlled.

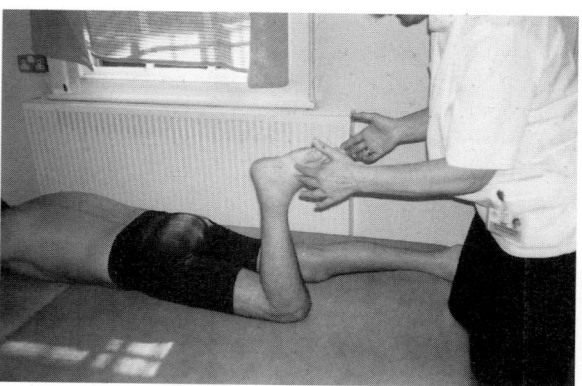

Figure 6.5   Hamstring strengthening in prone lying.

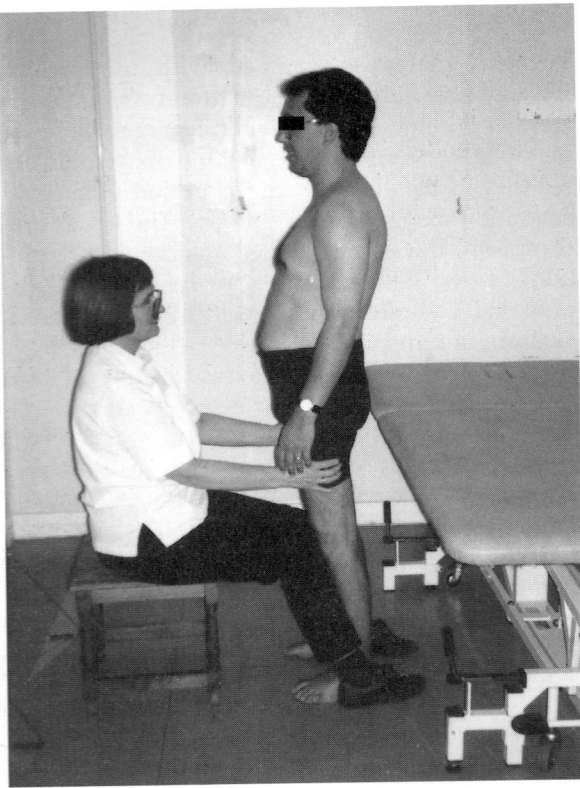

Figure 6.6 Standing with support from physiotherapist.

3. Bilateral back slabs were made of glass fibre material extending from the line of the hip joint to 1 inch above the malleoli. Hinged, ankle–foot orthoses (AFOs) were supplied to allow dorsiflexion but otherwise control the feet in the plantigrade position. (These were designed in such a way that they could be incorporated into a long leg caliper if this was felt to be appropriate at a later stage).

Walking using back slabs ensured full extension of the hips during stance phase of walking. This maintained the extensibility of the iliopsoas muscle and of the iliofemoral ligament. The patient utilised a four-point gait which, with the hinged AFOs, allowed for dorsiflexion but prevented loss of range into plantar flexion. Correct alignment of the legs and feet within the back slabs and AFOs maintained the feet in a neutral position, preventing inversion.

4. Overactivity of the upper body was not discouraged in that this was essential for independence in the wheelchair and for caliper walking. However, while facilitating active standing and sitting to standing, the emphasis was to ensure maximal activity of the legs. Progress was monitored by the reduction in upper limb activity in the maintenance and attainment of standing.

5. Bladder control was monitored by the urology department.

6. No specific intervention was carried out to facilitate sensory recovery. Increased activity and function improved the patient's lower limb awareness although he continued to be dependent on his vision to compensate for his sensory loss.

Treatment progression

Within 6 weeks the patient had achieved an independent gait using back slabs, hinged AFOs and a rollator walking frame. Throughout this period of gait re-education, an intensive exercise programme was continued to facilitate maximal activity of all muscle groups, most notably through sitting to standing and the maintenance of standing with support from the therapist. At this stage of his rehabilitation, he was discharged home and continued his treatment as an outpatient.

Having mastered an independent gait, the patient progressed to walking with only one back slab in postion; the slabs were removed alternately, the left first because the left leg was the stronger. The potential danger of this progression was shortening of the iliopsoas muscle due to the patient's inability to extend his hip during the stance phase of gait. Having grade 3 quadriceps on the Oxford Scale, the patient was able to maintain his leg in an extended position but only with the hip in a flexed position. This was discussed between the patient and therapist, the result being that walking with only one back slab in situ was always followed by a period of standing with both legs fully supported to ensure a full range of hip extension. In most instances this was carried out by the

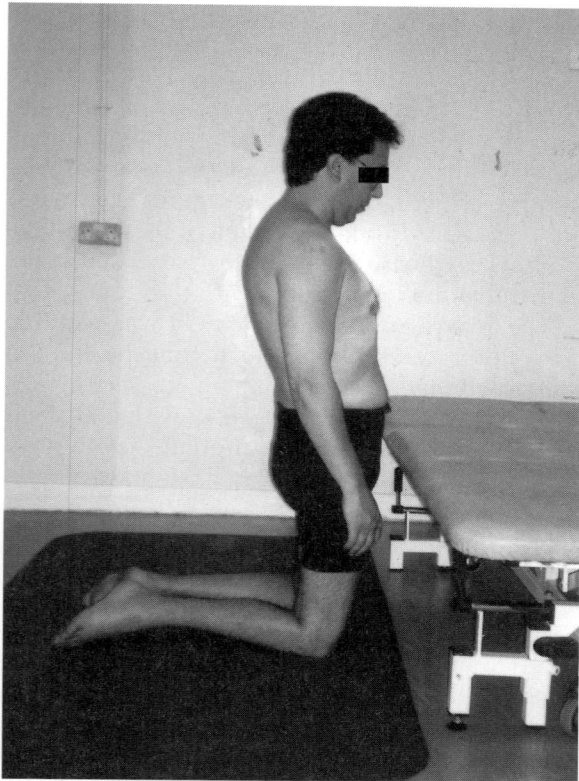

Figure 6.7   Kneel standing to facilitate hamstring activity and to maintain range of movement at the hip into extension.

patient on his return home. Kneel standing (Fig. 6.7) was recommended as an additional means of maintaining the length and extensibility of the psoas muscle.

3 months after the embolisation, in consultation with the patient, his wife, orthotist and consultant neurologist, it was decided to issue bilateral long leg calipers. There had been little recovery of the affected muscle groups and it was felt that wearing calipers would enable the patient to walk more consistently and functionally in his home environment. The patient's concern that this may reduce the potential recovery of the more impaired muscles was dispelled with assurances that his treatment sessions while in physiotherapy would be almost exclusively directed towards strengthening these muscle groups.

Summary

As with many patients following neurological damage, the prognosis for this patient in terms of functional recovery is uncertain. At worst, he is independent in his wheelchair and has the ability to 'walk' using long leg calipers and a four-point gait. The ethical dilemmas which play an increasing part in health care provision may well ultimately determine the outcome. For how long does, or can, therapy intervention continue? At what stage does further neurological or functional recovery become an impossible goal?

With continued physiotherapy intervention, combined with a home programme of exercises, this patient may achieve an independent gait with only AFOs as opposed to long leg calipers. Whatever the outcome, cessation of treatment must be agreed with the patient. In this instance, if there is insufficient recovery of the hip extensors to enable the patient to walk without long leg calipers, the patient must appreciate the need to continue with the calipers or standing in a frame. Were he to attempt to walk without this support following his discharge from treatment, contracture of the iliopsoas muscles would be the likely outcome. It is the therapist's responsibility to ensure that the patient fully understands the implications of his decision. The functional consequence of contracture of the hip flexors is the inability to stand in alignment. Additional stress is then imposed on the lumbar spine and lower limbs with increasing dependency of the arms to maintain an upright posture. However, it remains the prerogative of patients to decide whether or not they wish to accept this advice.

PATIENT FOLLOWING HEAD INJURY

This patient was admitted for rehabilitation 3 months after sustaining a head injury while living and working in America.

Due to the severe nature of his injuries, he had not yet been out of bed. He was in considerable pain and very aggressive towards all personnel including his family.

Following discussion between the patient, his wife and family, medical and nursing staff and therapists, the problems were identified as including:

1. reduced range of movement throughout the body with severe contractures of:
   a. both feet in plantar flexion and inversion
   b. the knees in extension
   c. the right hand, wrist and elbow in flexion
   d. the left hip fixed in 30 degrees flexion through heterotopic ossification
2. pain
3. inappropriate and aggressive behaviour
4. inability to sit unsupported due, primarily, to the immobility of his left hip
5. inability to stand or be placed in standing due to the deformity of his feet
6. dysarthria
7. total dependency on others for all activities of daily living
8. loss of short-term memory.

Treatment plan

1. Splints were made for the feet and right hand in an attempt to regain movement and prevent further deterioration in muscle and joint range. Below-knee casts made from glass fibre material were applied to the feet, maintaining the available 10-degree range of movement and controlling against inversion of the feet. The intention was to serially cast, changing the splint on a weekly basis, to support any increase in range. A cone-shaped SAN splint was applied to the right hand with a view to constant adjustment as the contracted tissues were lengthened. Use of these materials is described in Chapter 8.

Splinting was not used for the knees or right elbow as it was agreed that his increased level of activity should, in itself, result in an improved range of movement.

2 and 3. Pain management was instigated. This was felt to be an integral part of the behavioural problems. He associated therapy with pain and was therefore somewhat reluctant to participate in treatment, his initial reaction being one of aggression. Detailed discussion and explanation of the proposed procedures, analgesia prior to physiotherapy and a guarantee from the therapist that there would be no forcing of joint range resulted in almost immediate compliance. Feeling that he was now in control of his treatment, the aggressive behaviour ceased, with the exception of the occasional outburst which was rarely associated with difficulties arising in treatment.

The analgesia prior to treatment was required for only 1 week, after which time he himself suggested that it was no longer necessary.

3. The clinical psychologist provided support and advice on the most appropriate way to manage the patient's mood and behaviour, to all personnel involved in his care. This was of particular relevance for his wife and family who would often take the brunt of his outbursts of temper.

On admission, the patient had been described as being depressed. This was felt to be related more to his pain and general inactivity in being confined to bed than to clinical depression. From the moment that what he considered to be appropriate and purposeful intervention was instigated, depression was no longer a problem.

4. Radiography of his left hip revealed extensive heterotopic ossification fixing the joint in a position of 30 degrees of flexion. The patient had not been out of bed since his accident and his body reflected the position which earlier spasticity had dictated and enforced. This, according to his medical notes, was one of extension with flexion of the upper limbs. The extension of his left leg had been compounded by a debulking injury to the left quadriceps necessitating a skin graft.

Attempts to sit the patient, initially over the side of the bed, presented tremendous problems in that it was impossible to bring the trunk and pelvis forwards over the hips. In addition, the legs had to be supported, as the knees had a restricted range of movement from full extension to 20 degrees of flexion. This enforced posture at the hips with the pelvis in a position of posterior tilt resulted in the patient having to overcompensate with flexion of the trunk to prevent falling backwards (Fig. 6.8).

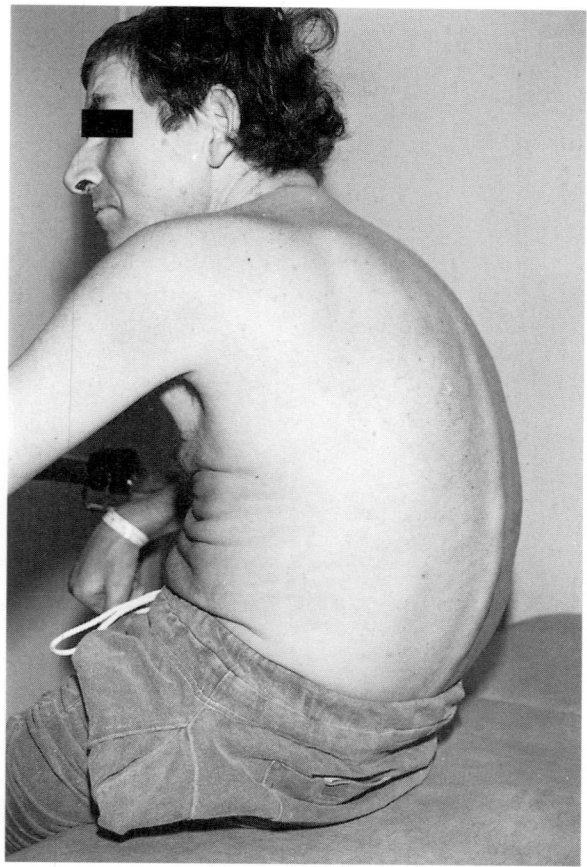

Figure 6.8 Sitting with excessive flexor activity to maintain balance.

For these reasons, active sitting without support was discouraged and a wheelchair provided which accommodated the deformities. The back of the chair was angled backwards with a wedged seat further reducing the hip angle. The legs were supported on elevating leg rests positioned at the maximum range of flexion which the patient could tolerate.

While recognising the limitations imposed by the immobility of his left hip, other restrictions in range of movement throughout the body, most notably of the trunk, were not of a permanent nature. An intensive programme of treatment was instigated to regain available range by means of mobilisation of the trunk in sitting and on the gymnastic ball (Fig. 6.9) and by positioning on alternate sides when in bed. Prone lying over a wedge was used to stimulate extensor activity within the trunk which would provide proximal stability to free the arms for function.

Although the patient was in a position of predominant extension, this was not enforced by excessive extensor spasticity. The patient had control of virtually all muscle groups but these were weak through disuse. In effect, the patient had become trapped within his own body as a result of the loss of range of movement which

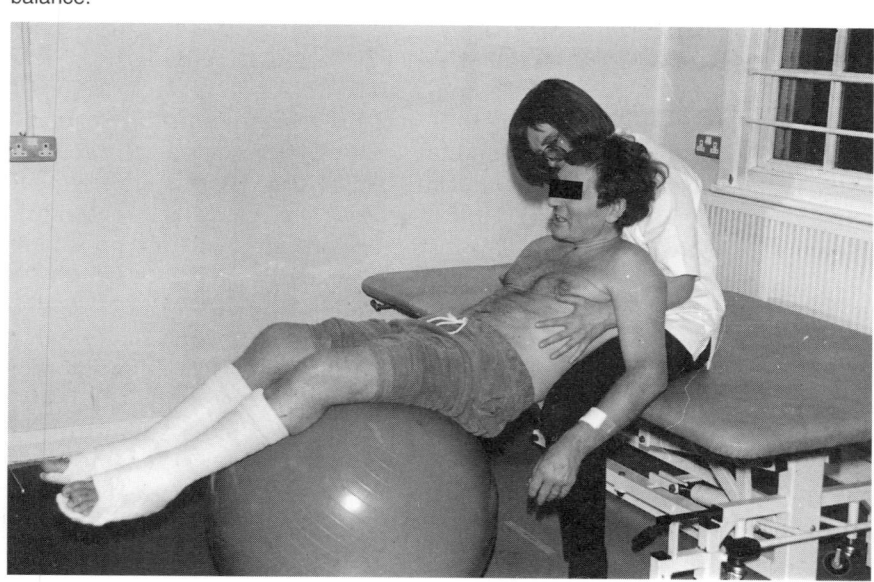

Figure 6.9 Mobilisation of the trunk using the gymnastic ball.

had arisen from his immobility and the earlier spasticity, now virtually resolved. As his awareness improved, attempts to move were dominated by flexion in his efforts to counteract his enforced extended position. It was therefore important to regain range into flexion but at the same time to stimulate extensor activity and reciprocal innervation.

5. Standing was considered to be an optimal means of stimulating normal extensor activity throughout the body. The below-knee splints provided stability at the ankles, albeit in a position of extreme plantar flexion. A heel wedge was positioned to accommodate the deformity. The Oswestry standing frame was used to provide additional stability, with two therapists lifting him up into standing by means of an Australian lift. This procedure was undertaken with great care, the patient feeling naturally apprehensive. This feeling of apprehension was compounded by the fact that, due to the lack of flexion at the knees, the patient was unable to transfer his weight forwards over his feet to stand, or be brought up into standing, in the normal way.

This position, as illustrated in Figure 6.10, was found to be most effective in facilitating trunk control and improved body awareness. Within 3 days the patient was able to lift his hands alternately off the table, demonstrating his improved proximal control and the inherent capability of his upper limbs. This demonstrated quite clearly that the movement impairment, although initially one of spasticity, was now one of disuse and subsequent weakness. The underlying tone was relatively normal, there being only minimal spasticity affecting the right side. Even in these early stages of rehabilitation it was felt that, with increased mobility and resolution of his contractures, the patient had the potential to achieve an independent gait and functional use of his hands.

6. The patient was severely dysarthric on admission and was assessed and subsequently treated by the speech therapist. However, his speech problems were compounded by both his behavioural state and his impaired respiratory control caused by his general immobility. As

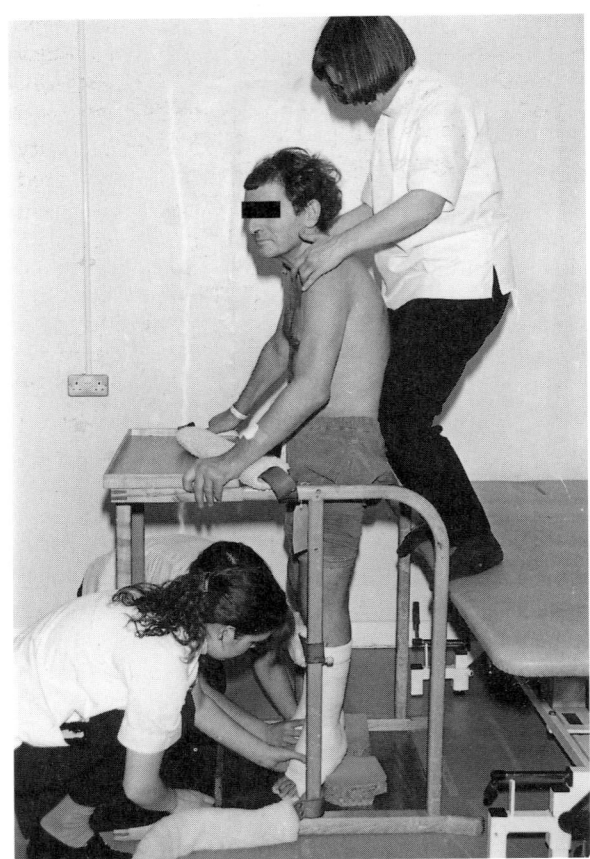

Figure 6.10 Standing in the Oswestry standing frame, wearing below-knee casts.

with all aspects of his care, although in this instance the speech therapist played a major role, all staff and his family contributed to the improvement in both his psychological state and mobility. The underlying speech impairment was significantly less than that initially thought.

7. The patient's total dependency on others for all activities of daily living resulted in tremendous frustration which was a causative factor of his inappropriate and aggressive behaviour. This provides a perfect illustration of how the environment can determine disability. For example, it was impossible for him to feed himself when lying in bed and yet, when sitting in a wheelchair, he was independent in this activity. He was unable to dress himself sitting unsupported but, when supported in the

wheelchair, he was able to put on and take off a T-shirt. These achievements, accomplished with no intervention other than providing the appropriate support, had a most dramatic effect in terms of the patient's attitude to his disability and to treatment. Much of his behaviour resulted from his lack of self-esteem and subsequent negativity in regards to possible improvement in his condition. Realisation that there were many things he could do for himself given the right environment created a more positive approach towards his treatment and management.

The attainment of function was dependent on restoration of range of movement. With improved mobility came an increase in functional achievement. The nursing staff and family were closely involved in utilising the gains made through the improved mobility. Transfers from the wheelchair to the bed, toilet and the car became much easier for the patient, staff and carers, with improved trunk mobility and as he became able to place his feet closer in towards his body. Within 4 weeks, the patient was able to transfer virtually independently with the use of a sliding board.

8. The loss of short-term memory was addressed by all staff and his family following advice from the clinical psychologist. The setting of short-term goals agreed with the patient, which were written down, provided a constant reminder to the patient as to what were the main objectives in terms of restoration of function. By breaking down the functional goal to the component parts, the patient was able to concentrate on specific aspects of everyday life, making continual reference to his written objectives. For example, when eating, his right arm was to be positioned forwards on the table whilst he fed himself with the left hand. All staff and his family were aware of this agreed objective and would ask him if he had forgotten something if the right arm was not on the table. In the early stages, the patient would often need to refer to his written instructions to find out what it was he had forgotten. With this constant reinforcement, a simple reminder became sufficient for him to ensure the correct positioning of the right arm.

The patient was very aware of this problem, which added to his frustration. All staff, and his family in particular, were encouraged to give him time and appropriate prompts to help him find his own answers, rather than responding for him immediately or telling him what to do.

The agreed long-term goal was that, in 3 months, the patient would return home independent in all activities of daily living and that he would achieve an independent gait using a rollator subject to the management of his foot contractures. (The ossification of his left hip would inevitably restrict activities such as putting on and taking off socks and shoes.)

Plan of action

1. To provide effective pain relief.
2. To influence his predominantly extended posture by providing appropriate seating.
3. To restore range of movement of the right hand and the feet by means of serial splinting.
4. To improve trunk and lower limb mobility to enable transfer as opposed to the patient having to be lifted into and out of the chair.
5. To maintain standing in the Oswestry standing frame for 10 minutes while lifting alternate hands off the support.

Three attempts were made to improve range of movement at the feet and ankles by means of serial splinting over a period of 3 weeks. No objective change was noted and it was apparent that this intervention alone would not be adequate to influence the established contractures. The patient was assessed by an orthopaedic surgeon who agreed to lengthen the Achilles tendon. This surgery was carried out 4 weeks after admission. The initial casts applied following surgery held the patient in 30 degrees of plantar flexion. Instructions were given by the surgeon that the casts should be changed on a weekly basis until plantigrade position was achieved.

Within 4 weeks this position was attained and the casts were then bivalved. The patient had continued to stand while in the casts within 1 week of the surgery. Following bivalving of the casts, progressive short-term goals were set for him to gradually increase the length of time he was able to stand without the support of the casts. This was carefully monitored, particularly in respect of pain and swelling. Analgesia was given as needed and support stockings used to control the swelling. The casts were discarded within 1 week.

This surgical intervention was the most significant factor in his rehabilitation in terms of his ability to walk. Being able to place the feet in the plantigrade position enabled him to transfer independently, bring himself from sitting to standing with minimal assistance from one person and initiate walking in the parallel bars, again with the assistance of one person. His standing posture is illustrated in Figure 6.11.

Within physiotherapy, continued mobilisation was specifically directed at improving his gait pattern. Although the range of movement in his knees had improved significantly – he now had 100 degrees of flexion – he was not yet able to

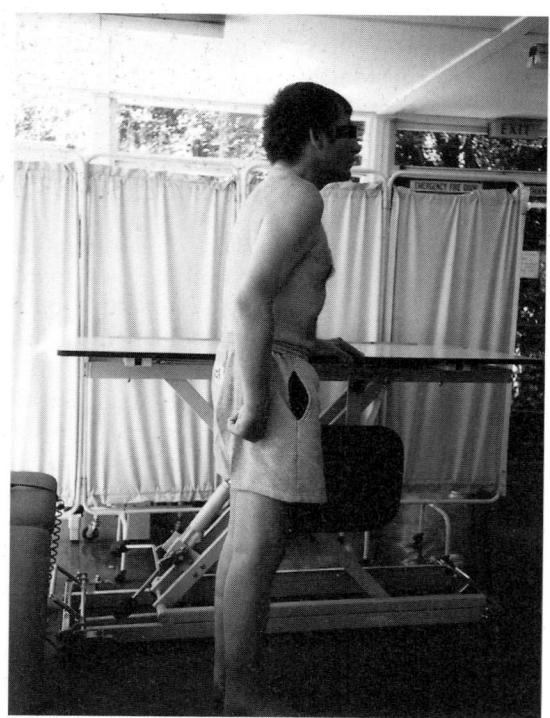

Figure 6.11   Standing with feet plantigrade.

utilise this increase of range in the release of the leg prior to stepping through. The patient had to be constantly reminded to bend the knee, which at this stage he was only able to do with active flexion as opposed to releasing the limb into flexion.

Summary

The patient was discharged home following 3 months of intensive rehabilitation. His status on discharge was full independence from his wheelchair and walking with a rollator with the supervision of one person. He still had the occasional outbursts of temper, most notably when he was challenged to do something with which he was not confident. His speech remained dysarthric but was intelligible to all if he spoke slowly. The problems with short-term memory persisted but, with written and verbal feedback, the patient felt that this had improved.

Following discharge, the patient attended for outpatient physiotherapy with the aim of further improving his gait. By this stage he was able to release his leg prior to stepping through, but this still required conscious effort. The potential to achieve a more fluent gait increased as the mobility of his feet and ankles improved. At this time there was a passive range of 5 degrees of dorsiflexion at his ankles.

No surgical intervention was contemplated for the heterotopic ossification of his left hip at this stage of his rehabilitation. At a later stage, surgical management may be contemplated with a view to removing the bony mass and potentially increasing the available range of movement. However, as surgery is also associated with the development of heterotopic ossification, there is understandably some reservation amongst surgeons to operate (Andrews & Greenwood 1993).

Unless this problem is addressed, it is inevitable that the patient compensates for the lack of range at the left hip, particularly when sitting. For this reason it is important that standing and walking become functional and are used on a frequent and spontaneous basis. Sitting with the pelvis in a fixed posterior tilt will result in increased flexor activity within the trunk and upper limbs for all functional goals. Constant reinforcement of flexion over a period of time, will be reflected in the patient's posture and a potential reduction in functional capability.

PATIENT WITH MULTIPLE SCLEROSIS

This patient had been diagnosed as having multiple sclerosis 6 years prior to her admission to the rehabilitation unit. Her initial symptoms had been those of weakness of the lower limbs with a gradual but severe increase in spasticity. On admission her problems were identified as including:

1. spastic paralysis affecting all muscle groups below the level of T4 making her wheelchair dependent; the right side was more affected than the left
2. scoliosis concave to the right
3. hip and knee flexor contractures
4. pain
5. frequency of micturition
6. inability to transfer independently from her wheelchair
7. increasing dependency on her arms for maintenance of balance
8. inability to walk further than 10 metres using a rollator walking frame.

These problems were agreed with the patient to be an accurate reflection of her current level of disability, which had deteriorated markedly in the previous 3 months. Prior to that time she was still able to walk functionally within her home, albeit with marked flexion of the legs and using a rollator (Fig. 6.12). The progressive increase in the severity of spasticity and pain had resulted in her becoming virtually dependent on a wheelchair.

The purpose of the admission was to find a means of controlling her spasticity, which was felt to be the major contributory factor to her pain, the development of contractures, increasing scoliosis and loss of functional ability. Her management at home had consisted of weekly visits from the community physiotherapist who admitted to feeling very ineffective given the

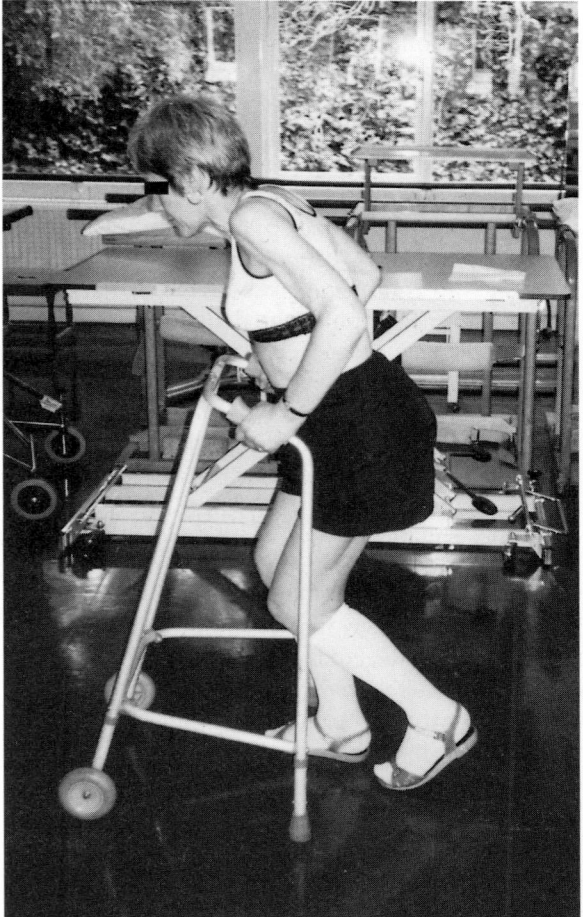

Figure 6.12   Walking with frame.

magnitude of the problems. The spasticity had in the patient's own words 'got out of hand' over the past 3 months.

A treatment plan was formulated in conjunction with the patient and all relevant personnel. This included the medical and nursing staff, the physiotherapist, the occupational therapist and the continence nurse. Full consultation was held with the local community services managing the patient at home. Figures 6.12, 6.13 and 6.14 illustrate her prevailing problems.

The aims and objectives of treatment were to provide effective control for her spasticity and thereby improve her functional capability. To this end, a review of her drug regime was to be implemented in conjunction with physiotherapy and occupational therapy.

The main focus for intervention was through the appropriate administration of antispastic drug therapy. The medical staff increased her oral dose of baclofen, but the patient felt little benefit in terms of a reduction in the level of spasticity and was unhappy with the side effects of drowsiness and increased weakness. The medical staff felt it was appropriate to try intra-thecal administration of the drug. The reason for this, which was discussed with the patient, was evidence suggesting that, with this more direct approach, the side effects would be lessened and the influence on the spasticity enhanced (Penn & Kroin 1985, Loubser et al 1991).

The response from the test dose was quite dramatic. The patient was able to move her lower limbs throughout her limited range and there was an immediate reduction in her pain. It was therefore decided to insert a pump in her lower abdomen for the controlled release of baclofen directly into the spinal cord as a more permanent measure for the control of her spasticity.

Problem 1, that of spasticity, was also addressed by the physiotherapist, since it was recognised as the direct causative factor of problems 2, 3 and probably 4, in addition to functionally giving rise to problems 6, 7 and 8.

1, 2 and 3. Initial intervention was aimed at restoring more equal weight-bearing in sitting to prevent further asymmetry. It was noted that the pelvis was being pulled upwards and back-wards on the right side due to the severity of the spasticity. Trunk mobilisations were used to try to inhibit the dominance of the right side and enable elongation with more equal weight-bearing through the ischial tuberosities. This intervention had to be performed slowly, allow-ing time for the patient to adjust to being moved and to consciously attempt to 'let go' of her spasticity. Great attention was paid to her sitting posture in her wheelchair by all members of the team to consolidate the small gains which were made in her symmetrical alignment.

Following this preparatory treatment, it was possible to stand the patient in the Oswestry

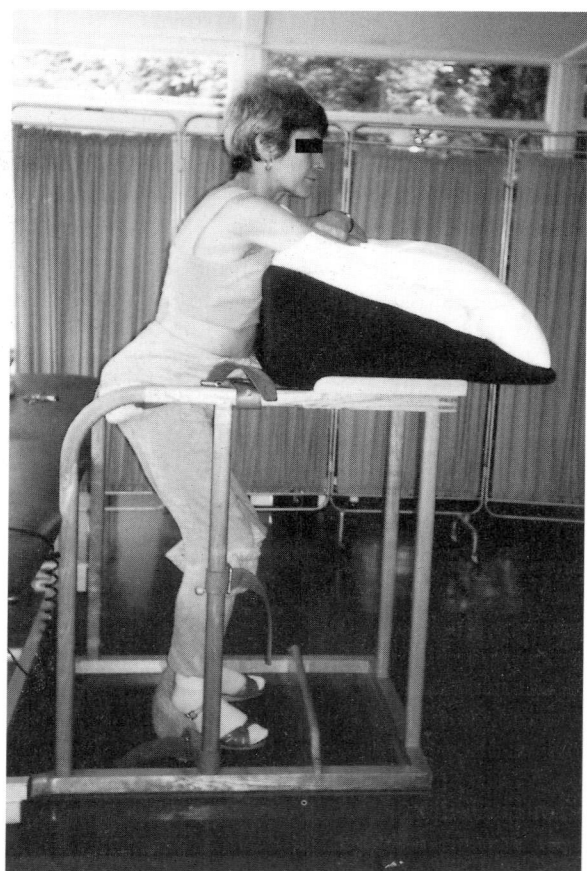

Figure 6.13 Standing in Oswestry standing frame.

standing frame, albeit with continued flexor dominance (Fig. 6.13).

The patient was also positioned in prone lying with a wedge to accommodate the hip flexor contractures (Fig. 6.14). It was essential that the wedge was of sufficient size to ensure that the patient was able to comfortably accept this position. The purpose of this intervention was to maintain and possibly regain some range into extension at the hips and knees.

Splinting was considered as a means of reducing the flexor contractures of the knees. This would have been in the form of drop-out casts as described in Chapter 8. The rationale behind this suggestion was discussed with the patient who was loath to proceed. She felt that

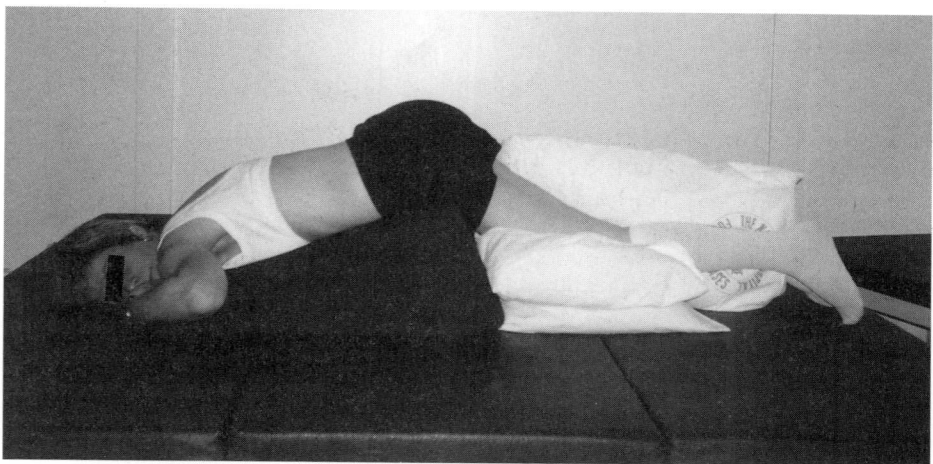

Figure 6.14   Prone lying with wedge to accommodate hip flexor.

enforced immobility of her legs might exacerbate her pain and preferred to try other interventions such as drug management and more conventional physiotherapy before resorting to the use of splints.

4. Pain was an unremitting problem. The patient was unable to sleep for more than 2 hours at a time, waking with a feeling of her legs being 'encased in steel'. Change of position by the nursing staff did little to alleviate her symptoms. Treatment in physiotherapy was also restricted. Pain increases spasticity and severe spasticity can give rise to pain. Any gains made during a physiotherapy treatment session were short-lived, due to the consistency and severity of the pain, perpetuating the vicious circle of increased spasticity. Analgesia had virtually no effect.

5. The patient's problem with frequency of micturition was managed by the nursing staff.

6, 7 and 8. These impaired functional tasks were considered to be a direct result of the spasticity and the consequent loss of range throughout the lower limbs. Treatment of the underlying spasticity was felt to be a prerequisite of any gain in function.

The progress made by this patient is illustrated in Figures 6.15, 6.16 and 6.17. The effective management of her spasticity by means of the intrathecal administration of baclofen provided the means whereby her pain

was reduced sufficiently to be no longer the restrictive factor it had been before. Of equal importance was the effect that this control of spasticity had on her movement and functional ability.

Physiotherapy prior to this intervention had shown little effect. Gains made during a treatment session, such as reduced tonus, improved posture in the wheelchair and her ability to be stood in the Oswestry frame, were not carried over in any functional context. The combined influence of the spasticity and the pain had dominated this patient's life and were continuing to do so.

Within 1 month of the insertion of the baclofen pump, this patient was able to independently:

- transfer to and from her wheelchair
- turn over in bed
- sit unsupported without the use of her arms for balance
- stand up from her wheelchair and maintain this position with the aid of a rollator walking frame
- walk, using a rollator for up to 2 minutes with a more upright posture.

Summary

In this instance the determining factor in the success of this patient's management was the

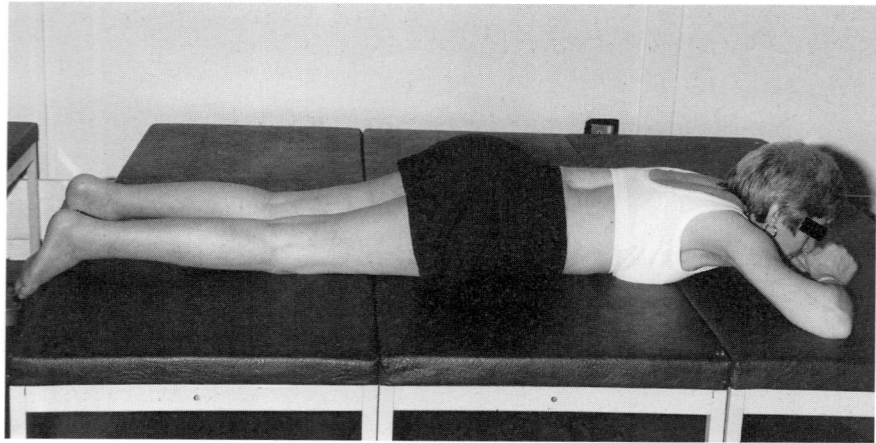

Figure 6.15 Prone lying following the administration of intrathecal baclofen.

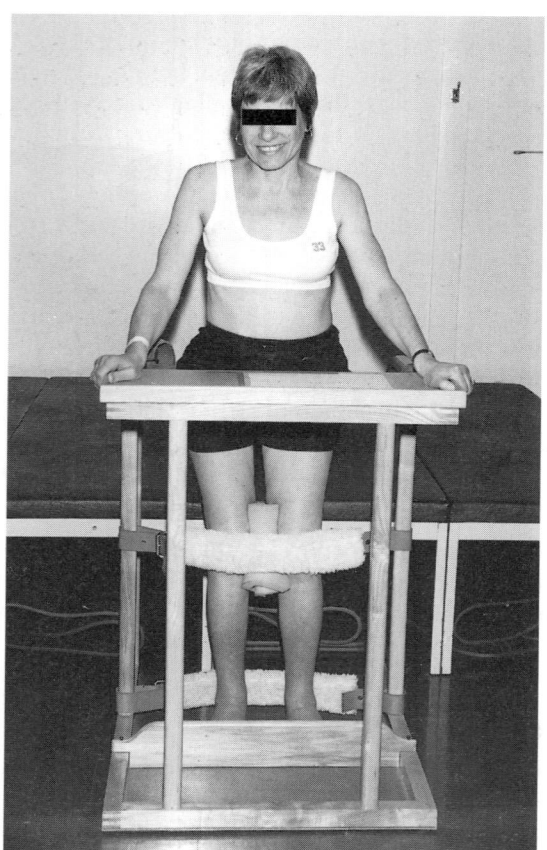

Figure 6.16 Standing following the administration of intrathecal baclofen.

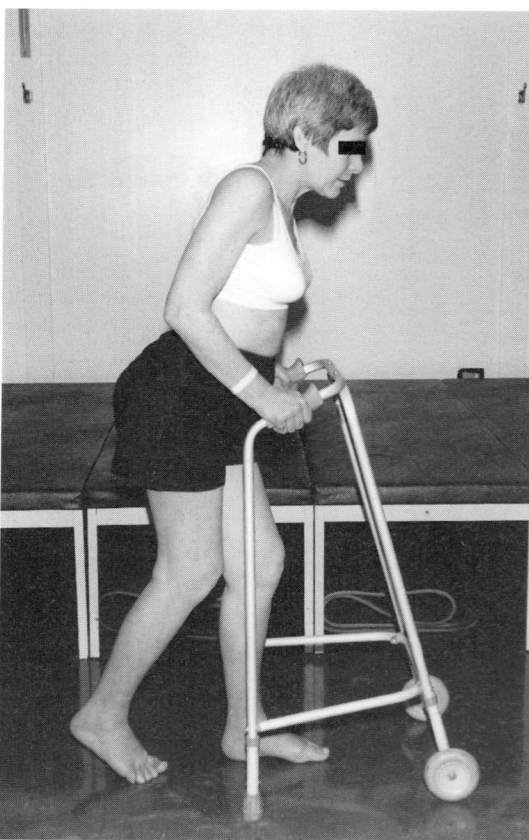

Figure 6.17 Walking following the administration of intrathecal baclofen.

control of her spasticity. The attainment of the aims and objectives was dependent upon this intervention.

Many patients with progressive neurological disease may suffer relapses in terms of their movement abilities or through perceptual and cognitive deterioration. It is all too easy to say that this is the natural progression of the disease and that nothing can be done. In this patient's case, she was fortunate that the community services identified a problem which they themselves were unable to resolve but about which they were prepared to seek further guidance. Without the described intervention, it is almost certain that this patient would have become bedbound within a very short space of time, with severe flexor contractures of hips and knees compounded by pain. The use of intrathecal baclofen with the subsequent improvement in her spasticity enabled therapy to be effective in the regaining of lost range of movement to the extent that she became fully independent from her wheelchair and able to walk functionally within her home.

DISCUSSION

Rehabilitation following an acute episode resulting in neurological impairment and subsequent disability is an accepted part of patient management in the western world. However, where this rehabilitation takes place and for how long will vary depending on the facilities available and increasingly on financial constraints.

In many instances, the neurological damage will give rise to permanent disability such as quadriplegia following spinal cord injury or residual hemiplegia following stroke. The restoration of normal movement is neither a realistic nor an attainable goal in these circumstances. The ultimate goal for all personnel involved in the rehabilitative process is to maximise the patient's level of function and, perhaps more importantly, to ensure that this optimal outcome is maintained.

REFERENCES

Andrews K, Greenwood R 1993 Physical consequences of neurological disablement. In: Greenwood R, Barnes M P, McMillan T M, Ward C D (eds) Neurological rehabilitation. Churchill Livingstone, London
Edwards S 1991 The incomplete spinal lesion. In: Bromley I (ed) Tetraplegia and paraplegia: a guide for physiotherapists, 4th edn. Churchill Livingstone, London
Kaye S 1991 The value of audit in clinical practice.

Physiotherapy 77(10): 705–707
Loubser P G, Narayan R K, Sandin K J, Donovan W H, Russell K D 1991 Continuous infusion of intrathecal baclofen: long-term effects on spasticity in spinal cord injury. Paraplegia 29: 48–64
Penn R D, Kroin J S 1985 Continuous intrathecal baclofen for severe spasticity. Lancet July 20: 125–127
Wade D 1992 Measurement in neurological rehabilitation. Oxford University Press, Oxford

CHAPTER CONTENTS

Introduction   135

Posture   136
Energy-conserving strategies   137
Posture as a prerequisite to movement   138
Learning postural control   138
Postural incompetence   139
Strategies adopted to maximise performance by
    the posturally disabled person   140
Complications associated with 'bad' posture   141
Measurement of postural competence   142

Biomechanics of the seated posture   142
Structure   142
Factors influencing stability   143
Primary areas vulnerable to deviation   145

Assessment   146
Purpose   146
Information required   146
Procedure   146
The sequence of assessment   147

Building a stable posture   149
Specific objectives of postural control   149
A step-by-step approach to a stable posture   149
Matching the level of ability to the support
    required   151

Specific problem solving   153

The art of compromise   156
Support versus freedom of movement   157
Supporting the feet   157
Support versus mobility   158
Client versus carer needs   158
Aesthetics versus efficacy   158
Check list to aid prescriptive practice   158
Counter-strategies   158

Conclusions   159

Acknowledgements   160

References   160

7

Postural management and special seating

Pauline M. Pope

INTRODUCTION

Posture as a subject is of particular interest to the physiotherapist and features prominently in many previous textbooks on neurology. Special seating, on the other hand, is a relative newcomer in the field of neurological physiotherapy. The linking of posture and seating in the same chapter serves to emphasise the relationship between them.

The population under consideration incorporates the relatively small numbers of motor and posturally impaired people who require a degree of external support to stabilise the posture of the body and its position relative to the environment. The problems presented by this group challenge the expertise of many experienced therapists.

Many reasons exist for the current interest in the relationship between the combined subjects of posture and seating. A brief historical perspective places the evolving field in context.

Posture in the able-bodied has occupied the minds of medical practitioners over the centuries. Faulty posture was thought to be responsible for a variety of maladies. Great emphasis was placed on correct postural habits, particularly in Victorian times. There are many who would agree with Zacharkow who stated in his comprehensive review (1988) that much of the literature of that period is equally valid and pertinent today.

Studies of posture in the able-bodied intensified in the 20th century culminating in more appropriate support for the body in a wide range of activities from sleeping to motor car racing. The disabled person unfortunately has not benefited in any comparable way.

Changes in the epidemiology of disease and injury have triggered a need to redress the balance. The advent of antibiotics increased the survival rate and longevity of those with disabling disease and injury, with the result that many have reached a level of disability not previously encountered.

The high-velocity activities characteristic of our 20th century lifestyle have increased the incidence of accidents which result in severe disability. Survival in these cases, and those of premature birth and birth injury likewise, owes much to advances in medical science and technology.

Policies of nursing care have also changed. Surveys conducted in the mid-20th century highlighted the prevalence and plight of the chronically disabled person: bedfast and suffering associated secondary complications (Asher 1947, Thomson et al 1951). As a result, the patient was encouraged to get out of bed.

These changes and the desire to improve the quality of life did not precipitate an immediate interest in the development of systems of postural control. A number of years passed before it was realised that the standard chair or wheelchair did not offer adequate support. The concept of a chair on wheels, the sole purpose of which was to increase mobility, had altered little since Victorian times. The 1970s saw a surge in new ideas and developments directed towards the resolution of postural incompetence.

In response to the changing epidemiology, the physiotherapeutic approach is also evolving from a position of treating the impairment to one of managing the physical condition (Condie 1991, Pope 1992). This concept incorporates control of body posture within the context of the whole environment and recognises the fundamental necessity of postural stability for effective functional activity.

Special seating in cases of neurological impairment is considered as a supplement to, or substitute for, mechanisms of postural control, with the purpose of reducing the secondary complications associated with the impairment while at the same time facilitating remaining functional ability.

It is important to emphasise that although this chapter is largely concerned with the analysis of problems associated with posture in sitting and the principles underlying their resolution, isolation of the subject in this way should never be considered in practice. It is imperative that postural management extends to all aspects of lifestyle. More damage to the body system is likely to arise from uncontrolled lying, than from uncontrolled sitting.

POSTURE

The word and the subject has suffered from imprecise definition and over-generalised application. Lack of precision is aggravated by association with adjectives such as 'good' and 'bad' without defining the terms of reference.

Whitman (1924) described man's erect posture as a constant struggle against the force of gravity. While acknowledging this, a more precise definition of postural competence is offered here in terms of the ability to:

- conform to the supporting surface in terms of symmetry and equality of load-bearing and contact surfaces
- select and adopt the alignment of body segments appropriate to the efficient performance of a chosen activity
- balance and stabilise the selected body attitude relative to the supporting surface
- adjust to changes within the body or support while maintaining balance and stability throughout the disturbance
- free from load-bearing those parts of the body required for movement
- secure a fulcrum about which the muscles can act.

'Good' posture is that body attitude which facilitates maximum efficiency of a chosen activity in terms of energy cost and effective performance, without causing damage to the body system.

Thus a 'bad' posture can be demonstrated in different ways; for example the unskilled lifting of a load which results in a lesion of the intervertebral disc, or the increased difficulty in writing when the arm is insufficiently supported.

It is fundamental to any understanding of posture that execution of a movement per se is not the concern of the organism, but the achievement of the objective for the minimum expenditure of energy.

Energy-conserving strategies

It is generally accepted that the so-called 'correct' postures in sitting and standing (Fig. 7.1A & B) cannot be sustained other than for short periods of time. They are energy consum-

ing and are rarely employed in everyday life. Postures such as those illustrated in Figure 7.2 are more usually adopted, conserving energy

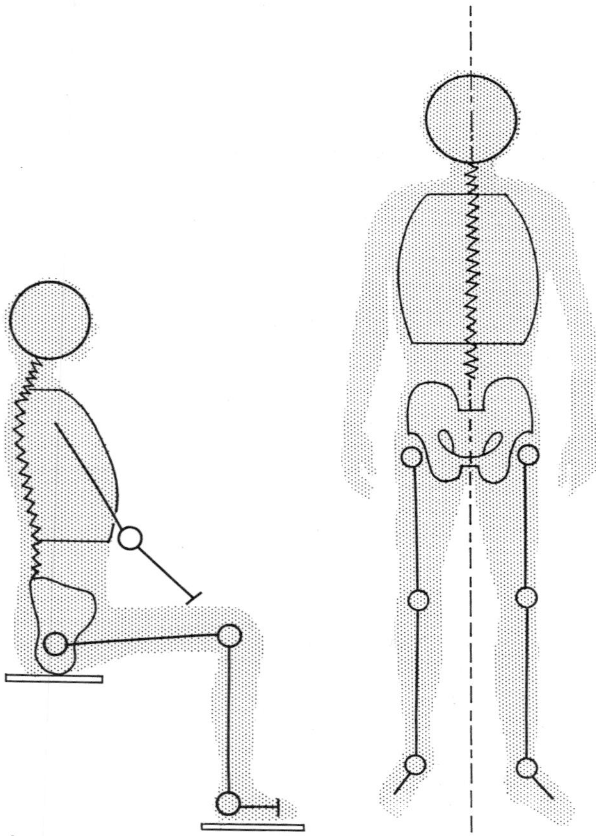

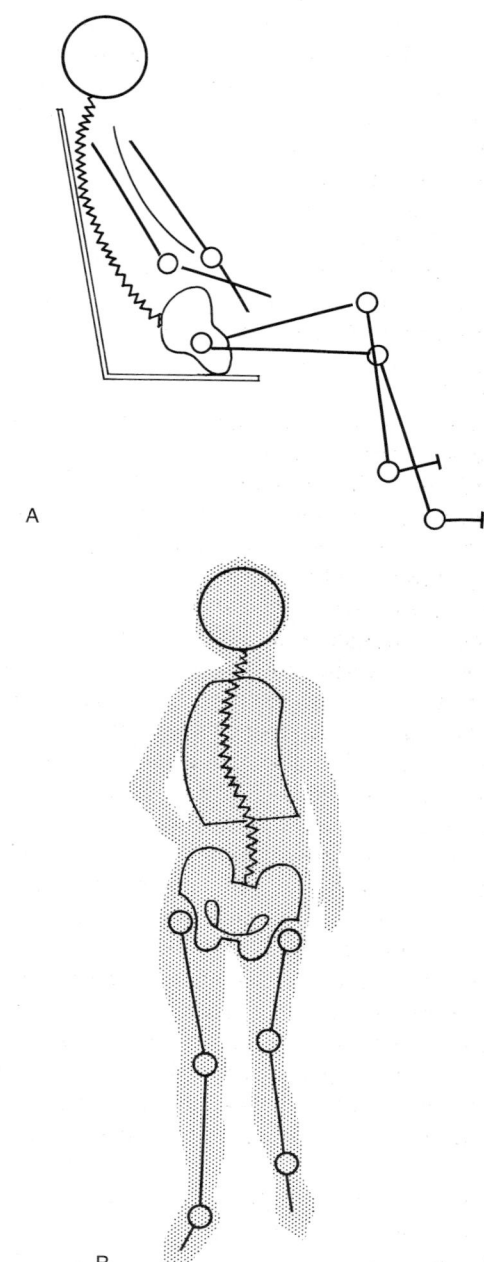

A

B

Figure 7.1 Anatomically aligned postures in (A) sitting and (B) standing.

Figure 7.2 Commonly used energy-conserving postures in (A) sitting and (B) standing.

and maintaining a balanced stable posture by astute use of the skeleton and soft tissues.

These postures are intrinsically 'bad'; they are potentially damaging to the system. However, damage is avoided as discomfort eventually signals overload and stress within the tissues, forcing a change of posture. Alternative tissues are then loaded until they too signal distress.

Posture as a prerequisite to movement

The number and amplitude of discrete movements of body segments is a function of the degree of control of the centre of mass over the supporting base area (Massion & Gahery 1978).

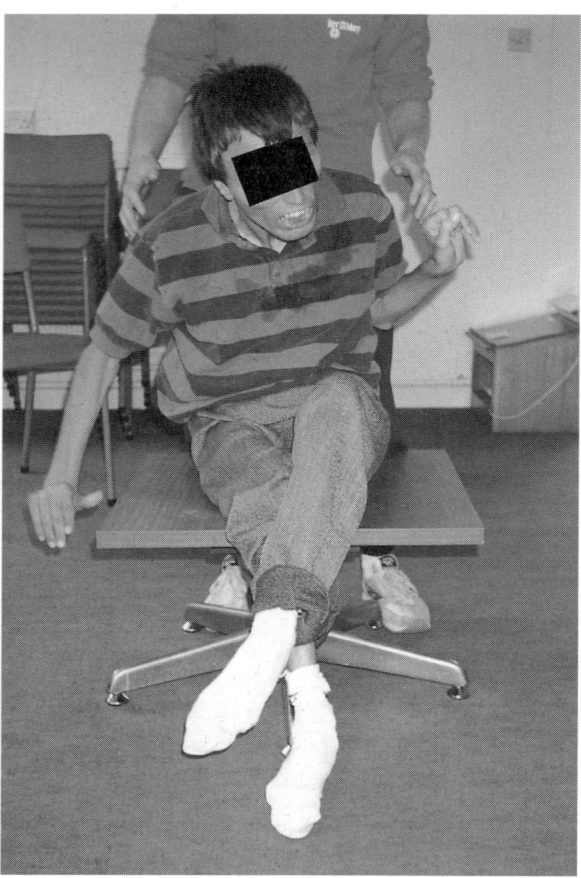

Figure 7.3 Typical posture demonstrating use of the limbs as an aid to balance in a man with cerebral palsy.

The gymnast and ballet dancer illustrate the ultimate in this control.

The anticipatory and preparatory nature of postural adjustments enhancing the efficiency of motor function is now well established and recognised as axiomatic. Preserving balance and stability of posture is considered to be a primary function taking precedence over other activities. When balance is threatened all body segments are recruited to maintain equilibrium. It is a familiar phenomenon; for example, when walking on a slippery surface, discrete movement of a limb is difficult if not impossible.

Figure 7.3 illustrates a comparable situation in the posturally impaired individual striving to maintain balance over a reduced area of support, in this case one side of the buttocks. An adequate base must first be established, if progress in terms of functional use of the limbs is to be realised.

Learning postural control

The basic components of the sensorimotor mechanism are present at birth in the healthy child. The integrity of these components, central activator and control mechanisms together with an intact effector and feedback apparatus, is essential to the learning of postural control.

Organisation of body segments develops sequentially starting with the ability to control the trunk, which acts as a stable base about which movement can occur (Pountney et al 1990). Associated development of purposeful movement appears to be the result of initial trial and error (Edelman 1993). 'Successful' random movements are reinforced, gradually achieving a level of efficiency consistent with the maturity of the body system and the needs and wishes of the individual. Efficiency results from a long-term process of learning to move within the external and internal constraints imposed by environmental conditions and those of the body itself (Massion 1992). The precise moulding of the intrinsic structures and mechanisms of posture and movement is governed by these constraints (Kidd 1980) in a manner analogous to that by which the magnitude and direction of the stresses and subsequent strains determine final bone structure. This knowledge is of profound significance when attempting to analyse so-called 'abnormal' movement such as that observed in the child with cerebral palsy. In these cases, initial impairment limits the ability to achieve an adequate postural base from which to move. As a result, the child develops strategies of movement designed to maximise efficiency from an inadequate base. Learning, therefore, may be considered in essentially the same way as in the healthy child, but resultant movement will differ in accordance with the prevailing, less advantageous, postural conditions.

The important point is to recognise that these movements are appropriate in the particular circumstances of the child. The imposition of a so-called 'normal' posture may well reduce performance, at least for a period of time. This is not to say that intervention directed to improve posture is inappropriate. Functional progress is dependent upon such intervention but a lengthy period of relearning may be necessary. A similar situation is very familiar to the able-bodied person who wishes to improve his performance of a given activity. A golfer, for example, may be advised to alter his technique. Initially, performance deteriorates but as remoulding of internal mechanisms occurs progress continues beyond a previous best.

Rapidly increasing knowledge of plasticity within the human system, the extent of this and the means by which it can be enhanced, support the view that appropriate intervention can be expected to improve performance in many cases. Experience suggests, however, that time and motivation are fundamental to a successful outcome. Radical change imposed on highly developed actions, however inefficient, in the older child or adult should be undertaken with caution. Some activities may have developed in a far from normal way but, as such, are relatively successful strategies overcoming the disadvantageous conditions operating at the time of learning. A notable example is swallowing in some cases of cerebral palsy.

Postural incompetence

Postural incompetence is recognised in the inability to organise the attitude of the body in terms of the earlier definition of postural competence (p. 136). It is manifest as follows:

- The body slumps or arches.
- The trunk rolls to one side. Lateral flexion is accompanied by rotation within the spine.
- The head falls forwards, sideways or backwards depending upon the direction of forces acting upon it.
- The trunk leans against the back support increasing the tendency to slide, predisposing to frictional damage to the skin. Where friction prevents sliding, shear and tensile stresses are high, deformation and mechanical damage occur within the tissue layers.

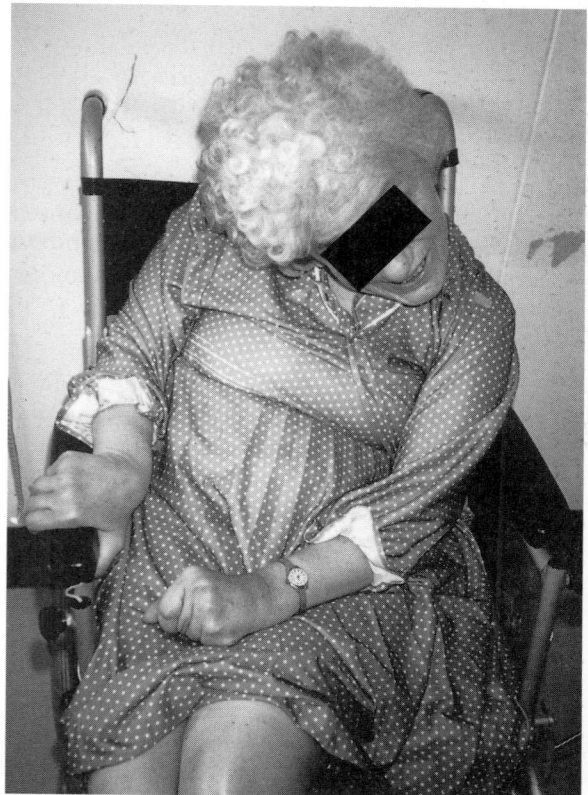

Figure 7.4 Buckling and bending of the spine stabilising one body segment against another.

- The tissues are subjected to unequal loading with resultant localised high pressures.
- Body segments buckle and bend, finding their own level of support (Fig. 7.4).

The precise attitude of the limbs and head may vary and is dependent upon the degree and location of impairment, released neural activity such as spasticity, spasms and some tremors, and the magnitude and direction of forces acting on the body. If these conditions are sustained, the tissues adapt, leading to 'preferred' postures and positional deformities (Fulford & Brown 1976, Pope et al 1991). The basic characteristics, noted above, are not exclusive to any particular neurological pathology, suggesting a strong environmental influence on their development (Pope 1992). If such is the case, it follows that the deleterious effects of the uncontrolled environment on the paralysed patient can be avoided or at least reduced.

Strategies adopted to maximise performance by the posturally disabled person

The ways in which performance may be enhanced are many and varied. The following examples illustrate two different but quite common strategies.

1. When postural paralysis or weakness increases the difficulty of independent feeding, the action may be enhanced in the following way. Stability is gained by slumping, using body structure for support. The overall height is reduced resulting in a lowering of the centre of mass, facilitating balance. In addition, the distance from plate to mouth is reduced (Fig. 7.5). Thus control of the action is maximised and energy consumption is reduced to a minimum.

2. The use of 'extensor thrust' as a basis for action (Fig. 7.6). In this, the shoulders and feet are used as the fulcrum about which movement strategies develop, in place of the more appropriate fulcrum for movement in sitting, i.e. the pelvis and thighs, when the inability to balance the trunk over the base exists.

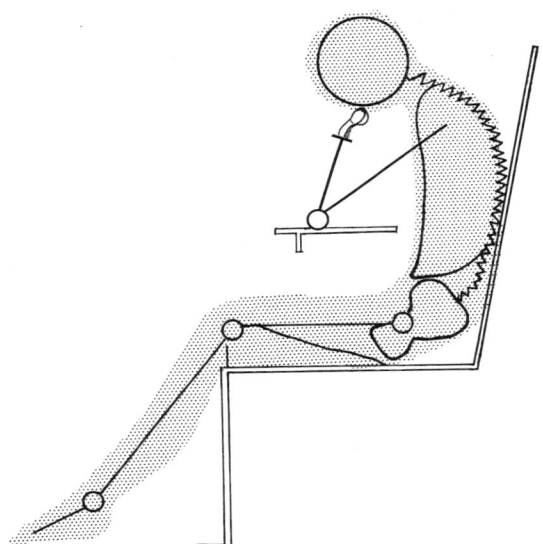

Figure 7.5 Strategy used to facilitate feeding, gaining segmental stability, lowering the centre of body mass and reducing the distance travelled.

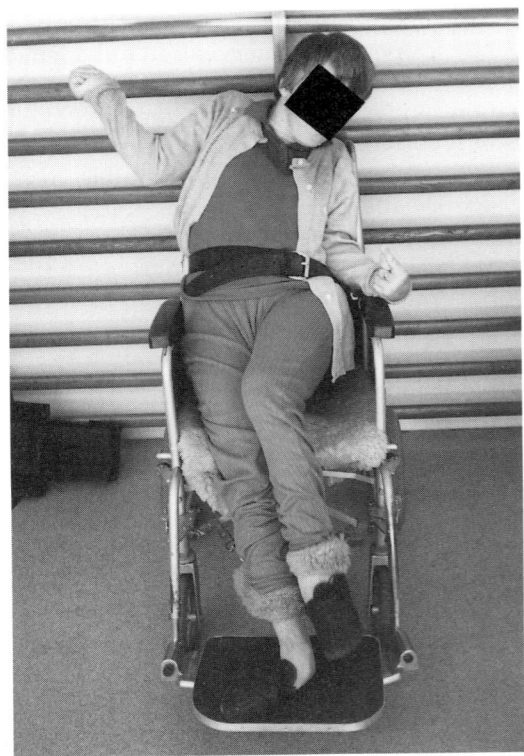

Figure 7.6 Action initiated by extensor thrust, using the feet as the fixed point replacing the normal fulcrum of pelvis and thighs.

The significant feature common to both these examples is the fundamental need to establish stability of position and a 'fixed point' about which to move.

It is not the postures per se which are 'bad'. In the first case, paralysis or fatigue prevents change of posture, thus predisposing to structural damage. In the second case, the inability to organise body posture more appropriately for the task reduces the efficiency of performance and limits the potential repertoire of functional activity.

The solution lies in the design of equipment which controls alignment, provides an appropriate base, and relieves loaded structures, while at the same time maximising remaining functional ability. A somewhat daunting task!

Complications associated with 'bad' posture

- Tissue adaptation leading to contracture and deformity.
- Tissue breakdown due to necrosis or mechanical damage.
- Reduced efficiency of performance.
- Respiratory distress.
- Discomfort.

In addition, spasticity, abnormal movement strategies and some forms of movement disorders

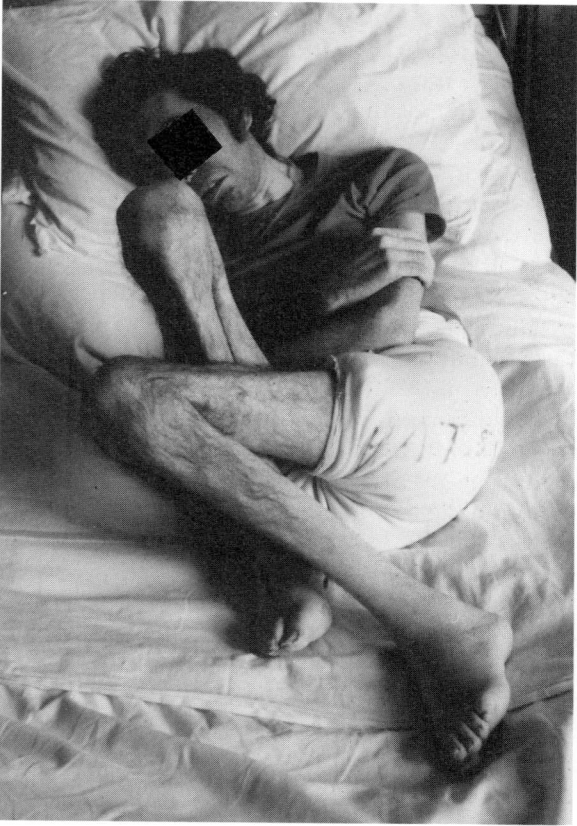

Figure 7.8   The bedfast state.

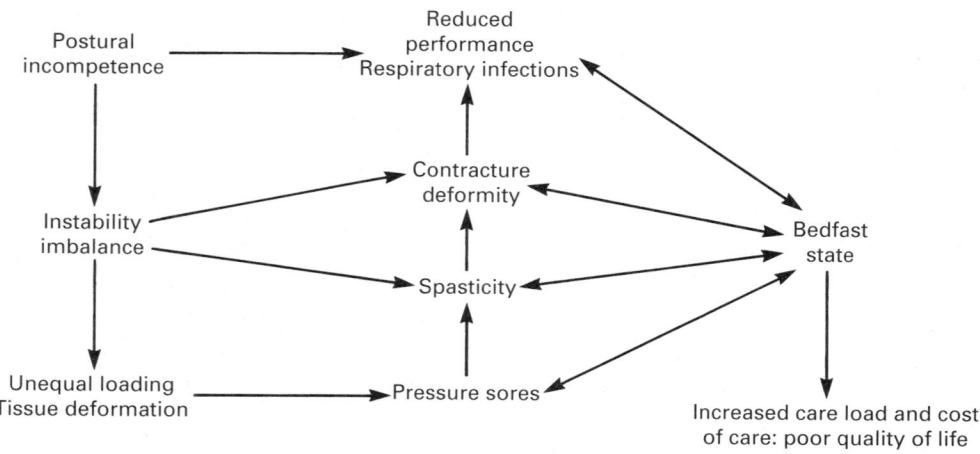

Figure 7.7   Development of complications associated with postural incompetence.

such as those frequently found in spastic and athetoid cerebral palsy, multiple sclerosis and following traumatic brain injury, appear to be functions of postural imbalance and instability. As such, these symptoms respond to positioning and postural control procedures (Pope 1992). Conversely, movement disorders such as dystonia, chorea and rigid syndromes found in Huntington's and Parkinson's diseases are less amenable, if not impossible, to control by these measures.

The sequence of development of complications may be represented as in Figure 7.7. The situation is self-reinforcing and, if left, the disabled person will eventually become bedfast (Fig. 7.8). It must be remembered that these complications arise from lack of postural control in both lying and sitting.

Measurement of postural competence

Quantification of postural competence is essential to effective evaluation of input.

The Physical Ability Scale (Mulcahy et al 1988), based on Hallett et al (1987), has been found useful. However, the quality of the posture is likely to be as important as the quantity in the identification of problems and the evaluation of outcome (McPherson et al 1991). The Scale has been modified to address this deficit (Pope 1993) (Fig. 7.9).

BIOMECHANICS OF THE SEATED POSTURE

Some understanding of the complexity of the body structure is essential prior to analysis of postural problems. A review of the main points is considered appropriate here.

Structure

The body is multisegmental and highly flexible. It is inherently unstable in the erect posture. The

Quantity (circle appropriate level)		Quality (tick correspondingly)	
Level 1	Unplaceable in sitting	Trunk symmetrical	
Level 2	Placeable with support	Head midline	
Level 3	Can balance, not move	Arms resting by side	
Level 4	Can move forwards within base, cannot reach sideways	Knees mid-position	
Level 5	Can sit independently, move arms freely and reach sideways	Feet flat on floor	
Level 6	Can transfer across surface, cannot regain sitting position	Weight evenly distributed	
Level 7	Can move into and out of sitting position	Score number of ticks	

Figure 7.9 Physical ability scale – measurement of quality and quantity (Pope 1993; based upon Mulcahy et al 1988).

degree of flexibility is readily appreciated when attempting to lift or support an unconscious or paralysed person, the feeling of which can be likened to lifting a fluid-filled balloon.

The body structure may be described as a series of segments of variable stiffness with linkages of varying mobility (Fig. 7.10A). The segments identified are the head, thorax, pelvis, thighs, lower legs and feet. The upper limbs are considered here as one segment. The linkages are the spine, hip, knee, ankle and shoulder joints.

Of the segments, the pelvis and head, together with the long bones, are relatively rigid components. The head is heavy in proportion to other segments and is balanced on the highly flexible cervical spine. The cage-like structure of the thorax and the multiple components of the feet render these segments more vulnerable to deviation, yielding readily under prolonged stress. The upper limb segment is additional weight carried by the trunk. The loading on the spine will increase or decrease according to the position of the arms at a given time.

Structure and movement of the linkages vary. The isolated spine is highly unstable and will bend and buckle under loads exceeding 2 kg (Morris et al 1961) and when subjected to eccentric loading (Koreska et al 1977). The result of sustained stress is irreversible damage within the disc and spinal ligaments.

The movements between vertebrae are complex, combining flexion, rotation and gliding. The particular combination depends upon the segment (Shirazi-Adl et al 1986). Shearing is resisted by facet joints and intervertebral discs. The structure can be likened to a complex helical spring, the plane and degree of movement varying with the segment. Although movement between adjacent vertebrae is small, even in the more mobile sections such as the cervical and thoracolumbar areas, the composite movement of the whole significantly extends the range.

The pivot joints at hip and shoulder allow extensive multiplanar movement controlled by muscle action. The shoulder joint linkage relies on the soft tissues for stability and, in cases of diminished or absent muscle control, these connecting tissues are particularly vulnerable to damage in handling. Knee and ankle joints are more limited in range and are predominantly uniplanar.

All linkages with the exception of the shoulder joint normally transmit load.

The base in sitting is formed by the pelvis and thighs. The superstructure above the pelvis is balanced on the rockers formed by the ischial and pubic rami, the whole rotating about the highly mobile pivot joint of the hip. Sagittal movement of the pelvis is limited only by contact of trunk with thigh in flexion and the tension of soft tissues in extension. In the absence of muscle control, the pelvis is free to rock forwards or backwards according to forces acting on it.

Kelly (1949) likened the erect posture above the pelvis to balancing a one-legged stool. Even worse, the one 'leg', the spine, is itself highly flexible and unstable!

Factors influencing stability (Fig. 7.10B)

The skeleton, connective tissue and the co-ordinated action of the muscles combine to give most of the support to the erect body posture.

The bones themselves together with the locking mechanisms of some joints, notably the facet joints of the spine, afford a degree of stability. The effectiveness of the support offered by the facet joints is reduced on certain movements, flexion and rotation of the spine particularly.

The connective tissues of the body, particularly the ligaments and tendons, assist in limiting movement at joints. They are most effective at joints that are subject to minimal movement, for example the pelvic basin. They are of limited value at joints which have a wide range of movement, being vulnerable to damage when subjected to rapid or strong forces and to lengthening under prolonged stress.

Muscle action is crucial to the intrinsic stability of the body structure. It provides most of the stability at linkages. The cervical spine relies heavily on coordinated muscle action in balancing the head on the shoulders. As muscles require a fixed point, a fulcrum, about which to

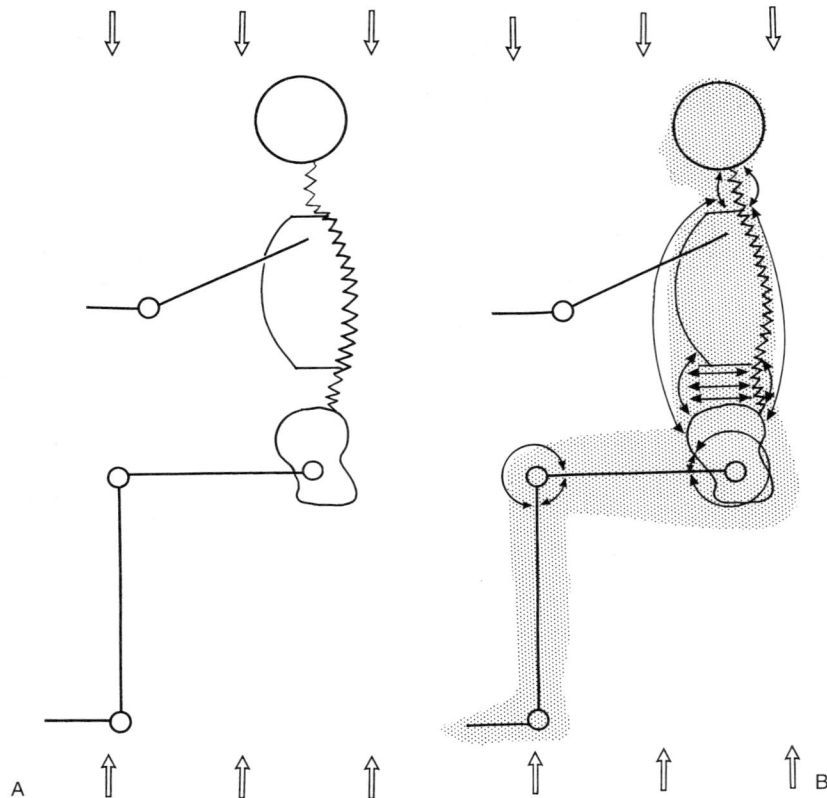

Figure 7.10 Diagrammatic representation of the structure of the body: (A) as a system of segments and linkages; (B) with the muscles, soft tissues and body cavity pressures involved in support and stability.

act at any time, head control can only be maximised if the upper trunk and shoulder girdle are stable.

Much of trunk stability is gained through the coordinated action of abdominal and erector spinae muscles (Zacharkow 1988). It is of interest to note that the isolated cadaveric spine held in the normal orientation at the base requires a loading of half body weight to assume the upright position. Without this loading, the lumbar spine tends to spring back into full lordosis (Deane 1982, personal communication), an observation made during investigation into idiopathic scoliosis. This feature is considered to conserve energy while maintaining an erect posture but emphasises the crucial role of the abdominal muscles in achieving and maintain-

ing balance and stability and in forward flexion of the spine.

Body cavity pressures provide a major contribution to the stability of the trunk. Abdominal cavity pressure, in combination with surrounding musculature, is responsible for the support of and prevention of damage to the spine (Morris et al 1961). Bartelink (1957) likened the abdomen to a fluid ball in which the pressure within and therefore the support are enhanced by muscular activity as effort increases. (Mechanisms of spinal movement and stabilisation are reviewed by Norris 1995.)

Distribution of body weight appears to be a significant factor influencing postural stability. Abdominal bulk has been observed to support the spine and stabilise the trunk in sitting in some disabled individuals. In addition, the centre of body mass is lowered and base stability appears to be increased. Conversely, amputation of a limb or the reduction of muscle bulk in paralysed lower limbs raises the centre of mass and increases the difficulty of balancing the trunk over the base.

The lower limbs and feet are said to contribute to stability in sitting (Son et al 1988). However, their effectiveness as stabilisers will be reduced when load transmission through the joints is not controlled by muscle action.

The achievement of a dynamic yet stable erect posture is a magnificent feat of structural design in combination with a perfectly synchronised cybernetic system responding to the changing demands of the body and environment.

Primary areas vulnerable to deviation

Where postural competence is inadequate, the body will bend and buckle between the opposing forces of gravity and the reaction of the supporting surface.

The areas observed to reflect initial postural incompetence are:

1. the pelvis about the hip joint
2. the mid-thoracic region of the spine
3. the cervical spine
4. the feet.

Due to its instability in sitting, the pelvis rocks forwards or backwards about the hip joint producing an anterior or posterior tilt of the pelvis (Fig. 7.11a), predisposing to malalignment of body segments above. Tilting is not necessarily symmetrical, as when severe restriction of flexion in one hip introduces a torsion element within the pelvis itself which predisposes to scoliosis and eventual structural deformity.

The mid-thoracic region of the spine between T6 and T9 is observed to be a point of high stress in the slumped sitting posture (Pope 1985). The forward position of head, shoulders and upper limbs exerts a large moment about the spine in this region; the ligaments stretch producing an exaggerated kyphosis (Fig. 7.11b).

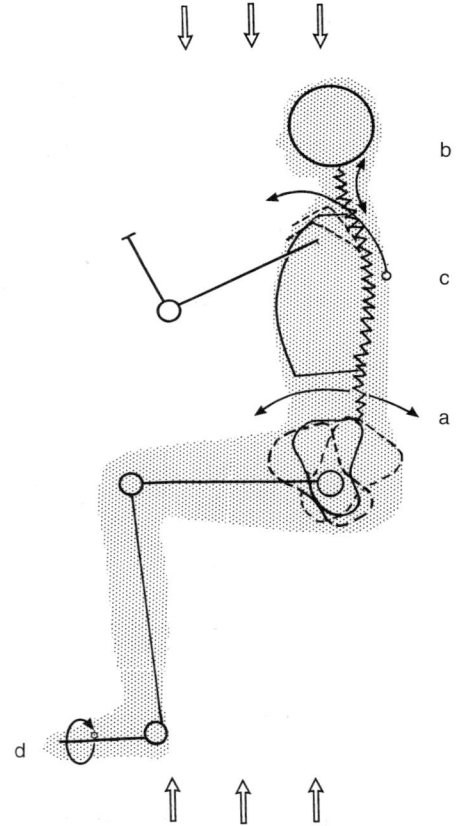

Figure 7.11   Primary areas of deviation: (a) pelvis about the hip joint; (b) cervical spine; (c) mid-thoracic spine; (d) feet.

Overstretched spinal tissues in the cervical region will reflect muscle weakness, fatigue and weight of the head. When some head control remains but trunk posture is slumped, the result is a compensatory cervical lordosis with tilting of the head (Fig. 7.11c). Head control under these conditions requires increased effort and is difficult to sustain. Swallowing and speech mechanisms are also compromised.

The delicate balance of loading through the feet is not easily achieved passively and without control of lower limb position. Any deviation from the normal line of weight-bearing will be compounded by the reaction of the supporting surface and will result in strained ligaments and, ultimately, deformity (Pope 1992).

ASSESSMENT

Purpose

Information is required in order to accurately identify the problems within the context of the particular clinical condition and lifestyle of the disabled person. With this information, realistic goals are set and recommendations made.

Assessment can be an effective means of evaluating practice.

Information required

Clinical data

- Medical: diagnosis, relevant signs and symptoms and past medical history, treatment (including medication or any proposed action such as surgery), overall prognosis.
- Physical: height and weight, presenting posture, joint range of movement, deformity, level of postural competence, location and degree of pressure on loaded areas, location and grade of current and past pressure sores, ability in activities of daily living including aids and strategies used, mode of transfer, mode of communication, level of fatigue.
- Psychological: comprehension, perception, behaviour. (This information is particularly relevant when considering powered equipment.)

Social data

- Home or institutional living: if assistance is needed, by whom and how often, frequency of change of carers, family needs and difficulties in relation to particular circumstances.
- Work or education: difficulties encountered.
- Leisure and social activities: frequency of outings, difficulties encountered.

Environmental data

- Access in and around the home and outdoors within the vicinity of the home.
- Access to work, education, leisure, and social activities.
- Means of travel and transport and any difficulties encountered.

Thorough knowledge of lifestyle and home circumstances is essential if errors in prescription are to be avoided. The assessment procedure will highlight the factors limiting the prescriptive options, for example the ability to stand transfer will influence the choice of seat and cushion. Ideally a home visit is arranged.

The assessment process may be represented as in Figure 7.12.

Procedure

Assessment should be carried out in a warm quiet room. The basic equipment required is as follows:

- standard assessment form
- variable-height plinth
- pillows and blankets
- boxes of differing height, to support the feet
- tape measure

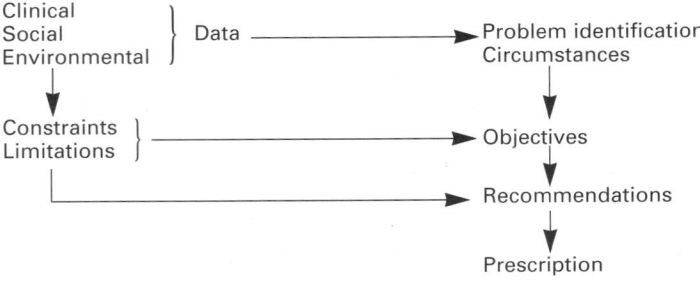

Figure 7.12 The assessment process.

- goniometer
- surface markers
- camera.

A suitable background is required against which photographs are taken. A consent form may be required for photographs.

The choice of measuring tools will depend upon the degree of accuracy required and the particular circumstances of the assessment. Sophisticated equipment, such as pressure monitors, may be necessary for research purposes but is not essential in general clinical practice, although some quantification of data whenever possible is recommended.

The exact composition of the assessment team will depend on circumstances, but usually includes therapist, doctor and engineer.

Where appropriate, the client should be accompanied by a person closely involved with his care.

Relevant information from other agencies and professionals not able to attend should be to hand.

As the resultant posture being examined is a reflection of the support or lack of it, the client should be assessed in the seat or chair which is most used. It is not satisfactory, although sometimes unavoidable, to see the client in, say, a transit wheelchair when he spends most of his time in an armchair.

The sequence of assessment

After making those attending welcome and comfortable, proceed as follows:

1. Check personal details and note date of assessment.
2. Ask the client and/or carer what they feel the problems are and how they would like them resolved. This information is extremely useful in establishing at the outset the perceived problems and whether the expectations are realistic.
3. Gather the relevant medical, social and environmental data.
4. Establish which solutions may have been tried in the past and what measures are currently used to relieve the problems.

5. While questioning, observe the client in his seat or wheelchair, noting the posture, any sign of discomfort, the degree of support, freedom and ability of upper limbs, areas of apparent loading, communication, comprehension and, not least, the relationship with the person accompanying him.
6. Observe independent mobility whether self-propelling or powered.
7. Photograph the presenting posture, from in front and both sides, without adjustment, removing articles only if they obscure the picture.
8. Examine in detail the quality of the presenting posture, without prior adjustment, in terms of body segment alignment, overall body attitude, contact surfaces and areas of support.

It may be helpful to superimpose this information on diagrams of the seated posture, an example of which is shown in Figure 7.13.

9. Transfer client on to a plinth.
10. Immediately observe the seat for signs of high loading.
11. Observe and note the body posture in lying without adjustment. The overall shape in lying will tend to reflect that observed in sitting.
12. Establish whether the presenting posture is correctable actively or passively. It is helpful to examine the trunk with hips and knees flexed as this allows the assessor greater control. Measure any asymmetry within the trunk, a simple method being the measurement of vertical and diagonal lines between coracoid process of the scapular and anterior superior iliac spines of the pelvis.
13. Measure joint range of movement, paying particular attention to hip, knee, ankle, foot and shoulder.

Hip flexion is tested with the pelvis in mid-position. If knee flexion contractures interfere with examination, the lower limbs are placed over the edge of the plinth. Knee extension is tested with the hip flexed to 90 degrees. (In general, hip flexion and knee extension are critical to the attainment of a stable seated posture.)

14. Examine the skin for signs of pressure.
15. Assess postural ability with the client seated on the edge of the plinth and feet

supported. Note if the arms or external support is required to maintain position.

16. Determine the degree of head control.

17. The client is then placed, and if necessary supported, in the optimum corrected sitting posture. Photographs taken at this stage are a useful reference when carrying out recommendations.

The amount of effort needed by the assessor(s) to hold and maintain the client in the corrected upright posture is a useful guide in determining where and what support is required and in what overall configuration. As an example, a hand required to hold alignment of the foot indicates that additional control is required when the foot rests on the footplate.

18. Transfer back to own seat.

When all data is gathered, the problems are identified within the context of the lifestyle and circumstances of the client. Realistic objectives are set and the limitations and constraints which may influence outcome are identified and recorded. The options are discussed and recommendations made.

Final prescription will depend upon consideration of the physical condition, the lifestyle, the constraints and limitations and the resources available. It will also depend upon what the client or carer can or will accept! Invariably the result will be a compromise.

It is strongly advised that recommendations based on the best clinical judgement be noted even when not possible or acceptable. Where recommendations and prescription differ, the

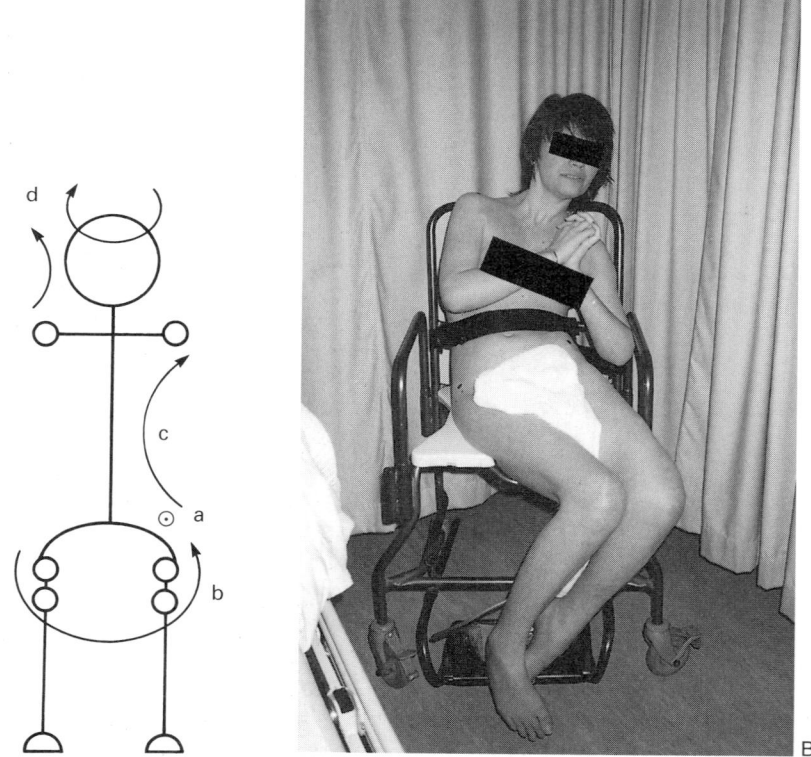

Figure 7.13 (A) Diagrammatic representation of anterior posture presenting in photograph of lady with brain injury (B) showing: (a) pelvis rotated forwards and elevated on the left side; (b) windsweeping of the lower limbs towards the left; (c) lateral flexion of the trunk towards the left; (d) side flexion and rotation of the head towards the right. The lateral profile can be represented similarly.

reason should be documented together with any anticipated problems arising from the prescription.

A review of the client should be automatic in order to evaluate outcome and prescriptive practice.

BUILDING A STABLE POSTURE

Given the inherent instability and complexity of the body system, the difficulty of substituting for even the smallest deficit in postural competence will be appreciated. The aim of intervention is to use the anatomical structure and intrinsic support where possible, applying external aid where it is likely to be most effective and least restrictive. Gravity is used to assist stability rather than using measures to counter it.

It is important that the result should be aesthetically acceptable.

Specific objectives of postural control

- Support and stabilise body segments and linkages in a symmetrical and appropriate posture for sitting.
- Minimise the load through the sections most vulnerable to deviation.
- Minimise tensile and shear stress within the tissues.
- Equalise pressures on loaded tissues.
- Facilitate function.
- Provide comfort.
- Provide for an easy change of position.
- Ease the care load.

There are times when it is not possible to satisfy all the criteria. Objectives may conflict, such as the need for adequate postural support and maximum functional activity.

It has already been noted that uncontrolled mobility of pelvis and hip joint, weight and position of the head, drag of the upper limbs and shoulder girdle and alignment of the foot give rise to problems when posture is impaired. Efforts are directed to control in these regions.

A step-by-step approach to a stable posture

At this stage and for purposes of description and clarity it is assumed that the client can be placed in anatomical alignment of the seated posture, that is, no significant tissue adaptation interferes with positioning.

Each body segment and linkage is controlled in turn. The extent of the support given will depend upon the degree of impairment.

It is logical to begin with the pelvis, as the orientation and location of the pelvis is 'a major controlling factor in attitude and motion due to its relationship to the centre of mass' (Reynolds 1978). The pelvis may be considered the keystone of the structure, the control of which is fundamental to balance, stability and alignment.

Step 1. Position a level symmetrical pelvis (Fig. 7.14a). Correct alignment is achieved after the client is seated by flexing the trunk about the hip joint in order to ensure an anterior tilt. The buttocks are then tucked as far back in the seat as possible. Check the position.

Step 2. The thighs are placed parallel and horizontal. The seat surface must accommodate the tapering shape of the thigh from buttock to knee thus preventing 'drag' on the seat position (Mulcahy et al 1988) (Fig. 7.14b).

Step 3. Feet are positioned in plantigrade and supported along the entire length of the foot (Fig. 7.14c). External control may be required to secure the position.

(The current tendency to design many wheelchairs with forward-positioned footrests is unsatisfactory for all but a small percentage of the more athletic wheelchair users. Any tightness in the hamstrings causes the feet to fall backwards off the footrest or, if strapped, to drag the hips forwards on the seat, predisposing to a slumped posture.)

Step 4. Knees are separated and flexed to 90 degrees, the lower leg hanging as near vertical as possible. The position is controlled, if necessary, by restraint exerting a force backwards downwards and outwards (Fig. 7.14d).

Knee and foot restraint can be considered complementary forms of control. It is rare that

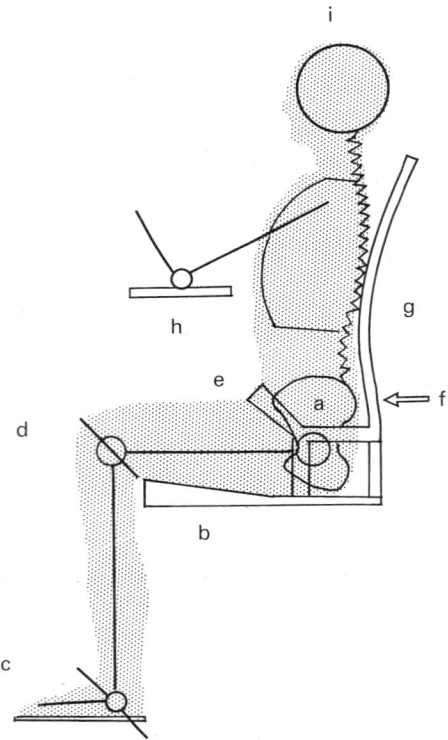

Figure 7.14   (a) Position of the pelvis; (b) accommodating the shape of the thigh; (c) feet in plantigrade, with control if necessary; (d) knees flexed and separated; (e) Y-shaped pelvic strap to assist in securing seat position; (f) posterior support for the pelvis directing lumbar curve; (g) profiling of upper and lower trunk segments; (h) support for the upper limbs; (i) head position – slightly posterior to midline.

the foot alone requires fixation as any tightness in the foot inverters will cause the knees to adduct. It is not unusual, however, to secure knee position alone.

Step 5.   Hip and pelvic position is secured by a strap with Y-shaped attachments exerting a force downwards and backwards, more effectively preventing posterior tilt of the pelvis (Letts 1992) (Fig. 7.14e).

Step 6.   Support is applied to the pelvis in the upper sacral region, to prevent posterior tilt, to direct the line of the lumbar curve and to act as a fulcrum on raising the trunk (Fig. 7.14f). A posteriorly tilted pelvis and flattened lumbar spine prevent extension of the upper trunk and alignment of the head on the shoulders.

Step 7.   The trunk is raised and supported against the backrest. The plane of the thorax differs from that of the pelvis; therefore support for the upper trunk should be angled to correspond with this difference (Fig. 7.14g). Contouring of the surface increases comfort and stability. A vertical backrest offers minimal support as there is little loading of the surface; the best this can achieve is to prevent falling backwards. It is interesting to note that the vertical backrest is a common feature of seating for the disabled person but rarely for the able-bodied!

Step 8.   Weight of the arms is taken by support anteriorly, thus preventing drag on the shoulders and rolling forwards of the trunk. The upper limbs are supported at a height which facilitates contact of the extended upper trunk with the back support (Fig. 7.14h).

In less severe cases, adjustment of height and widening of the arm rests may be sufficient, but it is quite inadequate for those with little postural control. A 'wrap-around' tray gives more effective support but must be level horizontally! It is important to stress that the arms are not used to prop the trunk.

Step 9.   Control of head position usually proves to be the most challenging task. Considering the weight of the head and flexibility of the cervical spine, this is not surprising. Effective control of the head is dependent upon satisfactory control of all other parts of the body first.

The optimum position for supporting the head is slightly posterior to vertical midline but maintaining horizontal vision (Fig. 7.14i).

Additional support may be necessary in the form of a neck collar or a head band. The latter is a last resort and if used should incorporate an elastic insert to prevent jarring the neck in instances of, for example, coughing. Both of these measures are aids to stability and are not the support itself.

Step 10.   Finally, the difficult question of the overall orientation of the whole support system must be addressed, that is, the position(s) most likely to meet the specification, taking into account the level of postural ability and

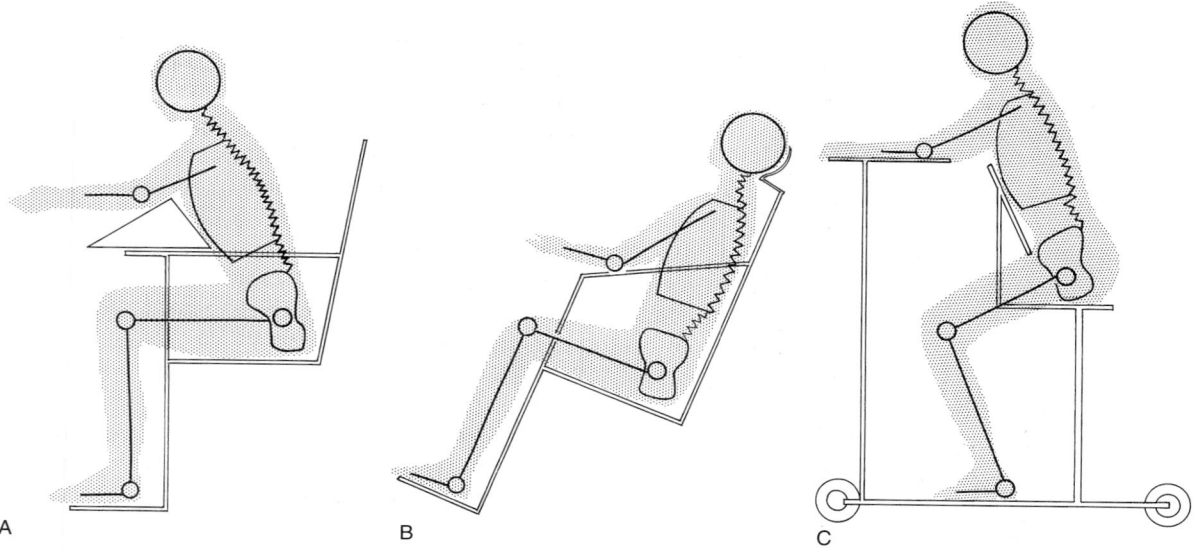

Figure 7.15   Stable postural configurations: (A) forward lean; (B) backward tilt; (C) straddle combined with forward lean.

circumstances of the client. The erect anatomically aligned seated posture in the posturally impaired person is difficult to secure over extended periods in spite of the means already outlined and addition of a variety of straps and harnesses. Bending and buckling occur over time in most cases. Thus, criteria such as postural stability, alignment, comfort, tissue viability and function are met by use of differing postural configurations and orientations (Fig 7.15). It is essential that the support is appropriate to each configuration. The detail of the support required and use of alternative postures has been described elsewhere (Pope et al 1988, Pope et al 1994).

Alternative configurations to the upright or erect posture are:

• Forward lean (Fig. 7.15A) – base stabilised as in steps 1–5. The trunk leans forwards pivoting about the hip joint, the knees are allowed to flex correspondingly, the trunk is supported anteriorly with the arms resting on a wedge placed on a tray.

• Tilted (Fig. 7.15B) – fully supported as in the step-by-step approach described above with the whole system tilted backwards. (Reclining the backrest without a corresponding adjust-

ment to the seat is contraindicated as it leads to base instability and a tendency to slide forwards.)

• Straddle/forward lean (Fig. 7.15C) resembling the posture of the conventional motorcyclist. The support given follows the principles of the segment-by-segment control of position outlined above but the means of support corresponds to the differing mechanical requirements of the configuration.

The ideal recommended, particularly in the severest cases, is a combination of forward lean, backward tilt and, where appropriate, upright. The latter is used only when some postural ability remains and for brief periods of time.

Matching the level of ability to the support required

Hard and fast rules dictating the amount of support required in a specific case cannot be given. Much will depend on the circumstances of the individual and, not least, what he/she or the carer will accept.

The categories below relate the amount of support to the Physical Ability Scale (Fig. 7.9) in terms of postural requirements. As such, they are not necessarily appropriate to the lifestyle of the particular individual (see 'The art of compromise', p. 156).

Level 1. Unplaceable; established contracture and deformity prevent alignment of body segments in, for example, scoliosis.

Custom seating is the preferred option, usually moulded in the optimum corrected alignment of the client. The upright position is not suitable as control of posture is then much reduced and progression of deformity continues. A tilting mechanism incorporated into the system offers the best compromise, allowing gravity-assisted positioning to maximise stability and segmental control together with brief periods in a more, but rarely full, upright position.

While the consensus opinion in the literature suggests that external supports do little to delay the progression or reduce the magnitude of scoliosis, it is the view of this author, based on experience, that containment and even some correction of deformity is possible, given appropriate and consistent postural management in both lying and sitting.

Level 2. Placeable with support. This level of postural ability requires the complete step-by-step build-up of support described above (p. 149). It is unlikely that the upright position can be used with any success for anything other than very brief periods. Gravity-assisted positions (Fig. 7.15) are required to maintain alignment and stability of body posture, preferably alternating between two positions for function and rest.

Level 3. Can maintain position when placed but the quality of the posture may differ from the normal seated configuration (Fig. 7.3).

A good stable base is fundamental for maximum holding of thighs and pelvis. Additional support will be required for trunk and arms. Upright sitting will be possible for short periods only. An alternative supported position, either leaning forwards or tilted, will be required to counter the effects of weakness and fatigue.

Level 4. Can maintain position and move forwards within the base. The support given is similar to that for level 3 but the trunk support needed may be less and the upright posture may

be tolerated for longer.

Level 5. Can sit independently, use either hand freely and can recover balance.

A firm, shallow contoured base, incorporating pelvis, thighs and feet, is the essential requisite, facilitating a wider range of postural adjustment and peripheral movement. A contoured backrest and support for the arms will be required for prolonged periods in sitting.

Levels 6–7. Sitting ability is sufficiently developed to allow movement out of position and to regain it.

Well-designed seating for the able-bodied is suitable, incorporating a firm contoured base and back support for extended periods of sitting. Similarly, the arms will require support, a table or desk to lean on, armrests or tray on a wheelchair. If this support is omitted, fatigue and 'drag' on the shoulder results in the slumped C-shaped spine and poking head, a posture not exclusive to the disabled person!

The higher levels of sitting ability may still require periods of rest in controlled postural configurations as a means of countering or preventing selective tissue adaptation. The necessity for 'therapeutic positioning' is judged by the ability of the individual to change his posture regularly.

The decision to use the upright position and the time for which it can be used, particularly with the lower levels of ability, depend largely upon the quality of the posture. Independent sitting achieved by deviation of alignment, asymmetrical loading and a lowering of the centre of body mass predisposes to established contracture and deformity and perpetuates use of the limbs in a postural role. The indication in these cases is for additional postural support rather than less. Further, it has been observed that the appropriate support does not prevent the development of independent postural control where the potential for this exists (Fulford et al 1982, Pope et al 1994) and may facilitate it.

The shape of the supporting components is important. The body itself is contoured in all planes. Much of seating for the able-bodied reflects this, with the result that comfort and stability of posture are improved. On the other hand, much of the seating for the disabled population incorporates flat surfaces or inappropriate contouring such as the 'hammock' seats of many folding wheelchairs. Comfort and support are thus compromised. Even the shallowest contouring will assist in 'channelling' or guiding body segments to the correct resting position, provided the overall shape conforms to that of the occupant. Contouring the seat helps secure alignment more effectively than a flat surface and a pommel. It must, however, be remembered that any contouring may well impede transfer and could be contraindicated in such circumstances. Contouring also demands correct positioning of the client in the system if it is to be effective.

To summarise, a secure base is essential for prolonged sitting in every case. Additional support is dependent upon the quantity and quality of sitting ability. The appropriate support will not necessarily interfere with development of intrinsic postural control. Access to alternative resting positions is necessary and reasonable, recognising that few of us can sit in one position for any length of time.

SPECIFIC PROBLEM SOLVING

Pelvic obliquity. The level of the seat should only be altered to compensate structural deficit such as amputation with disarticulation at the hip joint or when established deformity, as in severe scoliosis, makes compromise unavoidable. In all other cases the aim should be to achieve a level pelvis by correct alignment relative to a level surface. The technique when positioning the pelvis in cases of non-structural obliquity is to combine forward flexion of the trunk about the hip joint with bending into the concavity of the scoliosis. In this position, a level pelvis is achieved and held while the lower limbs are positioned. The trunk is then raised, maintaining alignment while the rest of the positioning is secured.

Reduced hip flexion. A minimum of a comfortable 90 degree angle at the hip joint is required if the upper trunk is to be aligned normally with the pelvis and thighs. If hip

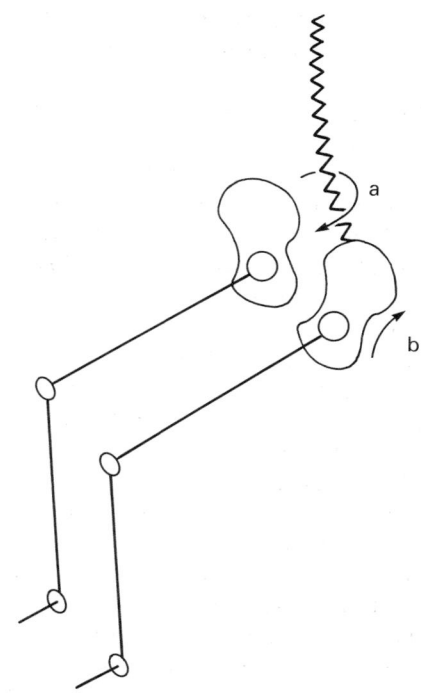

Figure 7.16   A seat-to-backrest angle greater than the available hip flexion angle induces (a) forward rotation on the side of the limited movement with (b) posterior tilting of the pelvis.

flexion is less than 90 degrees bilaterally and seat-to-backrest angle is more acute, the pelvis will tilt posteriorly and sliding and slumping occur. If hip flexion is limited on one side only, posterior tilting and rotation forwards of the pelvis on the side of limited flexion results (Fig. 7.16a & b), predisposing to scoliosis. A raised pelvis and scoliosis bending to the side of the reduced hip flexion are further developments frequently observed.

The existing hip angle determines the seat-to-backrest angle. If backrest alone is reclined to accommodate hip angle, sliding forwards will occur. The position is stabilised by ramping the seat without compromising the hip angle, or by tilting the whole system. Where appropriate, the ramp can be adjusted to accommodate any differential in hip flexion.

'Windswept' lower limbs. When established, these can lead to pelvic asymmetry predisposing

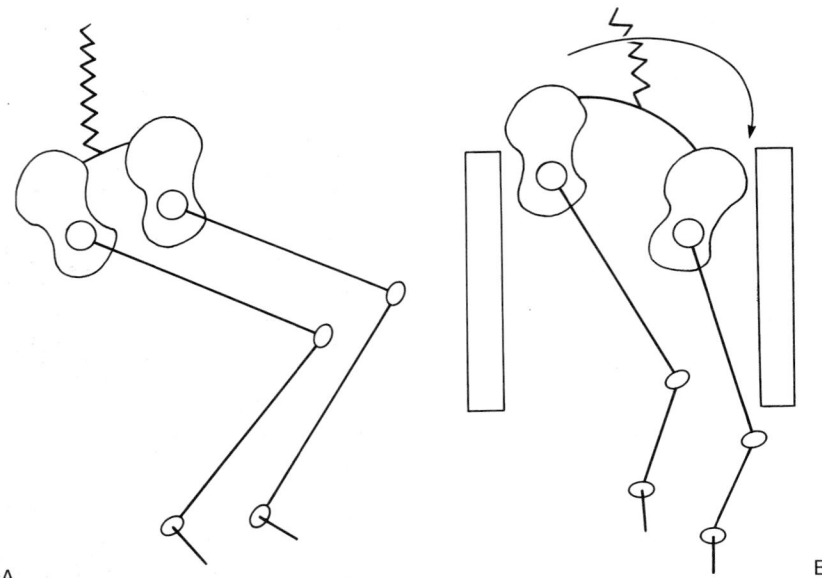

Figure 7.17 (A) 'Windswept' deformity of the lower limbs in lying. (B) When confined within the armrests of a conventional seat, the constraint imposed on the lower limbs rotates the pelvis.

to spinal deformity. When sitting in a conventional seat, the lower limbs are constrained in a forward direction; consequently the pelvis is rotated forwards on the side towards which windsweeping has occurred (Fig. 7.17). In general, maintaining pelvic alignment is the priority, and established deviation of the lower limbs must be accommodated.

Supporting the feet. Any bias of tissues towards plantar flexion and inversion will prevent the foot from maintaining alignment when placed on the footrests and will in general require additional control. The transmission of load when the foot is malaligned will compound the problem (Fig. 7.18A). Control should be applied as in Figure 7.18B; that is, proximal to the talocalcaneal joint.

Complete removal of support is recommended in some situations when the feet are used as the fixed point for movement and activity (Pope et al 1994). Under these conditions, harnesses and straps do little to secure an adequate base. Removing the point of fixation may encourage learning to sit, provided it is combined with an appropriately supported

postural configuration as in the SAM system (Fig. 7.19).

Knee flexion contractures. When very severe, knee flexion contractures can lead to the disabled person becoming bedfast. Even mild contracture is a major constraint on achieving a satisfactory stable balanced posture. The configuration of the conventional wheelchair seat, framework and footrests prevents accommodation of contracted lower limbs and feet. Feet will continually fall off the footrest when knee extension is limited. If prevented from doing so, the hips slide forwards, the pelvis tilts posteriorly, the spine flexes and a slumped posture results with all its concomitant problems (Pope 1985, Pope 1992).

Kyphosis. A round-shouldered posture of long-standing with overstretch of spinal ligaments yet still passively correctable may not be adequately controlled by the measures suggested in 'A step-by-step approach to stable posture'. A continuing tendency to roll forwards may be rectified by increasing the anterior tilt of the pelvis. The consequent increase in lumbar lordosis facilitates extension of the upper trunk.

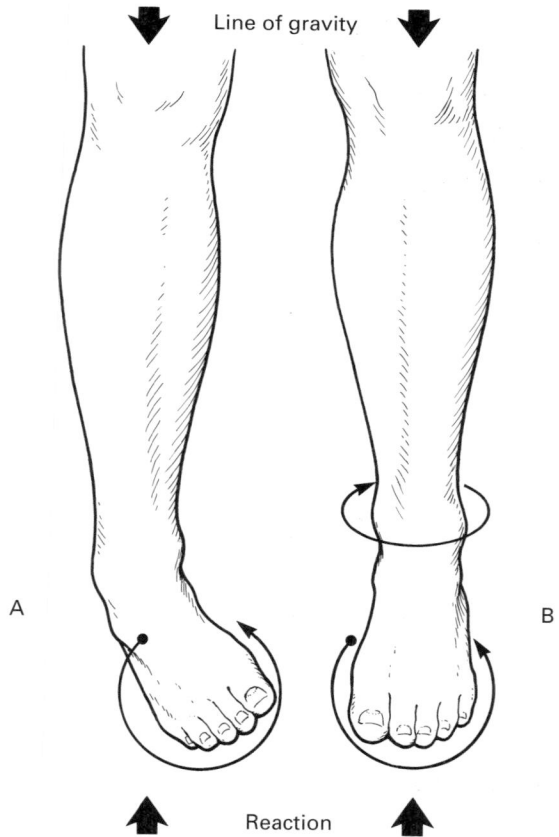

Line of gravity

A   B

Reaction

Figure 7.18 In (A) line of gravity falling medial to the normal compounds the deformity; (B) location and direction of control required to correct deviation.

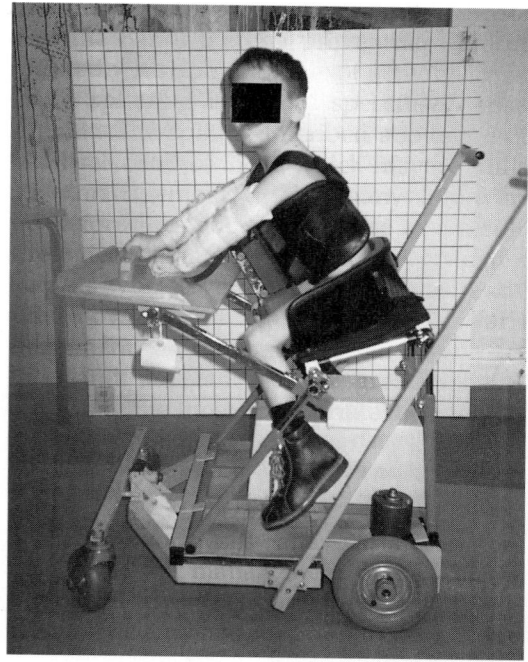

Figure 7.19 Child using the SAM system, feet unsupported to encourage action about a normal fulcrum or sitting base (Pope et al 1994).

In addition, it may be necessary to raise the support for the upper limbs. These measures will only be effective in combination with some degree of gravity-assisted positioning as in tilting.

An effective yet simple and comfortable means of countering a still mobile kyphosis is use of the forward lean posture, arms resting on a table or tray as in Figure 7.15A. An adequate range of shoulder elevation is, however, required.

An established structural kyphosis will require accommodation of the curvature posteriorly in order to bring the head to vertical midline, thus ensuring horizontal vision. If the backrest is reclined in order to achieve this,

sliding will occur. Tilting the system or increasing the rake of the seat is necessary.

In general, customised contouring of the backrest to the kyphotic trunk, combined with a degree of tilt, provides the most satisfactory solution.

Asymmetrical movement. Development of asymmetrical movement or asymmetrical recovery of movement as in cases of cerebral palsy or following brain injury can give rise to considerable postural problems in sitting. Each active movement tends to disturb balance and the body falls to the side of the movement. Because the person is unable to recover alignment, the posture is maintained. Further activity compounds the malalignment, increasing the curvature with eventual tissue and structural changes (Fig. 7.20). The problem is best managed by giving maximum trunk support, with particular attention directed to control at shoulder level on the side towards which movement occurs. Customised moulding is recommended.

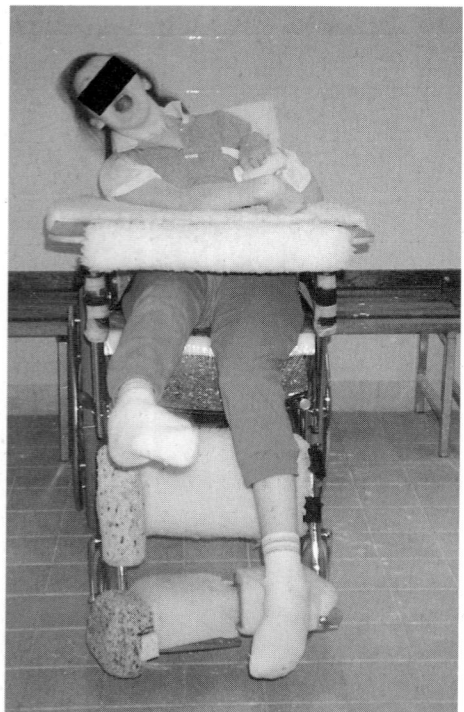

Figure 7.20 Lateral C-shaped posture characteristic of asymmetrical recovery of movement in the brain-damaged patient.

Spasticity and some movement disorders are problems associated with postural impairment. The symptoms are modified by treating them as a disorder of posture, directing effort to restore equilibrium, stability and alignment of body segments relative to the supporting surface as outlined earlier (p. 149).

THE ART OF COMPROMISE

There is rarely, if ever, any intervention related to the imposition of external means of postural control which does not have some disadvantage. Compromise is almost always inevitable.

It is, on the whole, relatively easy to analyse the condition, identify the problems and even to recognise the solution. The difficulty arises when the solution has to be applied within the context of needs, wishes, lifestyle and environment of the disabled person and those con-

cerned with his care. These are the factors setting the limits on intervention and preventing the establishment of a rigid prescriptive practice. The particular answer to a problem remains specific to that individual and his circumstances. It is never more delicate and challenging than in the circumstances of the home, as opposed to institutional, environment.

Clearly, this is the area which requires the greatest knowledge skill, experience and tact.

The art of compromise lies, first of all, in the recognition that compromise is necessary and acceptable. The skill lies in determining the priorities. Setting the priorities is an exercise in cooperation with the client and those most closely associated with him, which can be very demanding as each individual views the problem from a different perspective.

The data gathered at assessment is fundamental to the process of setting priorities and of compromise. Perhaps the most useful clue to the needs and wishes of the client and carers is the response to the initial questions at assessment – what is your problem and what would you like done about it? It becomes apparent during the assessment if the real problem has been recognised and whether the expectations are realistic and/or feasible. Where choices have to be made, the options are discussed, clearly identifying the advantages and disadvantages of each. The final decision should rest, as a rule, with the client and his carer.

There are cases in which it is advisable to accommodate the wishes of the client or carer against the better judgement of the professional, provided that safety is not compromised. As an illustration, the athletic young man suffering severe brain injury is confined to a wheelchair. He has little or no sitting ability. The understandable desire of parents/relatives is for a system which fits the premorbid image, i.e. 'sporty'; thus a lightweight wheelchair is requested. They may not be convinced that this is entirely unsuitable unless it is tried.

Any external support will, by definition, be restrictive to a greater or lesser degree. Best efforts in this respect are a poor substitute for inherent dynamic and highly sophisticated postural control mechanisms. Such support tends to attract attention, highlighting the disability.

It is not within the scope of this chapter to cover the whole area of compromise nor would it even be possible to do so. There are, however, situations which are frequent and difficult to resolve, no more so than when the solution calls for a 'trade-off' of movement or function. The following are a few frequently met examples of compromise.

Support versus freedom of movement

As a general rule, function takes precedence over preservation of postural symmetry. However, much can be done to satisfy both needs by judicious use of appropriate support together with alterations and adjustments to the environment, including angles and height of working surfaces.

There are occasions when restraint and control are desirable and permissible with the sacrifice of some movement.

High amplitude tremors are encountered in some cases of multiple sclerosis. These wild fluctuations of movement, particularly of limbs and head, result in damage to the body and are acutely distressing. Attempted functional activity is frustrating and futile. The symptoms are alleviated by giving the full support described earlier (p. 149). It is considered a measure of satisfactory control of central body segments when distal segments require minimal support.

Severe ataxia, such as in cerebellar disease. The dysmetria may be so severe that voluntary movement becomes functionally ineffective. The degree of dysmetria is a function of the number of intervening joints, the length of the limb to be moved and the distance to be travelled in execution of the task. Support and restraint applied to proximal segments and intervening joints, together with a decrease in the distance to be travelled, may enhance functional use of the distal segments. As an example, independent feeding may be possible if the disabled person leans forwards on a raised table, arms and shoulders well supported.

Spastic diplegia with inability to secure a satisfactory stable base (i.e. pelvis and thighs) above which to balance and control the trunk. These cases frequently require knee and foot restraint in addition to securing a stable base, which inevitably compromises movement of the lower limbs. Benefit is seen, however, in the facilitation of balance and functional activity in the trunk, upper limbs and head. In addition, learning to sit is probably helped rather than hindered, especially in the child.

Self-inflicted damage and mutilation as seen in cases of Lesch–Nyhan syndrome may require a system of total restraint. These conditions, together with the dystonias, are some of the least responsive to control through management of posture and are exceedingly distressing and frustrating for everyone concerned.

Supporting the feet

The feet and lower limbs contribute to the support and stability of the seated posture but this may be counterproductive in the following circumstances:

- The contracted foot – when alignment cannot be controlled by restraint, support through the foot will compound the deformity (Fig. 7.18A).
- The established 'pusher' – a strategy of using the feet as the initiating point of action seen in some cases of children with cerebral palsy and following brain damage. These people are unable to flex the trunk and bring body weight over the normal sitting base. It has been found useful to remove the support from under the feet by raising the seat, thus encouraging transference of base to thighs and pelvis and promoting movement about the new fulcrum (Pope et al 1994).

When not using the feet for support, particular attention must be given to the maintenance of a plantigrade foot by use of orthotic devices, supportive footwear and frequent stretching of tissues. A very effective means of stretching the tissues is the standing posture, provided the foot alignment is correct.

Support versus mobility

The addition of a ramp, wedge or contouring may impede transfer into and out of a seat, affecting the client or the carer. Adjustment is made in an attempt to satisfy mutually exclusive criteria, i.e. a secure postural base and easy transfer. In most cases the latter takes priority.

Support for the arms to relieve drag on the shoulders and upper trunk is frequently necessary. The client, however, may still wish or need to self-propel, in which case stability of the upper trunk is lost when the arms are not supported. The best compromise will depend on the individual case. Lever-type self-propulsion offers a solution to trunk instability and is ergonomically advantageous (Glazer et al 1980) but involves compromise of a technical nature.

Client versus carer needs

Solutions which significantly increase the time and effort of care are unlikely to be adhered to in the long term. Consultation between all parties will enable the prescriber to arrive at the most appropriate solution in the circumstances.

Aesthetics versus efficacy

Postural support or control is achieved in a number of ways, ranging from the simple and unobtrusive to the complex and obvious. There are few disabled people who wish to call attention to their disability. This may account for much of the non-compliance with recommendations when postural control is the issue. The following examples illustrate the point.

- The mother with a disabled child is content with a 'buggy' as it is commonplace for all small children. She is less able to accept a more conspicuous system, even while recognising the necessity for both the control of posture and promotion of function.
- The teenager, perhaps suffering from muscular dystrophy, with a collapsing spine, who wishes to be as functional and inconspicuous as possible in a wheelchair will reject additional effective, but necessarily restrictive, support.

Such cases require extreme care, sensitivity and delicacy in handling discussions. It is frequently necessary to proceed gradually, perhaps over a long period of time, in order to reach the best compromise.

Check list to aid prescriptive practice

The following questions have been found useful in helping to avoid inappropriate prescription of supportive equipment:

- Is it needed?
- Is it wanted?
- Do(es) he/she/they know how to use it?
- Can he/she/they manage it?
- Does it fit in with the home environment?
- Is it socially acceptable?
- Does it look good?
- What are the 'trade-offs' and are they acceptable?

Counter-strategies

There are times when, for one reason or another, intervention is not appropriate, possible or acceptable. In such cases, strategies are used to counter or minimise the deleterious effects of sustained 'bad' posture in sitting.

The stresses and strains in the spine may be relieved by the following:

- A period of time in prone lying with the arms elevated to mid-position and a pillow under the chest.
- Leaning forwards over a firm foam wedge or pillow placed on a tray or table, provided that the forward inclination is achieved by trunk flexion about the hip joint and not by flexion of the spine.
- Early signs of asymmetry within the trunk may be relieved by side-lying over a pillow or small roll. Care is essential to ensure the correction is being applied to the appropriate tissues. Surface marking of spinous processes will help to clarify this.

A programme of standing daily ensures a change of position, relieving pressure and

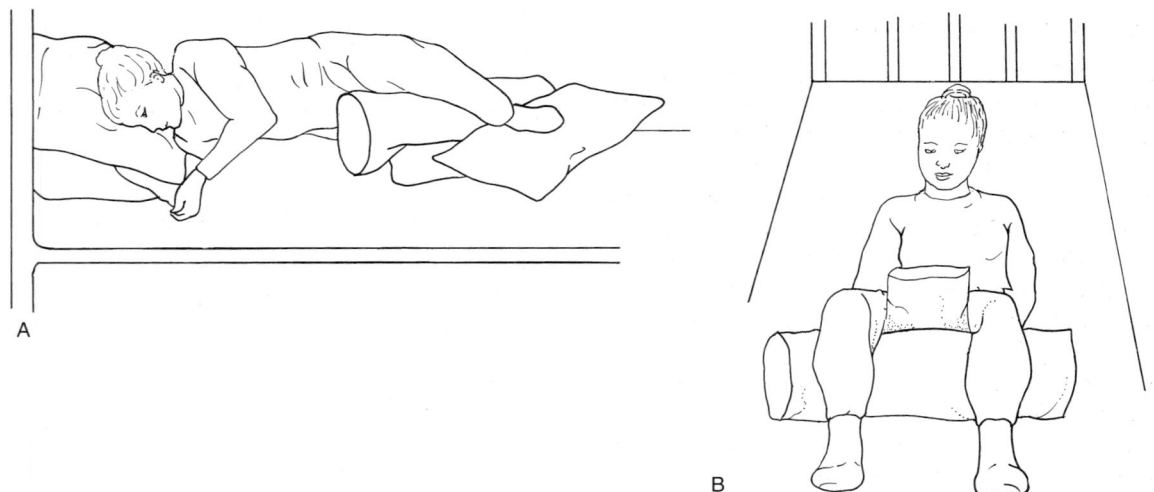

Figure 7.21   Control of posture in lying: (A) side-lying, trunk supported, roll between thighs to stabilise the position; (B) supine lying, feet supported, using a T-roll to stabilise position (Pope 1992).

maintaining length in those tissues which tend to shorten when sitting for sustained periods. The hip and knee flexors and plantar flexors of the foot are particularly vulnerable.

Perhaps the most effective counter-measure of all is control of posture in lying. The majority of the more severely disabled people spend a considerably larger proportion of time in lying than in sitting. It is here that many of the initial problems arise and tissue adaptation occurs as in the case of 'windswept' lower limbs.

Control of posture in lying is essential, even when the seated posture is supported adequately. It is a vital part of the overall physical management regime. The supported positions illustrated in Figure 7.21A & B offer a simple and effective means of postural control in lying (Pope 1992).

Corrective positioning to control posture in lying should be immediate in the acute stage of any disease or injury which threatens to incapacitate motor or postural ability, and certainly before any support for the seated posture is considered. Appropriate action at this stage will considerably lessen the problems associated with seating at a later time.

CONCLUSIONS

Successful outcome in terms of matching postural needs with lifestyle is dependent upon an in-depth understanding of problem development, comprehensive assessment, cooperative discussion and effort, judicious compromise and compliance with the recommendations.

Appropriate and consistent postural management can reduce or prevent secondary complications associated with postural impairment and do much to contribute to 'quality of life' (Pope 1994). Although initial outlay in terms of available resources may be comparatively large, effective intervention can reduce the cost and effort of care in the long term. In addition, effective postural management can enhance and reinforce recovery of function in those with the potential for this. In fact, it provides the 'platform' from which movement is encouraged and facilitated.

As a final word, problems presenting in the seated posture should not be treated in isolation. Consideration must be given to the management of body posture in all other positions and situations. However complex and diffuse the pathology, there are few, if any, who do not benefit from the appropriate management.

ACKNOWLEDGEMENTS

The author wishes to thank Gavin Jenkins, Mary Marlborough Centre Oxford, for the initial drawings, the Medical Illustrations Department of the John Radcliffe Infirmary Oxford for completion of the diagrams and family and colleagues for their comments during preparation of the manuscript.

The statement attributed to Deane on page 144 was made by Mr G Deane, Consultant Orthopaedic Surgeon, during a lecture at the University of Surrey in 1982, and confirmed in discussion with me thereafter.

REFERENCES

Asher R 1947 The dangers of going to bed. British Medical Journal 2(Dec 13): 967–968

Bartelink D L 1957 The role of abdominal pressure in relieving the pressure on the lumbar intervertebral disc. Journal of Bone and Joint Surgery 39B: 718–725

Condie E 1991 A therapeutic approach to physical disability. Physiotherapy 77(2): 72–77

Edelman G M 1993 Neural Darwinism: selection and reentrant signalling in higher brain function. Neuron 10(2): 115–125

Fulford G E, Brown J K 1976 Position as a cause of deformity in children with cerebral palsy. Developmental Medicine and Child Neurology 18: 305–314

Fulford G E, Cairns T P, Sloan Y 1982 Sitting problems of children with cerebral palsy. Developmental Medicine and Child Neurology 24: 48–53

Glazer R M, Sawka M N, Brukne M F, Wilde S W 1980 Applied physiology for wheelchair design. Journal of Applied Physiology 1: 41–44

Hallett R, Hare N, Milner A D 1987 Description and evaluation of an assessment form. Physiotherapy 73(5): 220–225

Kelly E D 1949 Teaching posture and body mechanics. Barnes, New York

Kidd G L 1980 The motor unit: a review. Physiotherapy 66(5): 146–152

Koreska J, Robertson D, Mills R H, Gibson D A, Albisser A M 1977 Biomechanics of the lumbar spine and its clinical significance. Orthopedic Clinics of North America 8: 121–133

Letts M R 1992 Principles of seating the disabled. CRC Press, Boca Raton, Florida 33431

McPherson J J, Schild R, Spaulding S J, Barsamian P, Transon C, White S C 1991 Analysis of upper extremity movement in four sitting positions; a comparison of persons with and without cerebral palsy. American Journal of Occupational Therapy 45(2): 123–129

Massion J 1992 Movement, posture and equilibrium: interaction and coordination. Progress in Neurology 38: 35–36

Massion J, Gahery Y 1978 The reflex control of posture and movement. Proceedings of IBRO Conference Pisa Italy 50: 219–226

Morris J M, Lucas D B, Bresler B 1961 Role of the trunk in stability of the spine. Journal of Bone and Joint Surgery 43A: 327–351

Mulcahy C M, Pountney T E, Nelham R L, Green E,

Billington G D 1988 Adaptive seating for motor handicap: problems, a solution, assessment and prescription. Physiotherapy 74(7): 531–536

Norris C M 1995 Spinal stabilisation. Physiotherapy 81(2): 64–79

Pope P M 1985 A study of postural instability in relation to posture in the wheelchair. Physiotherapy 71(3): 127–129

Pope P M 1992 Management of the physical condition in patients with chronic and severe neurological pathologies. Physiotherapy 78(12): 896–903

Pope P M 1993 Measurement of postural competency in the severely disabled patient. Booklet 5: Proceedings of meeting May 17th, the Hare Association for Physical Ability. Available from: The Education Officer, HAFPA, 3 Melton Grove, West Bridgford, Nottingham, England

Pope P M 1994 Advances in seating the severely disabled neurological patient. Physiotherapy Ireland 15(1): 9–14

Pope P M, Booth E, Gosling G 1988 The development of alternative seating and mobility systems. Physiotherapy Practice 4: 78–93

Pope P M, Bowes C E, Tudor M, Andrews B 1991 Surgery combined with continued post-operative stretching and management for knee flexion contractures in cases of multiple sclerosis. A report of six cases. Clinical Rehabilitation 5: 15–23

Pope P M, Bowes C E, Booth E 1994 Postural control in sitting, the SAM system: evaluation of use over three years. Developmental Medicine and Child Neurology 36: 241–252

Pountney T E, Mulcahy C M, Green E 1990 Early development of postural control. Physiotherapy 76(12): 799–802

Reynolds H 1978 The inertial properties of the body and its segments. NASA Reference Publication 1024. Anthopometric Source Book 1: 1–55

Shirazi-Adl A, Ahmed A M, Shrivastava S C 1986 Mechanical response of a lumbar motion segment in axial torque alone and combined with compression. Spine 11: 914–927

Son K, Miller J A, Schultz A B 1988 The mechanical role of the trunk and lower extremities in a seated weight moving task in the sagittal plane. Journal of Biomechanical Engineering 110(2): 97–103

Thomson A P, Lowe C R, McKeown T 1951 The care of the aged and chronic sick. E & S Livingstone, London

Whitman A 1924 Postural deformities in children. New York State Journal of Medicine 24: 871–874

Zacharkow D J 1988 Posture sitting and standing, chair design and exercise. Charles C Thomas, Springfield Ill

CHAPTER CONTENTS

Introduction   161

Physical principles   161
 Forces   161
 Clinical application   162

Classification of orthoses   163

LOWER LIMB ORTHOSES   163

Foot insoles   163

Ankle–foot orthoses (AFOs)   164
 Posterior leaf AFO   164
 The hinged AFO   166
 Below-knee calipers   167
 Anterior shell AFO   167
 Dorsiflexion bandage   168

Knee–ankle–foot orthoses (KAFOs)   169

Summary   172

Lower limb casts   172
 Prophylactic casting of the foot and ankle   172
 Casting of the foot and ankle for patients with
  residual spasticity   174
 Serial casting of the foot and ankle   175
 Back slabs to support the lower limbs in extension
  175
 Serial casting to correct knee flexion deformity
  177
 Drop-out casting   177

Summary   179

UPPER LIMB ORTHOSES   179

Shoulder supports   179
 The collar and cuff   180
 Cuff support   180
 The abduction roll or wedge   181
 Support using pillows or a tray/table   181

Elbow casts   181
 Serial and drop-out casting   182
 Back slabs   182

The wrist and hand   183
 Splinting for the spastic wrist and hand   184
 Splinting for the hypotonic wrist and hand   185

Summary   187

References   187

8

Splinting and the use of orthoses in the management of patients with neurological disorders

Susan Edwards
Paul Charlton

INTRODUCTION

The use of different types of splints and orthoses in the management of patients with neurological disorders has been, and remains, somewhat controversial, particularly for patients with hypertonus. As with all interventions, splints and/or orthoses should only be used after detailed assessment of the patient's problems, taking into consideration the effect that their application may have holistically.

An orthosis or splint is an external device designed to apply, distribute or remove forces to or from the body in a controlled manner to perform one or both of the basic functions of:

- control of body motion
- an alteration or prevention of alteration in the shape of body tissues (Rose 1986).

They may be used to compensate for weak or absent muscle function or to resist the unopposed action of spastic muscles (Fyfe et al 1993).

PHYSICAL PRINCIPLES

It is important to understand a number of physical principles when considering splinting for patients either as an aid to function or as an adjunct to treatment.

Forces

A force has magnitude and direction and when applied to a mass tends to result in movement in the direction of the force applied. Force may be defined as a physical action that always acts along a straight line and may be represented by a line, the length of which is proportional to the magnitude of the force, the beginning of which represents the point of application of the force and the direction of which corresponds to the direction of the force (Rose et al 1982). The graphical representation of force is known as a vector.

Ground reaction force

This is the force exerted by the ground to counteract:

- the vertical force of body weight
- the horizontal force in the line of propulsion
- the lateral force exerted as the body moves forward during the gait cycle.

These forces may be represented as a resultant vector which describes magnitude and direction. The vector origin represents the point of application of the resultant forces.

Moments

When a force acts on a body, the effect of the force is dependent upon the distance between the point of application and the turning point or joint. This effect is the moment of force which is equal to the magnitude of the force multiplied by the moment arm. The moment arm is the perpendicular distance of the line of action of the force from the joint axis (Galley & Forster 1987).

Pressure

This is the intensity of the force applied to a particular area and is the force per unit area. Pressure may be reduced by increasing the surface over which the force acts.

Clinical application

Motion may be caused or prevented by forces. In the human body forces are produced by muscle contractions. Patients with neurological disability often demonstrate impaired control of movement. Those with low tone are unable to generate sufficient force to maintain stability or produce movement. In this instance, the orthosis is merely required to oppose the weight of the limb, which may be achieved by a lively or sprung orthosis allowing use of any residual, purposeful movement. Those with hypertonus generate excessive but inappropriate force, often associated with abnormal stereotyped posture and movement. In this situation the orthosis is required to resist a much higher force and must be rigid to prevent unwanted movement by the pull of spastic muscles. In both instances, extrinsic support in the form of an orthosis may be required to facilitate stability and/or movement and thereby function.

The problem of an unstable knee illustrates the importance of these physical principles. In standing, the knee may be maintained in a position of extension in spite of minimal activity of the quadriceps muscle group, providing that the ground reaction force passes in front of the knee joint. In effect, the knee can be 'locked' in extension, often in association with flexion of the hip. The knee is protected in part by the anterior cruciate ligament and the posterior capsule of the joint, but, if this posture is maintained over a protracted period of time, these structures become lax, enabling the knee to move further into a position of hyperextension.

In this situation an orthosis may be recommended to provide stability and protect the integrity of the joint. The caliper is designed so that the line of force passes directly through the knee joint, thereby minimising the moment arm. Applied in this manner, the orthosis acts as a stabilising device with only small forces acting between the leg and the caliper.

Where there is a knee flexion deformity, the ground reaction force passes behind the knee joint. A flexion moment is produced, the magnitude of which rises as the degree of flexion increases. An orthosis may resist this moment by producing an equal and opposite moment through three point fixation (Fig. 8.1).

The pressure exerted by this resistance is determined by the length of the moment arm

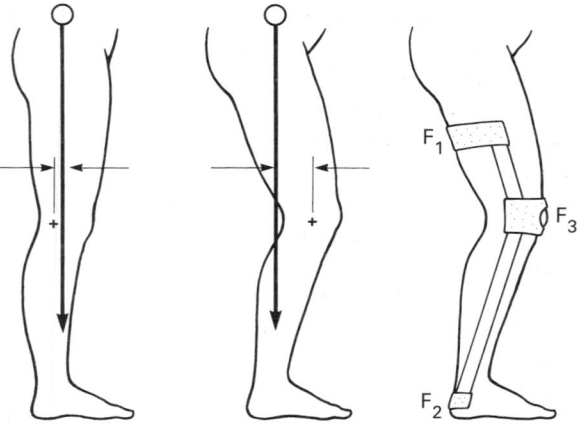

Figure 8.1 Three-point force application provided by long leg caliper (after Rose et al 1982).

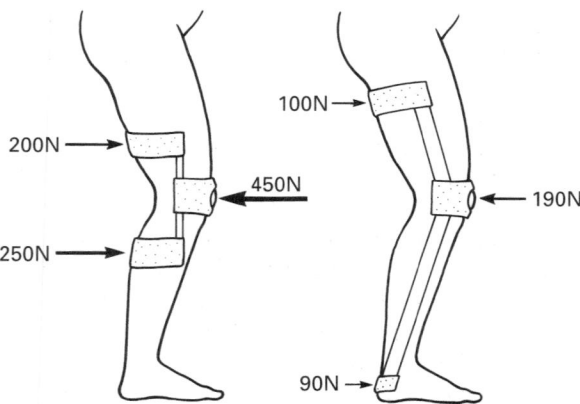

Figure 8.2 Comparative forces for a short knee support and a long leg caliper (after Rose et al 1982).

and the surface area over which it acts. For this reason the caliper should extend the full length of the leg, with a broad thigh band at the line of the hip joint, and attach into the shoe (Fig. 8.2).

CLASSIFICATION OF ORTHOSES

Orthoses are classified in relation to the parts of the body over which they act. Below-knee calipers or drop-foot splints are referred to as ankle–foot orthoses (AFOs), full leg calipers as knee–ankle–foot orthoses (KAFOs) and, if extending above the hip, as hip–knee–ankle–foot orthoses (HKAFO) (Training Council for Orthotists 1980).

LOWER LIMB ORTHOSES

FOOT INSOLES

Paralysis or an imbalance of muscular activity at the foot will compromise the normal transition of weight during the gait cycle.

Insoles may be used for two main purposes:

- to realign the foot by means of wedges and/or medial and lateral arch supports to provide a more even weight-bearing surface
- to unload painful areas.

There have been tremendous advances in the availability of moulded insoles which may be adapted to provide the total contact support required to ensure a more appropriate weight dispersal during walking. The texture of these supports varies, the more pliable being used for improved comfort whereas the more rigid give greater control.

There are many factors to consider in the design of insoles. They include:

1. *The height of the heel.* This should be low to provide greater stability. However, if there is shortening of the Achilles tendon (*tendo Achillis*; TA), this may be accommodated by increasing the heel height of either the insole or of the shoe. Where the objective of treatment is to regain this loss of range at the TA, gradual reduction in the height of the heel may facilitate this process. The width of the heel may be increased to improve either medial or lateral stability.

2. *Lack of mobility in the forefoot.* This may be compensated for by incorporating a raise at the level of the metatarsal heads. This will allow the patient to roll from heel to toe-off, with reduced movement necessary at the metatarsophalangeal joints.

3. *Muscle imbalance.* This may be either the primary or secondary problem in respect of foot deformity. In conditions such as hereditary motor and sensory neuropathy, the disease process affects the distal musculature, and the muscle imbalance at the feet and ankles is therefore the primary problem. The foot may be pulled into inversion with the weight being taken

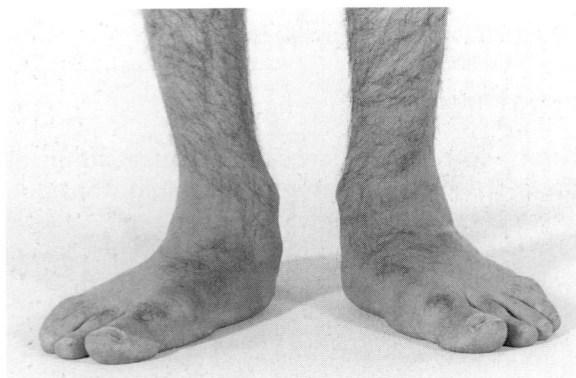

Figure 8.3 Pronated feet.

predominantly over the lateral border. Provision of an insole with a lateral wedge lifting the outer border and/or a post under the fifth metatarsal head may assist in the redistribution of weight over the full surface of the foot.

However, the changes which occur at the foot may be caused by muscle imbalance and malalignment of joints proximally, and as such are secondary complications. An example of this may be observed in the cerebral palsy patient with a spastic gait. The predominant flexed posture of the hips and knees and plantar flexion of the feet may lead to collapse of the medial arch and plantar fascia with resultant painful, pronated feet (Fig. 8.3).

Foot insoles may still be of value but it is important to recognise the primary problem and take steps to address this.

ANKLE–FOOT ORTHOSES (AFOS)

The purpose of the AFO is to effect control of the ankle and subtalar joints and maintain the foot in the plantigrade position or in a degree of slight dorsiflexion. In this way, the AFO has a direct influence on:

- the quality of the gait pattern
- the maintenance of range of the posterior crural muscle group and of the TA.

A patient with weakness or flaccid paralysis requires a less-supportive device to maintain the foot in plantigrade position, whereas a patient with spasticity pulling the foot into plantar flexion and inversion requires more rigid control.

Posterior leaf AFO

This is the most common type of AFO, made from plastic material which extends over the posterior aspect of the calf from below the fibula head to the metatarsal heads (Fig. 8.4).

Temporary stock AFOs are available in different materials and sizes and provide varying degrees of rigidity. Unless there is a significant deformity of the foot or excessive hypertonus, they may continue to be used by the patient in the longer term or until such time as adequate control of the plantigrade position is regained.

Temporary AFOs may be used to control the position of the foot when there is weakness or a

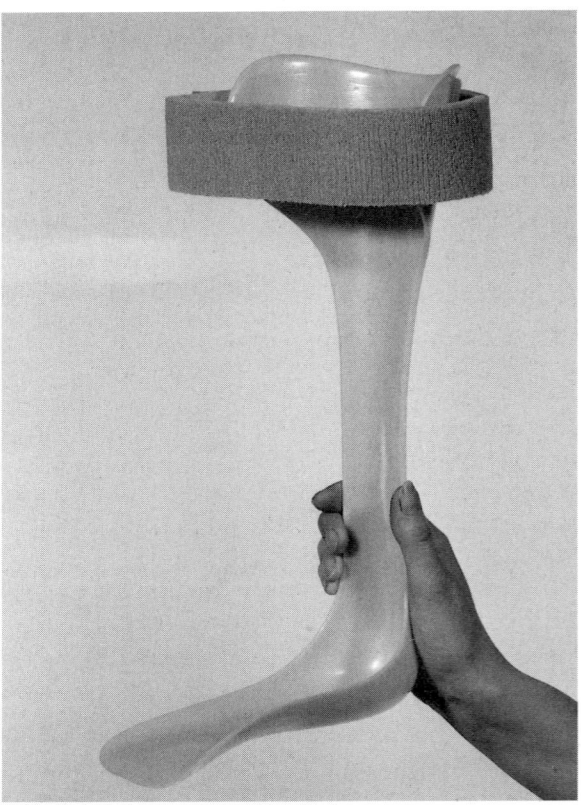

Figure 8.4 Posterior leaf ankle–foot orthosis.

flaccid paralysis of the foot and ankle musculature. If the patient has insufficient dorsiflexion, the walking pattern is altered, with compensatory strategies adopted to counteract this inadequacy. A high-stepping gait is used in order to ensure clearance of the ground when stepping through. Application of an AFO controls the foot position and enables a more efficient and effective gait pattern.

For patients with spasticity where the foot is pulled into plantar flexion and inversion, the compensations are more complex due to the holistic effects of this hypertonus. Where there is predominant extensor spasticity of the lower limb, the patient may attempt to hitch the leg through with overactivity of the trunk side flexors, there being inadequate release of the knee into flexion. Temporary AFOs are often ineffective in controlling the foot in the plantigrade position and may worsen the hypertonus with the pressure under the metatarsal heads. In this situation a more rigid, made-to-measure, polypropylene AFO may be required, incorporating the whole foot.

Transposition of weight during the gait cycle produces movement at the ankle joint into both plantar and dorsiflexion. However, in the event of fixation at the ankle joint, providing this is the only determinant of gait that is affected, increased flexion of the knee during the swing phase maintains the smoothness of the path of translation of the centre of gravity (Saunders et al 1953). This may be observed in a patient with a L4–5 or L5–S1 root lesion affecting the anterior tibial muscle group. The dropped foot corrected with a posterior leaf AFO, can be compensated for by increased flexion of the knee with little effect on the efficiency of the gait pattern. However, for many patients with neurological disability, the problem is rarely confined merely to the ankle joint and the compensatory strategies adopted are, of necessity, more extensive and diverse.

Considerations when prescribing AFOs

Splint flexibility. A more rigid AFO may be required for patients with severe spasticity or

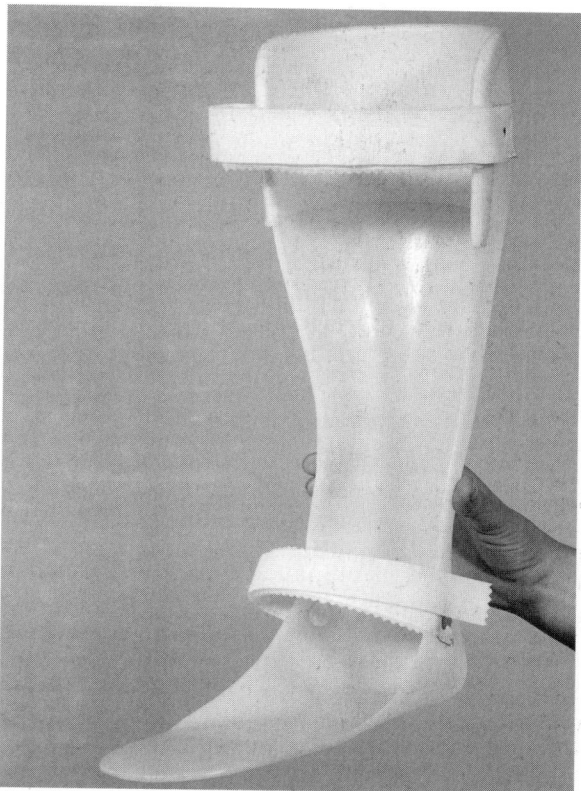

Figure 8.5   Rigid ankle–foot orthosis.

when there is already established deformity. The degree of rigidity is dependent upon the type and extent of the plastic material providing splintage. For example, a patient with marked plantar flexion and inversion spasticity may be supported in the plantigrade position or one of slight dorsiflexion with a rigid polypropylene AFO extending to include the toes and encasing the malleoli. A strap over the line of the ankle joint helps to ensure correct positioning of the heel in the splint (Fig. 8.5).

Established or predicted inversion deformity. A similar design is advocated for patients with established deformity, most commonly into inversion. Patients with hereditary motor and sensory neuropathy may develop such deformity unless there is appropriate, early intervention. The relative unopposed action of tibialis posterior will cause inversion of the foot, which in severe cases can create a deformity which resembles a club foot. A similar AFO to that described for the spastic patient is required to prevent further deterioration. Here, the purpose of the AFO is to exert pressure to prevent increasing inversion, and it is important that this pressure is dissipated away from the bony lateral malleolus. For this reason, the lateral border of the AFO from below the fibula head to just above the lateral malleolus is moulded inwards during the splint manufacture to redistribute pressure to this more fleshy part of the leg rather than over the more vulnerable malleolus.

The fixed position as provided by the posterior leaf AFO has both advantages and disadvantages.

Advantages

1. The fixed plantigrade position will facilitate the transference of weight over the full surface of the foot. (Where the initial contact is made with the forefoot, the weight tends to remain over the heel, which may result in compensatory flexion at the hips and hyperextension of the knees.)

2. More even transference of weight over the full surface of the foot tends to stimulate extension and abduction at the hips during stance phase of gait with the more forward placement of the centre of gravity.

3. If the foot is positioned in slight dorsiflexion, this tends to introduce an element of flexion at the knee through the mechanical stretch of gastrocnemius and thereby prevents or reduces hyperextension at this joint.

4. Forced maintenance of a spastic foot in dorsiflexion can be effective in decreasing extensor tone proximally to enable a more fluent swing phase of gait.

Disadvantages

1. The posterior leaf AFO prevents movement into dorsiflexion and plantar flexion. Many patients complain of difficulty in negotiating stairs due to the lack of dorsiflexion. If only one foot is splinted, the patient may compensate by always stepping down with the supported leg, but, where two AFOs are required, going downstairs may be impossible without assistance.

2. Patients with spasticity tend to be dominated by stereotyped postures and movements. Immobilisation of the foot and ankle will restrict potential postural adaptation within the foot and ankle and may lead to increased immobility of the intrinsic foot musculature. When used for patients with weakness, the support proffered by the splint may discourage return of function due to the lack of stimulation of muscle activity within the foot and of the muscles acting over the ankle and subtalar joints.

3. Where there is excessive spasticity, the foot may resist the splint, thereby exacerbating the increased tone. Splints that terminate at the metatarsal heads may stimulate a positive support response, but those which extend to include the toes restrict movement at the metatarsophalangeal joints.

4. Forced maintenance of a spastic foot in dorsiflexion may lead to increased flexion proximally and increasing difficulty in attaining extension during stance phase of gait.

5. This device is unsuitable for patients with oedema of the legs.

The hinged AFO

A hinge mechanism may be incorporated at the ankle joint to allow for dorsiflexion (Fig. 8.6).

This is an obvious advantage in terms of allowing movement into dorsiflexion during the gait cycle and in negotiating stairs, and is beneficial for most patients with flaccid paralysis. Those with spasticity often require the more rigid splint to eliminate the potential for clonus which may be stimulated by the movement.

Cusick (1988) advocates the use of a hinged 'crouch-control' ankle–foot splint whereby the patient is able to plantar-flex the ankle but dorsiflexion is restricted. This splint is recommended for children with excessive flexion of the lower limbs, this being the position referred to as 'crouch'. Although this relates to the management of foot deformity in children, the same principles may apply for adults. The most common cause of this posture is surgical

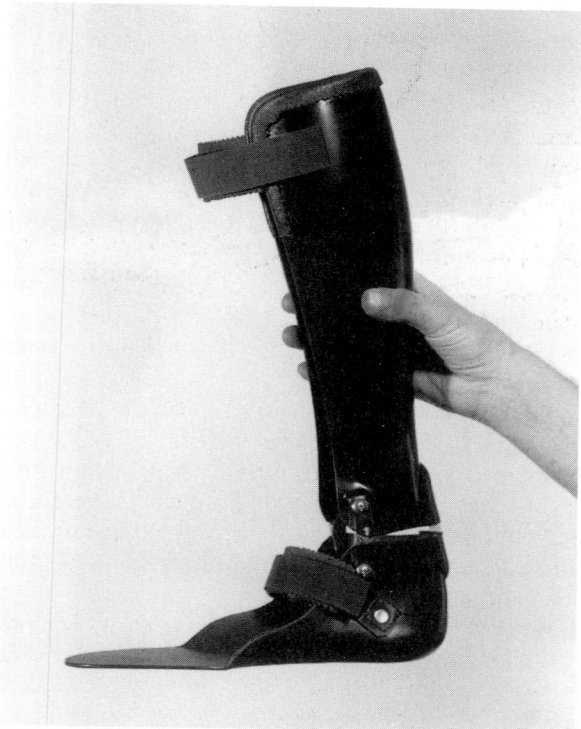

Figure 8.6   Hinged ankle–foot orthosis.

overlengthening of the Achilles tendons (Sutherland & Cooper 1978).

Below-knee calipers

Although now less frequently used, these calipers may be the support of choice when:

- there is oedema of the leg
- the foot is unable to conform to the rigid support of the posterior leaf AFO and resists the controlling force, thereby exacerbating the spasticity
- the predominant deformity of the foot is into inversion. A below-knee iron with an outside T- or Y-strap to control the foot in a neutral alignment may prove to be more effective than a posterior leaf AFO. The pressure exerted by the strap is often more tolerable than that provided by a rigid AFO.

It is important to ensure that the foot does not rotate within the shoe. It is not uncommon to find that the shoe itself deforms due to continued dominance of the spastic muscle groups.

These iron calipers with the socket fitted into the shoe are undoubtedly heavier than the plastic AFOs and this must be taken into consideration in respect of the effects on spasticity. In general, it would seem that most people prefer the appearance of the plastic AFOs, often referred to as cosmetic devices, rather than the metal irons.

Anterior shell AFO

This extends from an anterior band at the level of the patella tendon, laterally and downwards to terminate in a foot support similar to that of the posterior leaf AFO (Fig. 8.7). Carbon reinforcements may be required at the ankle to ensure adequate rigidity and a calf strap may be needed to prevent hyperextension of the knee.

The anterior shell AFO is of benefit for patients with weakness of the knee extensors but sufficient strength of the hip extensors to transfer the body weight forwards during stance phase of gait. The orthosis stabilises the knee in extension through the rigidity at the ankle and the anterior band preventing knee flexion as the hip extends.

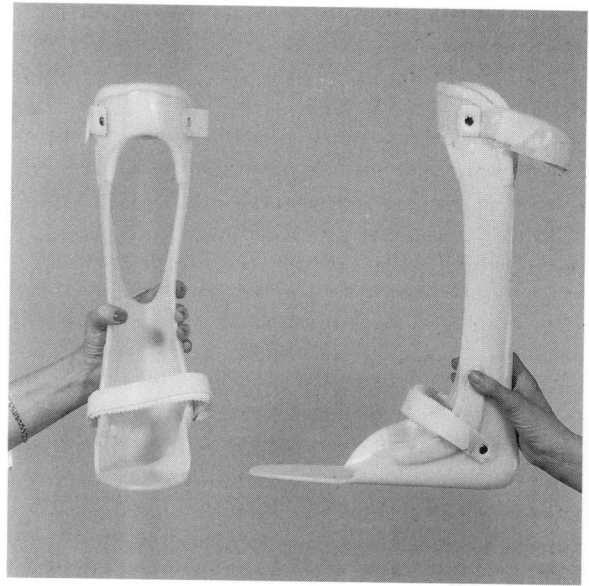

Figure 8.7   Anterior shell ankle–foot orthosis.

It is important to monitor the efficacy of this splint when supplied to patients with progressive neurological disorders. The anterior shell AFO becomes ineffective without the sustained control of the hip extensors.

Dorsiflexion bandage

A crepe bandage may be used as a temporary means of supporting the foot in dorsiflexion or the plantigrade position (Fig. 8.8).

Advantages

1. It enables movement into dorsiflexion whilst inhibiting plantar flexion.
2. For patients with hypertonus affecting the plantar flexors and invertors it may be applied with increased eversion to inhibit this increased tone.

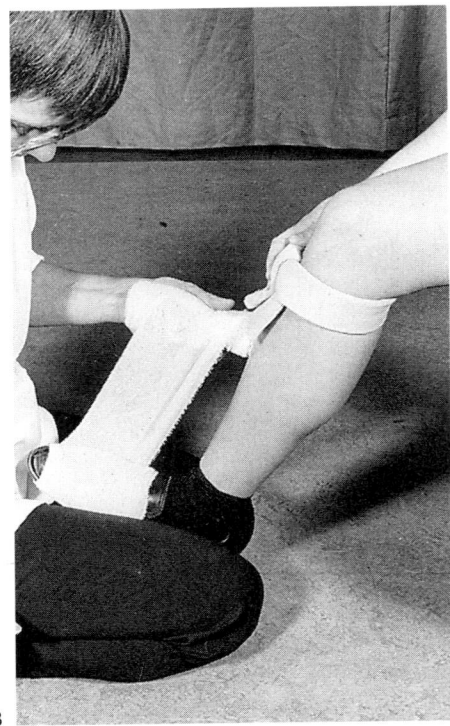

B

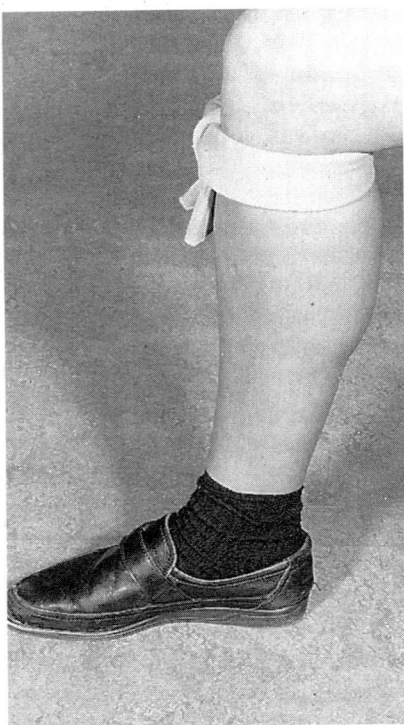

A

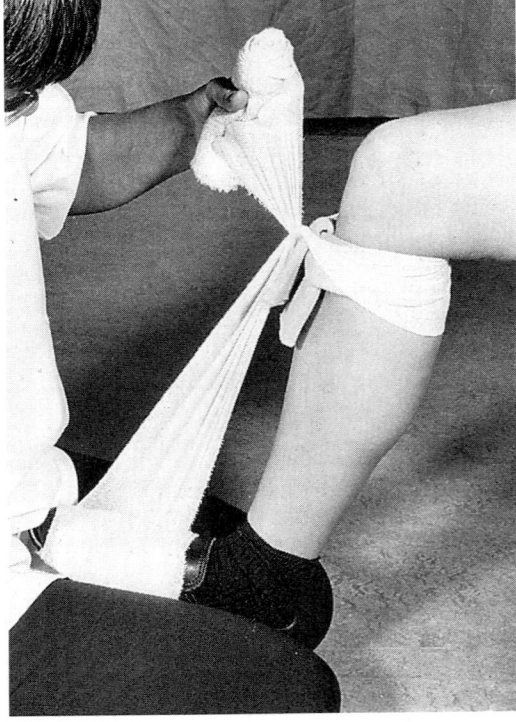

C

Figure 8.8 Application of bandage to hold foot in dorsiflexion and eversion. Note the small band of foam (A) to protect the skin from the pressure of the bandage. (Reproduced from Bromley 1991 with kind permission.)

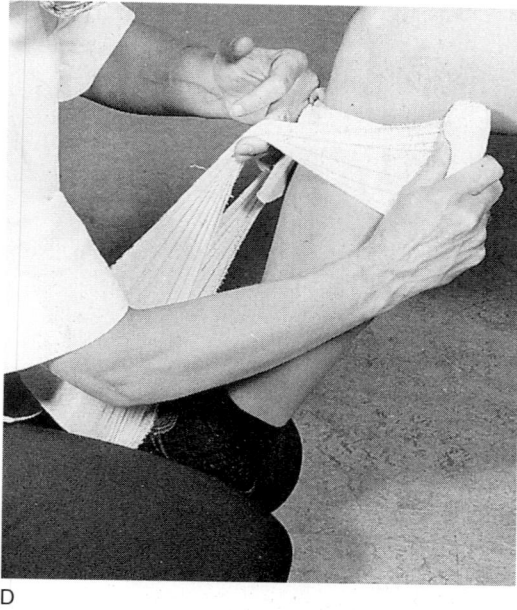

D

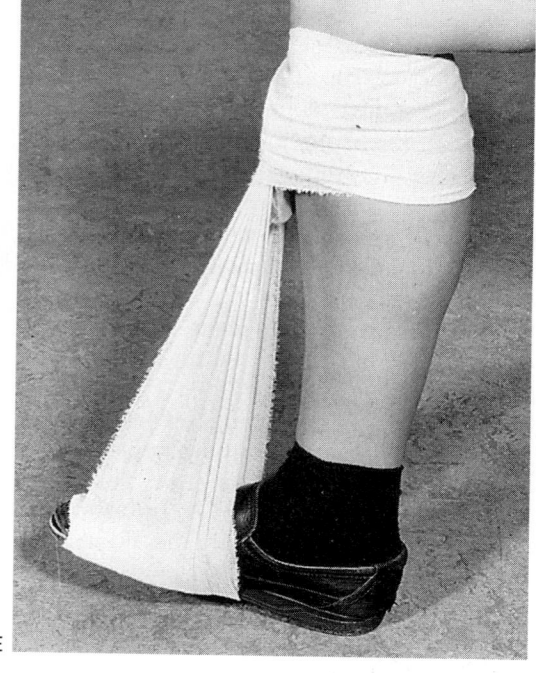

E

Figure 8.8   *(Cont'd)*

3. It improves stability, particularly where there is flaccid paralysis, in that it restricts posterior displacement of body weight. It also facilitates more normal alignment of the centre of gravity through the foot rather than through the heel during stance phase or when standing with the feet astride.

4. The foot itself maintains a greater degree of flexibility than with the more rigid AFO.

5. It serves as a means of evaluating the effects of a more permanent device.

Disadvantages

The main disadvantage of the dorsiflexion bandage is that it can only be used on a temporary basis due to the potential restriction to the circulation. A piece of foam circumventing the leg just below the fibula head goes some way to minimising the pressure applied around the leg and thus the circulatory effects. When used to control a flail foot, little pressure is required to maintain the plantigrade position. However, when it is used to inhibit strong plantar flexion and inversion spasticity, greater pressure is required to obtain the desired positioning with an increase in the potential risk of circulatory impairment. When this bandage is used in conjunction with a back slab, the effects on the circulation are minimised due to the hard shell reducing the constricting effect.

KNEE–ANKLE–FOOT ORTHOSES (KAFOs)

In normal stance, the line of force of the body weight passes in front of the knee (Galley & Forster 1987, Rose et al 1982) and minimal quadriceps activity is required to maintain the upright position. In the event of neurological impairment resulting in impaired lower limb control, various types of support need to be considered if the patient is to maintain or regain an independent gait.

The KAFO applies a three-point leverage system about the knee to support the leg in extension (see p. 163). It may be used to control either hyperextension or flexion of the limb.

Hyperextension of the knee

The knee may become hyperextended for several reasons which include:

1. To gain stability by 'locking' against the posterior structures of the knee if there is insufficient quadriceps activity to maintain normal stance.

2. Abnormal muscle tone whereby the quadriceps muscle group force the knee into hyperextension.

3. Weakness of the hip extensors whereby the pelvis is anteriorly tilted with subsequent hyperextension of the knees.

4. Weakness of the hamstring muscle group allowing unopposed action of quadriceps.

5. Mechanical shortening of the posterior crural muscle group and of the TA. In order for the heel to achieve contact with the floor, the knee is forced into hyperextension.

In each of these examples, the hyperextended position of the knee creates tension on the posterior structures of the joint, often leading to overstretching and pain.

The management and control of knee hyperextension varies depending on the cause.

1. The patient with weak and ineffective quadriceps control may benefit from an anterior shell AFO, providing there is adequate activity of the hip extensors. Alternatively, a KAFO may be required if there is more diffuse weakness preventing effective alignment of the pelvis and trunk.

2. A rigid AFO with the ankle held in dorsiflexion affects the knee position by virtue of the stretch applied to gastrocnemius. The greater the angle of dorsiflexion the greater the influence of flexion at the knee joint. It is important to recognise that the effect of this increase of flexion may render the spastic quadriceps ineffective as knee extensors, in which case a KAFO may be required. The use of a bandage, holding the foot in dorsiflexion is of particular value to assess the most appropriate orthosis.

3. A Swedish knee cage may prove effective in preventing hyperextension as a result of

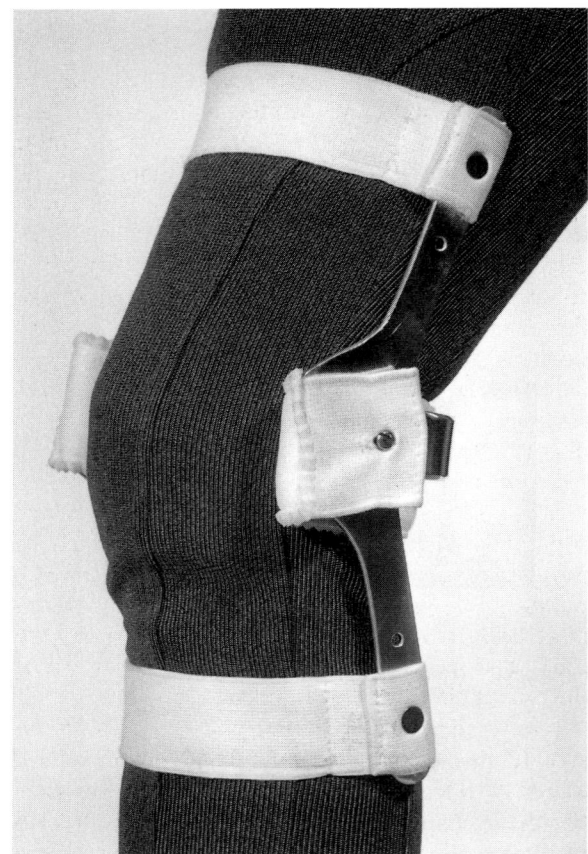

Figure 8.9 Swedish knee cage.

weakness or paralysis of the hamstrings (Fig. 8.9). This should be used with caution as the imposition of flexion at the knee may prevent full extension at the hip during stance phase of gait. This may lead to the development of hip flexor contracture.

4. Mechanical shortening of the calf muscles and TA may be accommodated for by provision of a heel raise, thereby reducing the tension of gastrocnemius. This maintains alignment of the body by preventing the otherwise necessary compensation of flexion at the hips to keep the centre of gravity within the base of support. Again there must be sufficient control of the quadriceps muscle group to stabilise the knee once forward from the hyperextended position.

Flexor spasticity of the lower limbs

This can severely impair or prevent an upright stance. Patients may stabilise using adduction and medial rotation of the hips, often with plantar flexion of the ankles. The consequence of this activity is usually that of increased extension at the lumbar and thoracic spine with retraction of the shoulders to generate sufficient anti-gravity control. Those with long-standing problems of flexor spasticity may walk in this way for many years. However, over time, the mechanical deficiencies of this means of ambulation may lead to joint damage and ultimately wheelchair dependence.

From a biomechanical viewpoint, early provision of KAFOs may be considered appropriate. However, maintenance of range of movement of the flexor muscle groups enables patients to use their extensor muscles more effectively and may prevent the need for such intervention. In this way, the compensations described above may be minimised.

Inevitably there are some patients with flexor spasticity of the lower limbs who have inadequate underlying extensor activity to maintain themselves upright against gravity without excessive use of trunk and head extension. In this instance, the patient must be given the choice of continuing to walk in the way described above, with the possible long-term consequences of muscle and joint problems, or to use KAFOs.

Patients with a more acute onset of flexor spasticity of the legs should be encouraged to use mechanical support to effect extension of the knees and to maximise recovery of the extensor muscle groups. The severity of spasticity will dictate the intervention. If the patient has severe flexor spasticity, mechanical support should be used with caution in that forcing the legs into extension may exacerbate the spasticity. Inhibitory techniques such as mobilisation of the trunk and pelvis and controlled gentle stretching of the affected muscle groups may prove effective in enabling the patient to accommodate to the support.

It is important that the patient is able to accept the support in that, if there is ongoing resistance, the flexor spasticity may manifest itself in other areas of the body. For example, if the knee is held rigidly in extension but the flexor spasticity persists, it may shunt into the hip flexors and abdominal muscle groups, preventing normal alignment of the body in standing.

Patients with paralysis or weakness of the lower limbs

Standing patients with insufficient extensor activity of the lower limbs has been discussed in Chapter 5. The use of various standing frames and standing the patient between two or more therapists relates to the unconscious or more severely disabled patient. Patients with persistent or progressive weakness may require a KAFO to enable them to become or remain ambulant. For example, a patient with a spinal cord lesion of the low thoracic or lumbar area and complete paralysis of the legs, requires full leg support to stand and walk using a four-point or swing-through gait (Bromley 1991).

There are various types of KAFO, which differ primarily in the material from which they are made and the locking mechanism of the knee. The KAFOs made from plastic materials are generally lighter in weight and are moulded to the contour of the leg. They terminate in a plastic foot piece which inserts into the patient's shoe. The metal KAFOs are not as close fitting and are therefore preferred where there is oedema or potential changes in muscle girth. A socket is inserted into the heel of the patient's shoe (Fig. 8.10).

For patients who hyperextend but are stable in flexion, with good quadriceps activity, a free knee joint with an extension stop is required. This allows for full range of movement at the knee joint throughout the gait cycle while preventing hyperextension of the joint.

If the knee is unstable in flexion, with inadequate quadriceps activity, the knee must be locked into extension to effect weight-bearing. There are two main types of locking mechanisms:

- manual, where the patient must lock and unlock the device by hand with the knee in the extended position

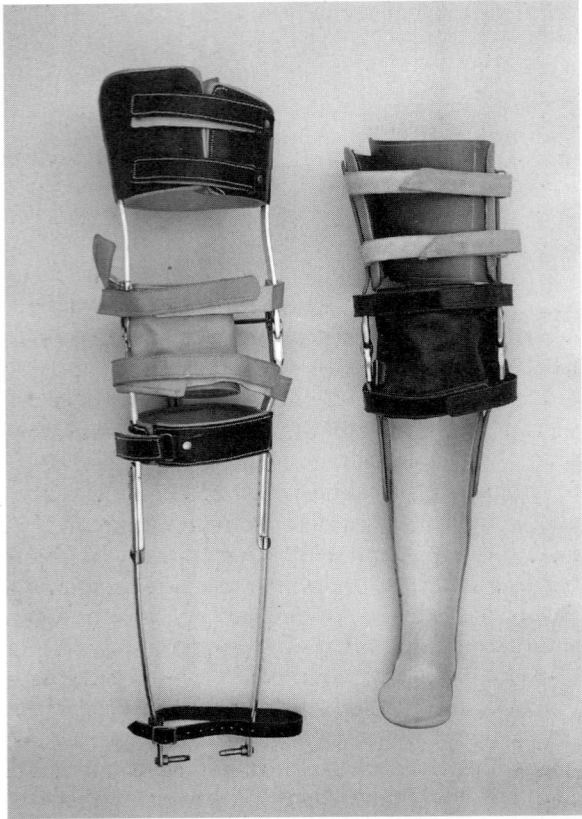

Figure 8.10 Knee–ankle–foot orthoses.

- semi-automatic, where the KAFO locks automatically by means of a spring device when the leg is fully extended but which requires manual release into flexion.

Determining factors in the choice of locking mechanism include hand function and the ease of knee extension.

SUMMARY

The orthoses described above are by no means exclusive. Patients with more extensive paralysis or movement impairment may require additional control extending above the hip. Examples of what may be considered 'walking systems' include the 'para-walker' (hip guidance orthosis) (Nene & Patrick 1990) and the reciprocal gait orthosis (Beckman 1987).

Temporary orthoses are useful in assessing their effect and patient tolerance and compliance before proceeding to a definitive orthosis. The patient must be fully involved in the assessment procedure. The most mechanically appropriate orthosis may, for some patients, be cosmetically unacceptable and it is essential to establish that the splint will be worn before embarking on what is a costly intervention.

LOWER LIMB CASTS

Various materials are available for use in casting. Plaster of Paris (POP) is often recommended as it moulds more readily to the contour of the limb (Sullivan et al 1988, Booth et al 1983). Glass fibre casting tape with polyurethane resin, hardens more quickly than POP and POP or other synthetic materials with a more rubberised texture may be used in conjunction with glass fibre strengthening. Two people are required to apply the cast; ideally a therapist to hold the limb in the optimum position and a technician or therapist experienced in the use of the chosen materials.

When making casts, a protective cover over the working area, aprons for the therapists applying the cast, *blunt-ended* scissors and a bowl of tepid water are required. Rubber gloves are essential when working with synthetic materials. A plaster saw must be readily available to remove any cast which encases a limb. Routine monitoring must be carried out to ensure that there are no pressure or circulatory problems. If there is any suspicion that the cast may be causing such problems, it must be removed immediately.

The use of glass fibre materials is described for each of the following casts.

Prophylactic casting of the foot and ankle

Patients with spasticity pulling the foot into plantar flexion and inversion are in danger of developing shortening of the posterior crural muscle group and of the Achilles tendon. This is a recognised complication following head injury where spasticity may become a dominant feature (Yarkony & Sahgal 1987, Kent et al 1990). The severity of the spasticity may be such as to produce shortening of the calf structures within days or even hours of onset. In this situation, the early use of casting to maintain the plantigrade position of the foot and ankle is recommended (Sullivan et al 1988, Conine et al 1990).

Ideally, the cast should be applied before the onset of spasticity, enabling the therapist to maintain the optimal position of the foot without force. However, not all patients develop spasticity and it is therefore important to establish criteria to identify those patients most likely to do so. The patient's score on the Glasgow Coma Scale (GCS) indicating the severity of injury is a determining factor, but even this measure does not predict which patients will develop severe spasticity. When a patient is weaned off ventilatory support and paralysing agents have been withdrawn, spasticity may become evident. Readministration of the paralysing agents provides an opportunity to apply the cast without contending with the spastic forces.

Application

The cast should be applied with the knee flexed to reduce the stretch on gastrocnemius and with the foot held in plantigrade position or in slight dorsiflexion. Providing the patient is medically stable, the cast should be used in conjunction with standing and it is therefore important to ensure that the angle is such as to permit the patient to stand in alignment. The medial arch of the foot should be supported and the cast moulded around the contour of the leg, particularly at the Achilles tendon to prevent movement within the cast.

The materials which are required for below-knee casts include:

- 2 mm felt padding or foam
- 7.5 cm or 10 cm stockinet
- under-cast padding
- 2 or 3 × 10 cm glass fibre bandages
- 1 slab (5 thicknesses) of glass fibre material (this is only required for additional reinforce-

ment if there is severe, or potentially severe spasticity)
- 1 wet crepe bandage.

The application of the cast is illustrated in Figure 8.11. The patient is in supine as, in the immediate aftermath of head injury, patients may be unable to be placed in an alternative position due to medical instability.

Felt padding is applied over the sole of the foot, the shaft of the tibia, the medial and lateral malleoli and across the metatarsal heads. Self-adhesive felt may be used but non-adhesive is preferred, particularly for those with sensitive skin. This is attached by means of non-allergenic tape.

A piece of stockinet is applied from the knee line to include and extend beyond the toes. A strip of felt padding is applied over the stockinet circumventing the leg just below the head of fibula.

Under-cast padding is applied from below the head of fibula, each turn overlapping the previous turn, extending to the metatarsophalangeal joints. Excessive padding is not recommended in that this allows for greater movement within the cast.

A 10 cm glass fibre bandage is soaked in the tepid water, gently squeezed and applied, without pressure, from below the fibula head to the metatarsal heads. Each turn of the bandage covers half of the preceding turn and a figure of eight is used around the ankle joint to ensure that the heel is covered.

The slab of glass fibre is positioned at the back of the leg, extending from below the fibula head to include and support the toes. The slab is cut at either side of the heel to provide a smooth contour. The stockinet is pulled back to be secured within the cast by the second glass fibre bandage. Throughout the application of the bandages and slab the therapist moulds the cast around the TA and under the medial arch. (If the full slab is not required, a slab of 5 thicknesses must be placed under the sole of the foot.)

A wet crepe bandage is applied to ensure lamination of the layers of glass fibre, with a

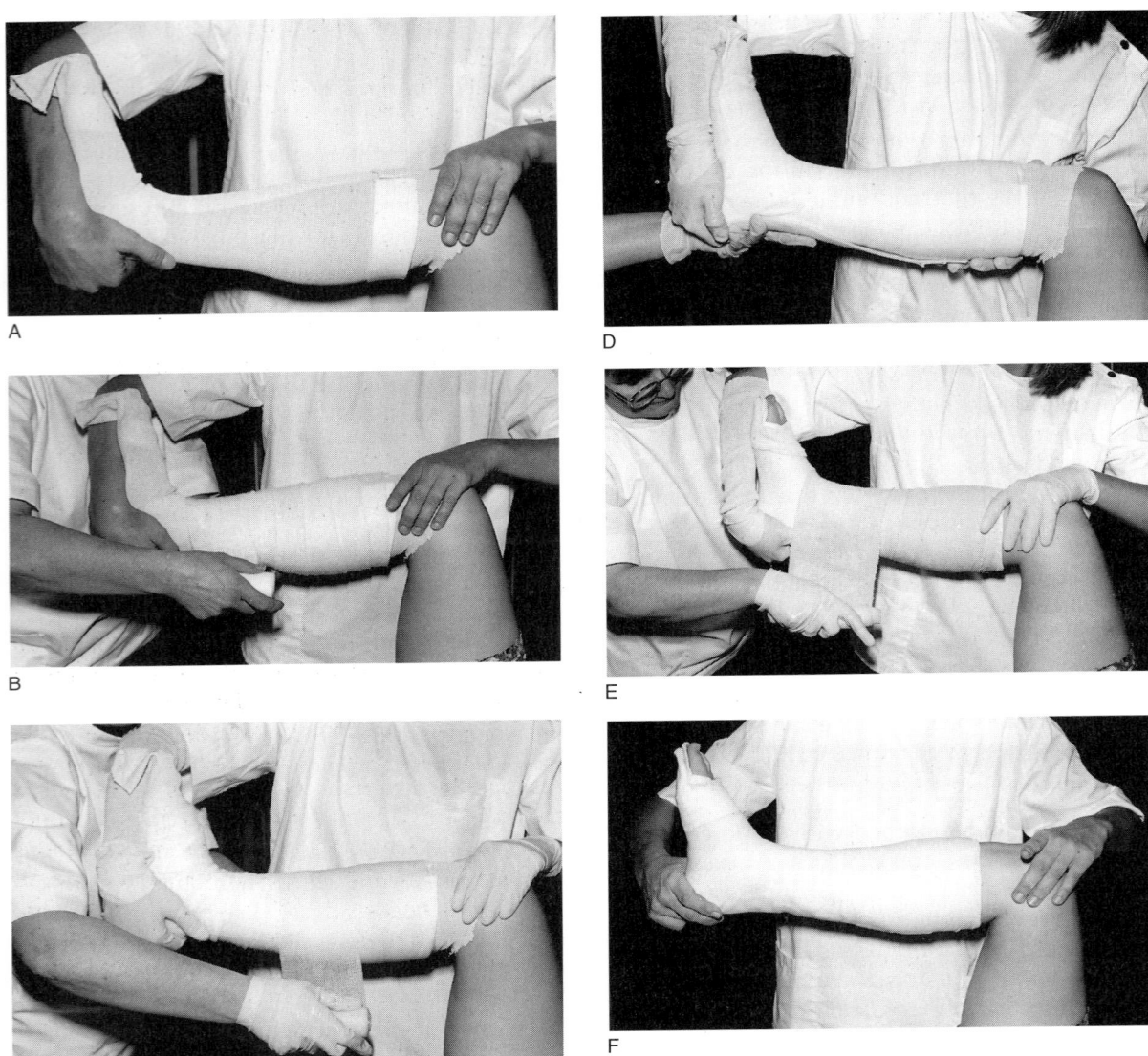

Figure 8.11 Below-knee cast: (A) holding position; (B) application of under-cast padding; (C) application of glass fibre bandage; (D) back slab extending the length of the cast to include the toes; (E) securing the cast with wet crepe bandage; (F) completed cast.

board placed under the foot to ensure a flat surface for subsequent weight-bearing.

Casting of the foot and ankle for patients with residual spasticity

This cast may also be of value when used for

patients with residual plantar flexor spasticity but without contracture. In this situation, the cast may be applied with the knee bent to 90 degrees and with the patient either in sitting with the foot supported on the floor or on a stool (Sullivan et al 1988) or in prone lying using a board (Moseley 1993). These positions allow for maximum dorsiflexion by stretching soleus while relieving pressure on the gastrocnemius component of the posterior crural muscle group.

Slight dorsiflexion is often desirable, particularly if the patient is ambulant. The dorsiflexed position may alter the gait pattern in that the patient requires less effort to clear the foot during swing phase. Glass fibre is the material of choice when used for patients with residual spasticity. POP takes a minimum of 36 hours to harden sufficiently for weight-bearing, during which time the pressure exerted by the spasticity may weaken the cast. The majority of glass fibre materials are ready for weight-bearing approximately 30 minutes after application and are also significantly lighter than POP.

Serial casting of the foot and ankle

Where there is established shortening of the posterior crural muscle group and of the Achilles tendon, serial casting may be considered. The cast may be applied with the patient either in sitting, as described above, or in prone with the knee flexed to 90 degrees. The calf structures are stretched to their maximum range. If plantigrade is not achievable, the heel is built up to ensure even weight-bearing over the full surface of the foot. Care must be taken to ensure that the force applied to gain the maximum range at the ankle does not create excessive strain over the medial arch of the foot.

The cast should be changed approximately every 7 to 10 days. The foot and ankle are mobilised and then recast to maintain any further increase in range. If no increase in range is obtained after three applications, it is most unlikely that any further casting will be of benefit. Surgery may then be necessary to regain the plantigrade position.

Back slabs to support the lower limbs in extension

The advantages and disadvantages of back slabs to secure the knees in extension have been discussed in Chapter 5 in relation to patients with varying levels of disability. They may be used for patients with either increased flexor or extensor tone or for those with inadequate extensor activity to maintain the legs in extension. They are invariably a temporary measure and may be used:

- to determine the patient's ability to utilise this support in a functional way prior to supplying more permanent KAFOs.
- to achieve a more normal alignment in standing with improved pelvic, trunk and head control
- to stimulate extensor activity of the hips
- to maintain or regain range of movement of the hip flexors
- to attain a plantigrade position of the foot by controlling the position of the knees and mobilising the patient over the base of support.

Application

The patient is positioned in prone lying with the feet extending over the end of the bed. This is to ensure that the bulk of the posterior crural muscle group is arranged similarly to when the patient is standing. If the feet are in plantar flexion, the contour of the leg is significantly altered. The legs are positioned in neutral in respect of medial or lateral rotation. For those patients with complete flaccid paralysis, a small bandage may need to be positioned under the ankle to prevent hyperextension of the knee. The back slab extends from the line of the hip joint to at least 2 cm above the malleoli. The slab provides a shell which extends laterally to encompass just less than 180 degrees of the leg circumference to enable the splint to be put on and taken off.

The materials which are required for back slabs include:

- 15 cm stockinet
- 4 × 15 cm glass fibre bandages arranged to a pre-made paper template of the leg
- 2 wet crepe bandages
- zinc oxide tape.

The application of back slabs is illustrated in Figure 8.12.

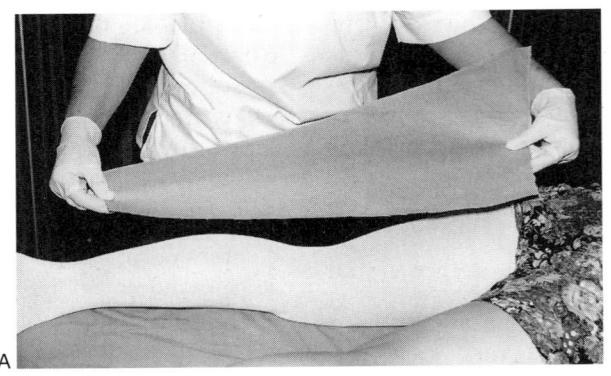

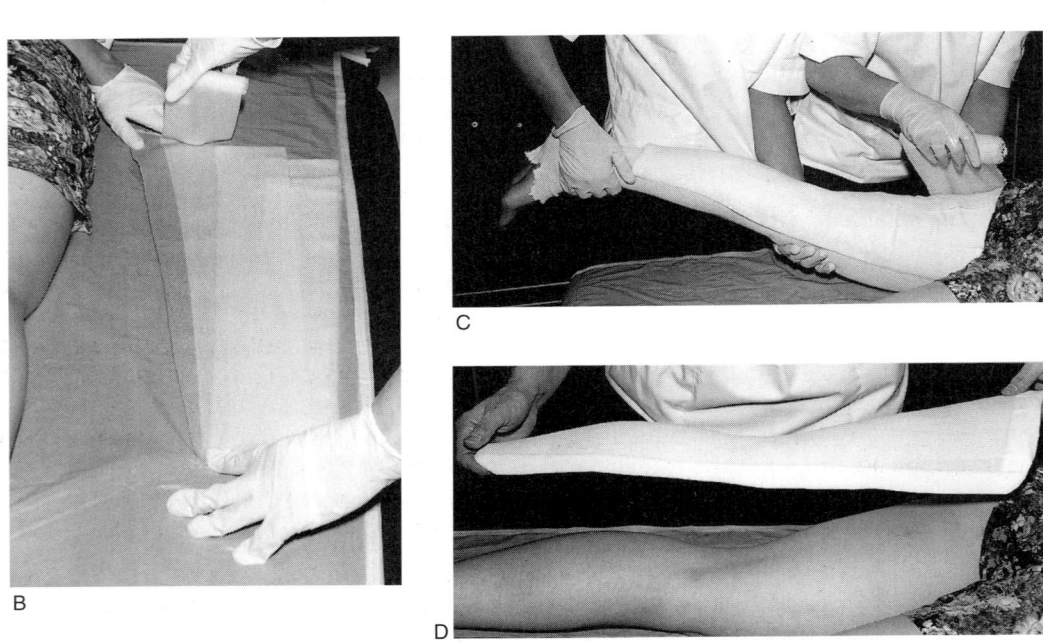

Figure 8.12 Application of back slab: (A) paper template cut to shape of leg; (B) glass fibre bandages arranged to shape of template; (C) back slab secured by means of wet crepe bandage; (D) completed back slab.

The stockinet extends from above the line of the hip joint to below the heel.

The glass fibre slab is applied following immersion in the water and moulded around the contour of the leg.

The material is trimmed while still wet and malleable to follow the line of the hip joint and to ensure a uniform edge above the malleoli.

The wet crepe bandages are applied to laminate the material and to secure the slab in place. The glass fibre hardens sufficiently to remove the splint after 5 minutes.

Rough edges are sanded down and zinc oxide tape applied around the borders of the splint to provide greater comfort. The splint may be used within 30 minutes of being made.

The important aspects of the back slab are that:

• It extends up to and follows the line of the hip joint to enable full extension of the hip with a slight posterior tilt of the pelvis. This allows for full range of movement of the iliopsoas muscle and of the iliofemoral ligament.

- It finishes at least 2 cm above the malleoli to prevent pressure over these bony prominences.
- It maintains the knee in full, but not hyper-, extension.

Serial casting to correct knee flexion deformity

This has been advocated as a means of regaining range of movement at the knee (Booth et al 1983, Davies 1994). A POP or glass fibre cylinder is applied with the leg held in the maximum degree of extension. It extends from the line of the hip joint to at least 2 cm above the malleoli. The cylinder is removed after approximately 1 week to 10 days and immediately reapplied, where possible, with an increased range of extension.

The rationale for this method of splinting is twofold:

1. If the cause of the loss of range is flexor spasticity, by maintaining the limb in the maximum available range of extension, the flexor spasticity may be reduced through prolonged stretching. This enables an increased range of movement when the splint is changed.
2. If the limb is contracted into flexion with residual changes in the property of the muscles, serial casting may regain range within the contracted structures by applying a prolonged stretch.

Drop-out casting

This provides a more dynamic and less forceful means of regaining range of movement. The leg is extended to its maximum range and the cylinder then applied with the knee 5 or 10 degrees less than the full available range. This reduces the stress on the spastic flexors or on the contracted structures. Once the cylinder has hardened, a section of the cast is cut away as illustrated in Figure 8.13D which, while preventing further flexion, allows for increased range into extension. For those patients with less

than a 30 degree flexor contracture, this form of splinting may be used in conjunction with standing, the lower portion of the splint moving away from the calf as the patient achieves a more upright position.

This type of cast is only effective if the available range is greater than 60 degrees (Booth et al 1983). If the knee cannot be extended to an angle of greater than 60 degrees, the pressure over the cut-out section above the patella is too extreme and sores may ensue. For this reason serial casts are advocated until such time as 60 degrees is attainable.

Application

The application of the cylinder is similar for both serial and the drop-out casts. The patient is positioned in supine with the physiotherapist holding the foot and applying steady traction to obtain the maximum range of knee extension. Rotation at the hip is controlled to obtain a neutral position. For patients with severe spasticity or contracture, two therapists may be required to control this position of the leg, one applying pressure from the foot and the other controlling from the hip to obtain neutral alignment.

The materials which are required for a long leg cylinder include:

- 15 cm stockinet
- 2 or 3 × 15 cm bandages of under-cast padding depending on the length and size of the leg
- 2 or 3 × 15 cm glass fibre bandages
- 1 slab (5 thicknesses) of glass fibre material extending over the posterior surface of the leg (this is only required if there is severe, or potentially severe spasticity)
- strip of 2 mm sticky-backed felt
- 2 wet crepe bandages
- zinc oxide tape.

The method of application is illustrated in Figure 8.13.

The stockinet extends above the line of the hip joint to below the malleoli.

The under-cast padding is applied to cover the length of the leg, each turn of the bandage

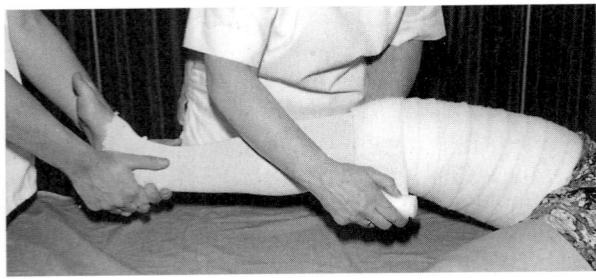

A

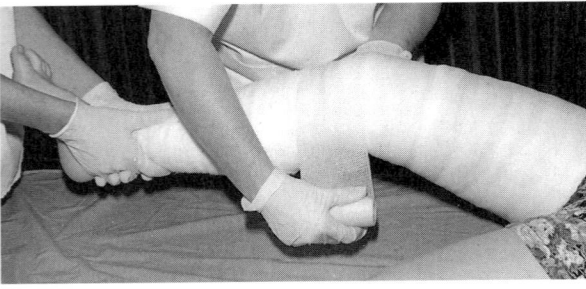

B

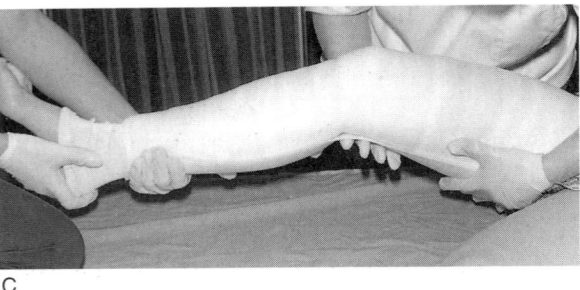

C

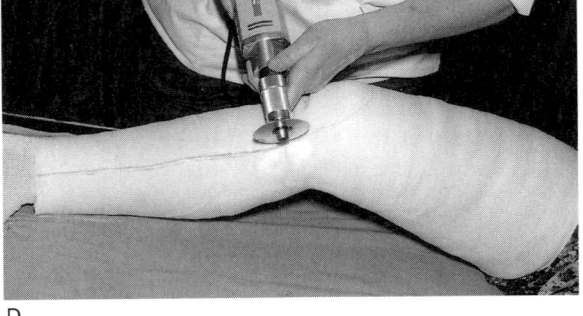

D

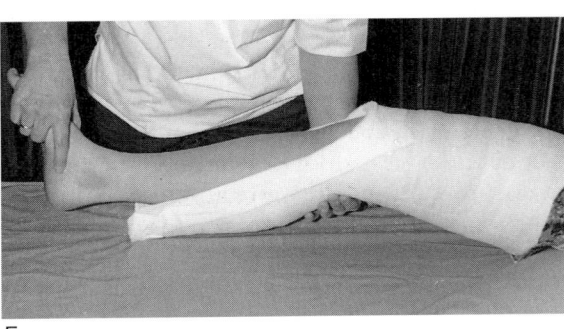

E

Figure 8.13 Drop-out cast for leg: (A) application of under-cast padding; (B) application of glass fibre bandage; (C) back slab positioned over posterior aspect of leg; ((D) plaster saw used to remove section over anterior aspect of tibia; (E) completed cast.

covering half the width of the preceding one, giving two thicknesses throughout. Excessive padding is not recommended as this allows for excessive movement within the cast.

One 15 cm glass fibre bandage is soaked in water and applied, without pressure, from as high up the leg as possible, to at least 2 cm above the malleoli (two bandages may be required to extend the length of a longer leg).

The slab of glass fibre material is positioned on the back of the leg extending from as near to the line of the hip joint as possible to at least 2 cm above the malleoli. This is secured in place by the second glass fibre bandage which also secures the stockinet and pad-

ding over the upper and lower borders of the cast. With drop-out casts, the lower border is not secured until removal of the front section.

The wet crepe bandages are applied over the cast to ensure lamination of the material.

Once the cast has hardened, the front section over the tibia, extending laterally from each malleolus to above the patella, is cut away using the plaster saw.

The stockinet and padding are cut and secured with zinc oxide tape around the border of the cut-out section. The 2 mm sticky-backed felt is applied to the border of the cast above the patella.

Summary

There are many different types of splints and orthoses which may be used to obtain the desired support or maintenance of range of movement of a limb. New materials are continually being developed which provide alternative options. The rubberised texture of the 3M softcast bandages reinforced with glass fibre is an example of these new developments. The soft cast can be cut with scissors to remove the splint and then rivets attached to enable its re-application (Fig. 8.14). The rigidity of this splint is comparable to those made from glass fibre, fully encasing the limb, but is not dependent on a plaster saw for removal. This type of splint is of particular value when nursing or medical staff are concerned about the possibility of pressure sores developing within the cast.

POP has long been the casting material of choice for patients with neurological dysfunction. Sullivan et al (1988) consider plaster to be the preferred material in that 'it is strong, inexpensive, easily moulded, reinforced or repaired once dry, and does not splinter leaving sharp edges, as may occur with fibre glass'. However, glass fibre and other synthetic materials, are strong, slightly more expensive than POP (on average half the quantity of glass fibre is required to that of POP), easily moulded, rarely need reinforcement, and sharp edges may be avoided with the appropriate use of padding. An additional advantage of the glass fibre materials is that there is considerably less mess and therefore reduced time spent clearing up.

In our opinion, glass fibre and other synthetic materials have developed to such an extent that they are now the material of choice when casting patients with neurological dysfunction.

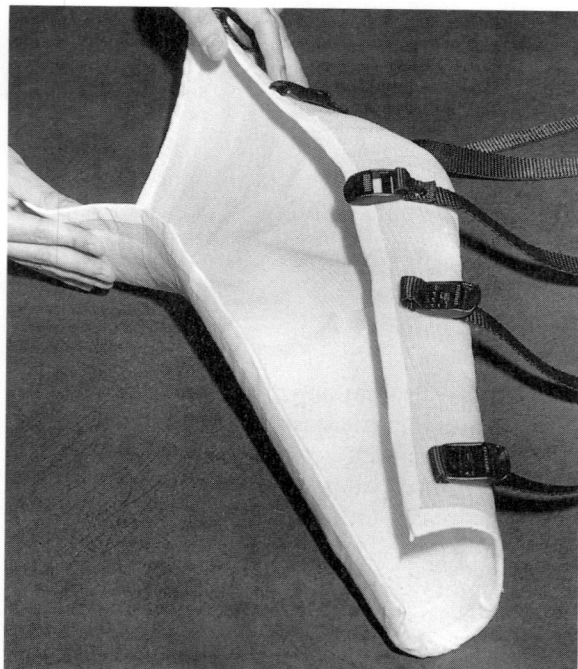

Figure 8.14   Softcast long leg cylinder.

UPPER LIMB ORTHOSES

Upper limb supports or casts may be of value in the management and treatment of upper limb dysfunction, particularly in improving joint alignment and in preventing trauma. This section considers different types of splints and materials which may prove effective in achieving these objectives.

SHOULDER SUPPORTS

The mechanics of the shoulder joint and subsequent problems which may arise following neurological impairment have been discussed in previous chapters. This section considers the different supports which may prove of benefit to patients where there is either insufficient tone or increased tone affecting the shoulder musculature.

Subluxation of the shoulder is a not uncommon sequela to changes of tone affecting the muscles that provide stability around the shoulder joint (Williams et al 1988, Bobath 1990, Davies 1985). Patients with a complete brachial plexus lesion demonstrate this complication in the extreme whereas those with less severe weakness or spasticity retain some, if inadequate, control. The different types of support which are available for the shoulder include:

- the collar and cuff
- cuff support
- the abduction roll or wedge
- support using pillows or a tray/table.

The collar and cuff

This may be used to support the arm at the elbow and the hand. It passes around the shoulder as opposed to round the neck and is fitted so as to maintain alignment of the glenohumeral joint with the elbow at 90 degrees or slightly less.

Advantages

1. This provides full support for the limb and therefore protects against overstretching of the structures around the shoulder.

2. The hand is supported level with the elbow and there is therefore less likelihood of the limb swelling.

Disadvantages

1. The fully supported, flexed position discourages active movement and, for those patients with increased tone, this posturing tends to reinforce the spastic flexor pattern.

2. This positioning does not allow for any balance response of the upper limb and therefore affects postural adjustments within the trunk.

3. Patients with sensory problems or neglect of the affected side have less stimulation to use the arm if it is fully supported.

Cuff support

This is advocated particularly in the management of patients with hemiplegia where the disadvantages of the collar and cuff are most relevant (Bobath 1990, Williams et al 1988). This is attached around the upper arm and attached by means of a sheepskin-lined strap in a figure of eight around the other shoulder (Fig. 8.15). The weak or flaccid arm tends to hang in

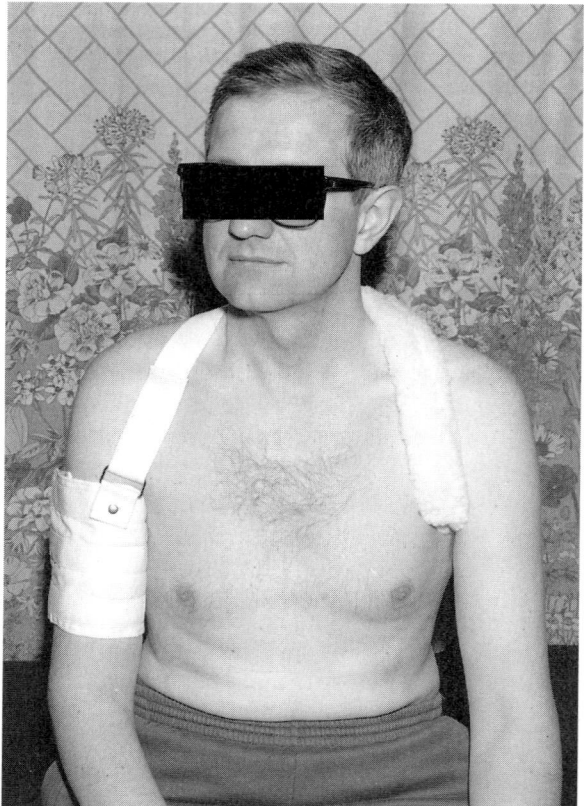

Figure 8.15 Cuff support.

adduction and medial rotation and the spastic limb is often pulled into this position. For this reason, the strap should be secured anteriorly to encourage lateral rotation.

Advantages

1. Williams et al (1988) noted a significant reduction in the degree of inferior subluxation. However, there is some debate in clinical practice as to whether the cuff does in fact achieve this end.

2. The support around the upper arm does not interfere with distal movements and potential return of active movement.

3. The arm is able to respond more appropriately to postural adjustments occurring in the trunk and in the maintenance of balance.

4. The patient and all personnel involved in the care of the patient are constantly reminded that this is a vulnerable joint.

Disadvantages

1. The flaccid arm hangs dependently by the side and is prone to swelling.
2. It is difficult for the patient to apply this support unaided.

The abduction roll or wedge

This is used for patients with increased tone and was first advocated by Bobath (1978). Following a CVA, the pattern of spasticity affecting the upper limb is usually one of predominant flexion (Rothwell 1994). The roll/wedge is placed in the axilla, attached by means of a strap passing across the back and around the opposite shoulder in a figure of eight (Fig. 8.16). The size of the roll/wedge is determined by the severity of spasticity.

Advantages

1. The bulk afforded by the roll/wedge brings the arm away from the body. This places the arm in a position of slight abduction, thereby

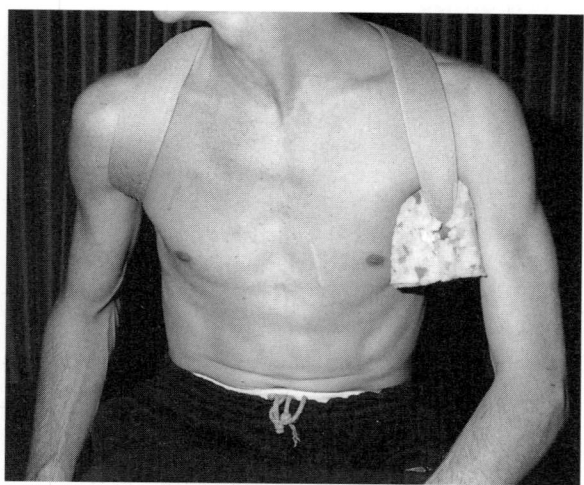

Figure 8.16 Abduction roll/wedge.

inhibiting the dominance of adduction and medial rotation.

2. Placing the roll/wedge in the axilla and removal of it ensure that the upper limb is moved away from the body on a regular basis and thus improves hygiene. All personnel involved in this procedure should be trained to handle the limb with care to prevent traumatising the joint.

Disadvantages

1. Positioning of the arm in slight abduction may create greater mechanical instability due to the effect on the locking mechanism (see Ch. 5).
2. Movement of the arm into abduction by untrained personnel may traumatise this vulnerable joint.
3. It is difficult for the patient to position the roll independently.

Support using pillows or a tray/table

The chair-bound patient may have the shoulder joint supported by means of pillows or resting the arms forwards on a table or on a tray attached to the wheelchair. Attention must be paid to the arrangement of the pillows and the alignment of the shoulder girdle, particularly in terms of protraction/retraction. Many patients utilise this means of support, but in some instances, the pillows are inappropriately positioned and serve more as 'leg warmers' than as support and protection for the shoulder joint.

ELBOW CASTS

Contracture of the elbow joint is a not uncommon sequela of increased tone affecting the flexor muscle groups. Flexor spasticity is the most prevalent synergy following CVA and is frequently observed in patients following traumatic brain injury or disease. Other patients who are susceptible to flexor contracture of the elbow joint are those with cervical cord lesions where biceps is unopposed by triceps. Various types of splints or casts made from different materials may be utilised to prevent or correct these contractures.

Serial and drop-out casting

This is similar in function to that described for the lower limb. The cast extends the length of the arm from just below the axilla to include the wrist and hand up to the palmar crease. The lower border may be extended to form a platform to maintain the fingers in extension, and a thumb spica may be used to maintain its position. The arm is extended to 5 or 10 degrees less than the maximum available range of elbow extension with the forearm in neutral. The position of the wrist is determined by the degree of flexion or extension and ulnar deviation. For the drop-out cast, the section over triceps is cut away to allow for extension.

Application

The cast is applied with the patient in supine or in sitting depending upon the medical condition and positional effects on tone. Glass fibre material is again preferred due to its lighter weight and quick setting properties.

The materials which are required for an arm cylinder include:

- 7.5 cm stockinet
- 1 or 2 × 7.5 cm bandage of under-cast padding
- 2 or 3 × 7.5 cm glass fibre bandages
- 1 × 7.5 cm slab (3 thicknesses) glass fibre material (this is only required for additional reinforcement if there is severe, or potentially severe, spasticity)
- 1 wet crepe bandage
- 2 mm felt padding
- zinc oxide tape.

The method of application is illustrated in Figure 8.17.

The stockinet extends from the acromion process to below the metacarpal heads. The stockinet is cut to free the thumb. Felt padding is applied over the ulnar styloid and around the base of the thumb.

The under-cast padding is applied to cover the length of the arm, each turn of the bandage covering half of the preceding one. Excessive padding is not recommended as this allows for movement within the cast.

A glass fibre bandage is soaked in water and applied, without pressure, from just below the axilla to include the wrist. The slab is placed over the flexor aspect of the arm and secured in place by the remaining bandage. Care must be taken to ensure that the thumb is free and that the splint allows for flexion of the metacarpal heads. The stockinet and padding should also be secured over the upper and lower borders of the cast unless the cast is to be made into a drop-out in which case only the hand section is secured.

The wet crepe bandage is applied over the cast to laminate the materials.

Once the cast has hardened (after 10 minutes), the section over the triceps muscle extending to below the olecranon process is removed, using the plaster saw.

The stockinet and padding are cut and secured with zinc oxide tape around the border of the cut-out section.

Some patients with severe flexor spasticity affecting the arm may have relatively low tone proximally at the shoulder. For this reason, *POP is not recommended for serial or drop-out casts of the upper limb* as it tends to be very heavy. Patients are usually encouraged to stand and, with these splints, the excessive weight applied to the arm may contribute to subluxation of the shoulder.

Back slabs

These may be made out of either thermoplastic, glass fibre material or POP. When using either glass fibre or POP it is best to make a full cylinder and then bivalve the cast, securing it in place by means of crepe bandages. The combination of 3M softcast and glass fibre as described on page 179 provides a further option.

These slabs are of particular value for patients with unopposed muscle activity such as those with cervical cord lesions. If there is a danger of biceps becoming shortened, these splints may be used at night allowing functional use by day.

Patients with severe and persistent spasticity may find it difficult to accommodate to the back slab and generally respond better to the full cylinder or drop-out cast.

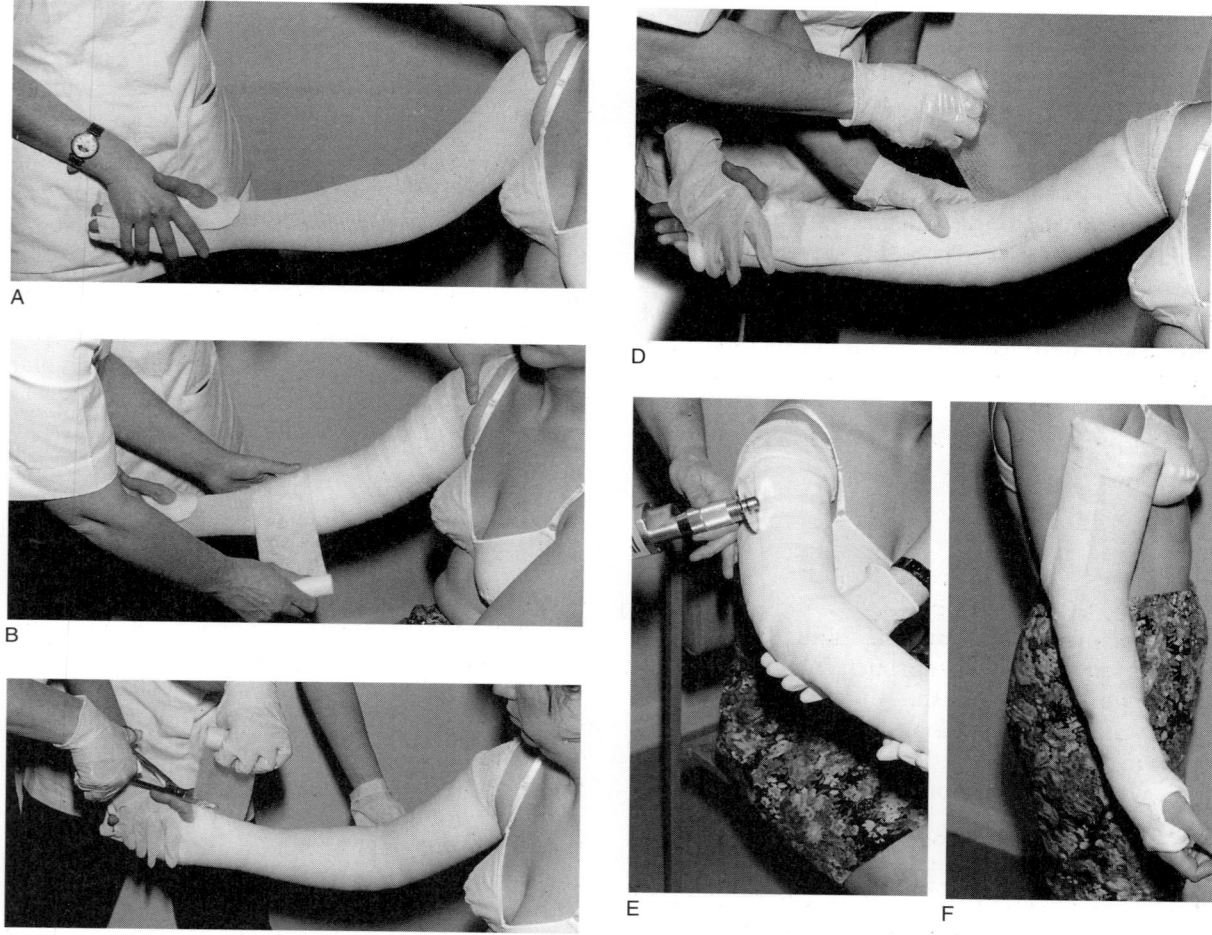

Figure 8.17   Drop-out cast for elbow: (A) holding position; (B) application of under-cast padding; (C) application of glass fibre bandage – the bandage is partially cut to ensure freedom of movement of the thumb; (D) back slab secured with glass fibre bandage; (E) plaster saw used to remove section over triceps; (F) completed cast.

Myositis ossificans or heterotopic ossification is a complication which may affect various soft tissues and joints of the body, particularly following head injury (Garland & Keenan 1983). The elbow joint is often affected, and splinting for these patients should be used with caution. Forcing of range may lead to an increase in the severity of symptoms and must be avoided. For this reason the drop-out cast is preferred in that

this does not need to be applied with the arm in its maximally extended position.

THE WRIST AND HAND

There are many different types of splints which may be used to maintain or improve hand function. This section includes a selection of splints or casts which may be used for patients with spasticity and resting splints for patients with hypotonus.

Splinting for the spastic wrist and hand

Splinting patients with hand dysfunction as a result of spasticity remains a controversial treatment technique because of the paucity of research and contradictory results from investigations (Langlois et al 1989). The types of splints which are advocated for the treatment of spasticity include:

- the volar splint
- the dorsal splint
- the finger spreader
- the cone.

The volar splint

This is one of the earliest splint designs that attempted to reduce spasticity by applying a prolonged stretch to the affected musculature. It attaches over the flexor aspect of the forearm and fingers (Fig. 8.18). It is designed to maintain the wrist in extension with slight flexion of the interphalangeal joints and flexion of the metacarpophalangeal joints to approximately 80 degrees. The thumb is positioned in abduction.

If the patient is able to accommodate to this position, this splint may be appropriate in controlling spasticity. However, if there is established shortening of the wrist and hand structures following prolonged spasticity, the patient may resist the splint, reacting against the flexor contact.

The dorsal splint

This splint is designed to facilitate the extensor musculature of the forearm, through cutaneous stimulation of the dorsal aspect, and inhibit the flexor muscles. Consequently, the degree of flexor spasticity is reduced (Louis 1962). However, it has a finger platform which, with the straps to secure the splint to the forearm, also provides cutaneous stimulation to the flexor aspect (Fig. 8.19).

The aim of the splint is to maintain or regain range of movement as described with the volar splint. Various thermoplastic materials are used in the manufacture of both the volar and dorsal splints.

The finger spreader

The use of a foam finger spreader was advocated by Bobath (1978) as a means of effecting inhibition of finger flexion and adduction and thereby facilitating the extensor muscles. It was hypothesised that, as part of a reflex inhibiting pattern, this may decrease spasticity proximally. Doubilet & Polkow (1977) adapted this spreader into a more durable form using a low-temperature bioplastic material, and Snook (1979) incorporated the principle of finger abduction with extension of the wrist and interphalangeal joints into a dorsal platform (Fig. 8.20).

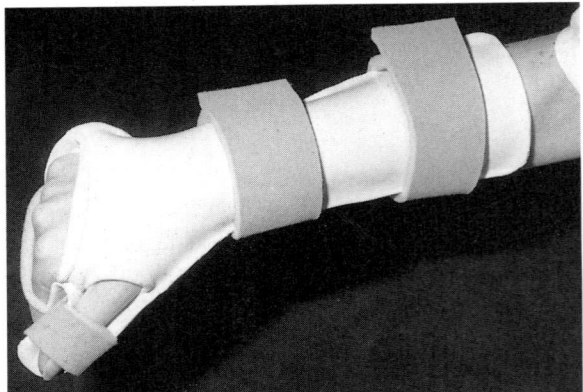

Figure 8.19 Dorsal splint.

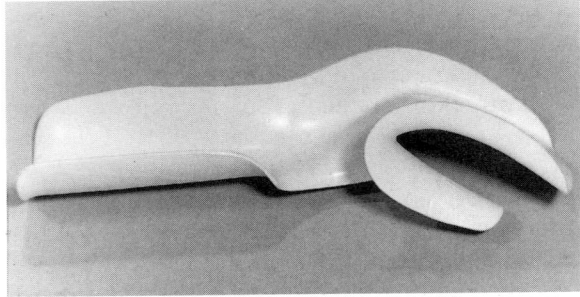

Figure 8.18 Volar splint.

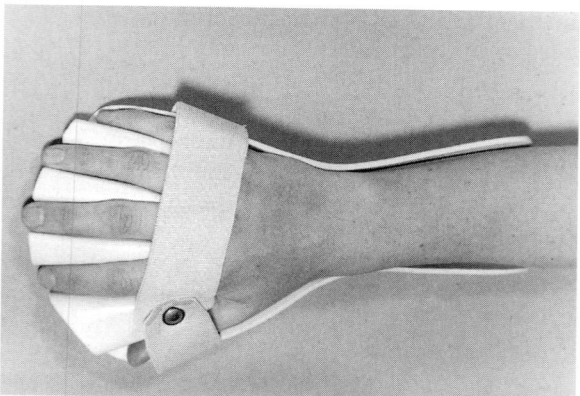

Figure 8.20 Finger spreader.

The latter modifications, using more rigid materials, deviate from the dynamic principles of the foam spreader but each have demonstrated a decrease in flexor tone (Doubilet & Polkow 1977, McPherson 1981).

The cone

The use of a firm cone placed in the palm of the hand was first introduced by Rood (1954). The constant pressure over the full flexor surface was believed to be inhibitory to the flexor muscles (Stockmeyer 1967). This principle has more recently been incorporated into a modified volar splint with cone attachment (Fig. 8.21).

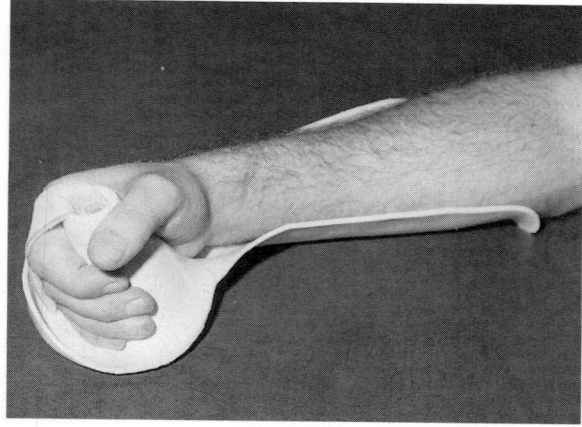

Figure 8.21 Cone/volar splint.

These are some examples of splints which may be used in the management of spasticity affecting the hand. Modifications to each of these designs continue to be developed. In clinical practice, it is often a case of trial and error to determine the most effective splint for the management of spasticity of the hand. Investigations to date, however, do not indicate for whom hand splints may produce beneficial effects in reducing or limiting the effects of spasticity (Langlois et al 1989).

Splinting for the hypotonic wrist and hand

Flaccid paralysis of the wrist and hand may result from neurological impairments such as cervical cord damage, brachial plexus lesions or neuromuscular disorders. Passive movements of the affected joints to maintain full range of movement should be instigated, but optimal positioning during the remaining time is of paramount importance in preventing shortening of soft tissue structures.

Splinting is often advocated as part of treatment as a means of maintaining range of movement. It tends to be less controversial than when used for patients with spasticity, and application is generally easier. However, although there is less danger of contracture than when there is stereotyped spastic posturing, splinting is often necessary to prevent loss of range of muscles and joints through enforced immobility. Four different forms of splinting will be discussed:

- the volar resting splint
- the boxing glove splint
- taping to maintain appropriate positioning of the fingers where the patient is, or will be, dependent on a tenodesis grip
- thumb opposition splint.

The volar resting splint

This splint design has been described above in the management of the spastic wrist and hand. The wrist and fingers are positioned in what is often termed a functional position. The web space between the thumb and index finger must be preserved with the thumb in abduction. It may be advisable to alternate the different forms of splintage, using the volar resting splint for 4 hours and then applying a boxing glove splint for the following 4 hours. In this way the position of the wrist and hand is constantly altered, thereby reducing the risk of shortening of soft tissue.

The boxing glove splint

This splint was initially designed by Cheshire (Cheshire & Rowe 1970/71) and was advocated by Bromley (1991) for the prevention of swelling and the maintenance of a good functional position for patients following cervical cord lesions. Cheshire considered that swelling could be prevented if the collateral ligaments of the metacarpophalangeal joints are kept at their maximum tension, i.e. when the joints are kept in 90 degrees flexion. The proximal interphalangeal joints should be held in 90 degrees flexion with the distal interphalangeal joints extended (Fig. 8.22).

In some older patients following cervical cord injury, oedema followed by contracture of the metacarpophalangeal and interphalangeal joints occurs in spite of regular and intensive treatment. The joints often resemble rheumatoid arthritic joints and are red, shiny and swollen (Bromley 1991). The development of oedema is thought to be due to impairment of vasomotor control but the aetiology of this hand condition is still obscure.

A modification of the boxing glove splint is to use a crepe bandage placed in the palm of the hand. This is only recommended if the wrist extensors are intact or in conjunction with a wrist cock-up splint.

Taping

This is the current method of choice at the National Spinal Injuries Centre, Stoke Mandeville Hospital, for both reducing oedema and developing a tenodesis grip for patients with a C6 cervical cord lesion (Curtin 1993). The positioning of the fingers is as with the boxing glove splint. Taping is usually instigated overnight, allowing the patients to use the hands functionally by day. It is often used in conjunction with a wrist support to obtain the optimum position for functional use.

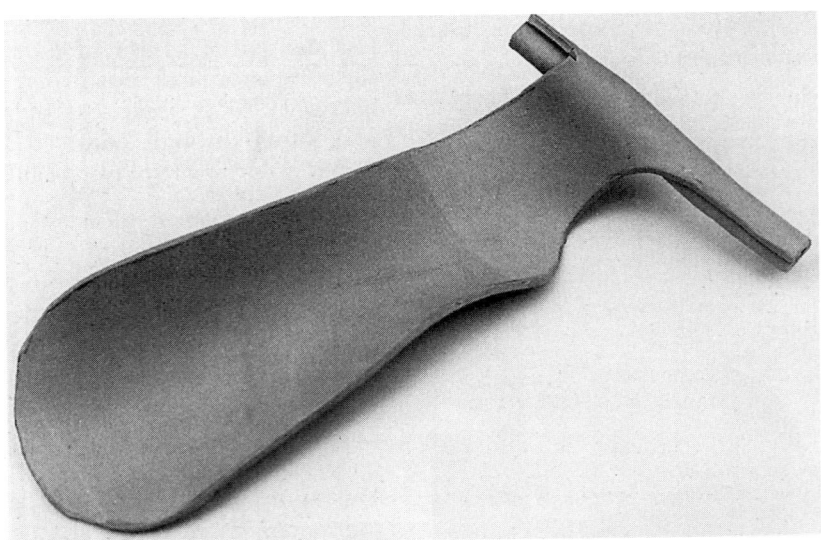

Figure 8.22 Unpadded cock-up support for the boxing glove splint (reproduced from Bromley 1991 with kind permission).

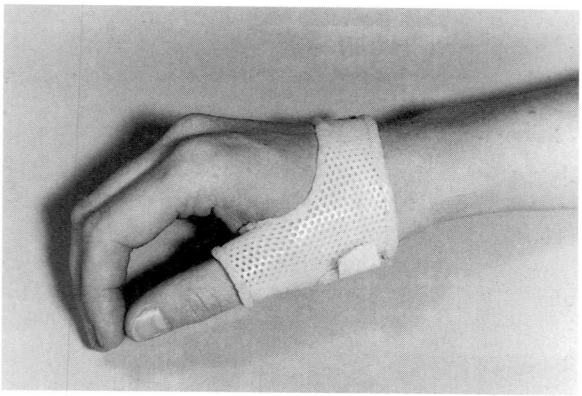

Figure 8.23   Thumb opposition splint.

Thumb opposition splint

This splint is of value for patients with weakness of the intrinsic hand musculature. The thumb opposition splint or thumb post may be used to maintain the thumb in opposition, thereby allowing a pincer grip with the index finger (Fig. 8.23).

Patients with weakness or paralysis of the intrinsic hand musculature resort to gross hand function using finger flexion as opposed to opposition. The use of the thumb opposition

splint enables more appropriate and functional use of the hand, thereby preventing deformity associated with dominant flexor activity.

Hand splinting is a very specialised area of treatment. The splints described above are only a small selection of those which may be utilised in the management of the many and varied hand deformities which may arise as a result of neurological damage. It is often the occupational therapists who have greater experience and in-depth knowledge of available materials for the management of the neurological hand. Their advice and assistance is of great benefit in determining the most appropriate intervention.

SUMMARY

The use of orthoses and casts can prove beneficial in the management of patients with neurological dysfunction. However, this is a complex speciality and, in order to avoid adverse effects, advice should be sought from staff experienced in this field. When casting, the therapist must be familiar with the chosen materials and practice is recommended on normal subjects prior to attempting this intervention on patients.

REFERENCES

Beckman J 1987 The Louisiana State University reciprocating gait orthosis. Physiotherapy 73(8): 386–392

Bobath B 1978 Adult hemiplegia: evaluation and treatment. 2nd edn. Heinemann Medical Books, London

Bobath B 1990 Adult hemiplegia: evaluation and treatment, 3rd edn. Heinemann Medical Books, London

Booth B J, Doyle M, Montgomery J 1983 Serial casting for the management of spasticity in the head-injured adult. Physical Therapy 63(12): 1960–1966

Bromley I 1991 Tetraplegia and paraplegia: a guide for physiotherapists, 4th edn. Churchill Livingstone, Edinburgh

Cheshire D J E, Rowe G 1970/71 The prevention of deformity in the severely paralysed hand. Paraplegia 8: 48–56

Conine T, Sullivan T, Mackie T, Goodman M 1990 Effect of serial casting for the prevention of equinus in patients with acute head injury. Archives of Physical Medicine and Rehabilitation 71(5): 310–312

Curtin M 1993 The management of the C6 quadriplegic patient's hand. British Journal of Occupational Therapy 56(12): 455

Cusick B D 1988 Splints and casts: managing foot deformity in children with neuromotor disorders. Physical Therapy 68(12): 1903–1912

Davies P M 1985 Steps to follow: a guide to the treatment of adult hemiplegia. Springer-Verlag, Berlin

Davies P M 1994 Starting again. Springer-Verlag, London

Doubilet L, Polkow L 1977 Theory and design of a finger abduction splint for the spastic hand. American Journal of Occupational Therapy 32: 320–322

Fyfe N, Goodwill J, Hoyle E, Sandles L 1993 Orthoses, mobility and environmental control systems. In: Greenwood R, Barnes M P, McMillan T M, Ward C D (eds) Neurological rehabilitation. Churchill Livingstone, London

Galley P M, Forster A L 1987 Human movement: an introductory text for physiotherapy students, 2nd edn. Churchill Livingstone, London

Garland D E, Keenan M-A E 1983 Orthopaedic strategies in the management of the adult head-injured patient. Physical Therapy 63(12): 2004–2009

Goldspink G, Williams P 1990 Muscle fibre and connective tissue changes associated with use and disuse. In: Ada L,

Canning C (eds) Key issues in neurological physiotherapy: physiotherapy foundations for practice. Butterworth-Heinemann, Oxford

Kent H, Hershler C, Conine T A, Hershler R 1990 Case control study of lower extremity serial casting in adult patients with head injury. Physiotherapy Canada 42(4): 189–191

Langlois S, MacKinnon J, Pederson L 1989 Hand splints and cerebral spasticity: a review of the literature. Canadian Journal of Occupational Therapy 56(3): 113–119

Louis W 1962 Hand splinting: effect on the afferent system. American Journal of Occupational Therapy 16: 143–145

McPherson J 1981 Objective evaluation of a splint design to reduce hypertonicity. American Journal of Occupational Therapy 35: 189–194

Moseley A M 1993 The effect of a regimen of casting and prolonged stretching on passive ankle dorsiflexion in traumatic head-injured adults. Physiotherapy Theory and Practice 9(4): 215–221

Nene A V, Patrick J H 1990 Energy cost of paraplegic locomotion using the Parawalker–electrical stimulation 'hybrid orthosis'. Archives of Physical Medicine and Rehabilitation 71: 116–120

Rood M 1954 Neurophysiological reactions as a basis for physical therapy. Physical Therapy Review 34: 444–449

Rose G 1986 Orthotics: principles and practice. Heinemann, London

Rose G K, Butler P, Stallard J 1982 Gait: principles, biomechanics and assessment. Orlau Publishing, Oswestry

Rothwell J 1994 Control of human voluntary movement, 2nd edn. Chapman & Hall, London

Saunders J B, Inman V T, Eberhart H D 1953 The major determinants in normal and pathological gait. Journal of Bone and Joint Surgery 35A(3): 543–558

Snook J 1979 Spasticity reduction splint. American Journal of Occupational Therapy 33: 648–651

Stockmeyer S A 1967 An interpretation of the approach of Rood to the treatment of neuromuscular dysfunction. American Journal of Physical Therapy 46(1): 900–955

Sullivan T, Conine T, Goodman M, Mackie T 1988 Serial casting to prevent equinus in acute traumatic head injury. Physiotherapy Canada 40(6): 346–350

Sutherland D H, Cooper L 1978 The pathomechanics of progressive crouch gait in spastic diplegia. Orthopedic Clinics of North America 9(1): 143–154

Training Council for Orthotists 1980 Classification of orthoses. Department of Health and Social Security. HMSO, London

Williams R, Taffs L, Minuk T 1988 Evaluation of two support methods for the subluxated shoulder of hemiplegic patients. Physical Therapy 68(8): 1209–1214

Yarkony G M, Sahgal V 1987 Contractures: a major complication of craniocerebral trauma. Clinical Orthopaedics and Related Research 219: 93–96

CHAPTER CONTENTS

Introduction   189

Non-progressive impairment   190
   Persistent vegetative state (PVS)   190
   Cerebral palsy in adulthood   193

Progressive neurological and neuromuscular
   disorders   195
   Multiple sclerosis (MS)   196
   Hereditary motor and sensory neuropathy
      (HMSN)   199

Discussion   203

References   205

9

Longer-term management for patients with residual or progressive disability

Susan Edwards

INTRODUCTION

There is little dispute that people sustaining neurological damage or disease with resultant disability should receive a period of physical treatment and management following the initial onset of that impairment. The duration and timing of interventions vary considerably and are determined not only by the prognosis and perception of need but to an increasing extent by the resources available to support health care. The purpose of this chapter is to discuss the optimal level of care which should be provided for people with residual or progressive disability and handicap and to consider those factors which relate to management.

The main emphasis for patients with chronic and progressive conditions, where functional recovery is limited, is to prevent secondary complications and maintain function at an optimal level. Compensation for neurological disability is often considered to be undesirable, the aim of treatment being to 'restore normal movement'. However, where there is diffuse, irreversible damage to the central nervous system or progressive deterioration, this aim may not be realistic and compensatory strategies which are appropriate for the patient should be encouraged in order to maximise function.

There are two categories in which patients may be considered when looking at long-term management:

- non-progressive impairment
- progressive impairment.

The first category includes patients following cerebrovascular accident (CVA), head or spinal injury and those with cerebral palsy. For these patients, although the impairment itself is non-progressive, the disability and subsequent handicap may increase over time (Bax et al 1988). The second category of progressive impairment includes patients with a wide range of conditions such as multiple sclerosis, Parkinson's disease, cerebellar degeneration and neuromuscular disorders.

To illustrate the problems encountered by patients and their long-term management, two examples from each category will be discussed.

- In the non-progressive category: persistent vegetative state (PVS) following head injury; and cerebral palsy in adulthood.
- In the progressive category: multiple sclerosis; and hereditary motor and sensory neuropathy.

NON-PROGRESSIVE IMPAIRMENT
Persistent vegetative state (PVS)

Introduction

Severe brain injury or disease may result in such irrevocable damage to the central nervous system that functional recovery becomes an unattainable goal and patients remain dependent on others for the rest of their lives. This condition is often referred to as persistent vegetative state (PVS) (Jennett & Plum 1972). The vegetative state is a clinical condition of complete unawareness of the self and the environment, accompanied by sleep–wake cycles, with either complete or partial preservation of hypothalamic and brain stem autonomic functions. In addition, patients in PVS show no evidence of sustained, reproducible, purposeful or voluntary behavioural responses to visual, auditory, tactile or noxious stimuli; show no evidence of language comprehension or expression; have bowel and bladder incontinence and have variably preserved cranial nerve and spinal reflexes. PVS is a diagnosis which implies a prognosis. It can be judged to be permanent if it persists for 12 months after a traumatic injury and 3 months after non-traumatic damage. Recovery may still occur, but it is rare and at best associated with moderate or severe disability (Multi-Society Task Force on PVS 1994).

The management of patients in PVS offers the sternest challenge to all personnel involved in their care and there is a lack of agreement of the focus that long-term management should take. Vogenthaler (1987) stated that 'obviously living and vocational rehabilitation are not relevant' but Pope (1988) asks the question 'if not, then what is?'. The main criteria for determining a successful outcome is the promotion of both physical and mental recovery but, for those in PVS, this will never be realised. For these patients, it is inappropriate to evaluate success or failure using these performance indicators. The patient who remains free from contracture and pressure sores, and with the positive release phenomena under control, can be considered as a static success (Pope 1988).

In some instances, it may be possible for a patient to be cared for at home, provided adequate support is available from the community services. In others, long-term management of the patient in some form of institution where constant nursing care is available, is necessary. Irrespective of the ultimate placement, the immediate family and friends must be considered as part of the team and be involved in the decision-making process at all stages of the patient's management.

The term 'silent epidemic' has been used to describe people who survive brain injury in PVS (Klein 1982, Freeman 1992). Despite the preservation of hypothalamic and brain stem function, the severe neurologic injury necessary to produce the vegetative state reduces the life expectancy to approximately 2 to 5 years. Survival beyond 10 years is unusual (Multi-Society Task Force 1994). Irrespective of this bleak prognosis in terms of life expectancy, it is the remit of all staff to ensure that the optimal level of care is provided to maintain the patient's dignity and hygiene.

Ethical considerations

Advances in medical science and technology are enabling many more people to survive even the most severe trauma, which may lead to PVS. The British Medical Association (BMA) Medical Ethics Committee (1992) states that treatment can only be justified if 'it makes possible a decent life in which a patient can reasonably be thought to have continued interest'. However, in the immediate aftermath of severe brain damage, it is often difficult for medical staff to assess the probability of meaningful recovery. It is debatable what a meaningful recovery is. Whatever the satisfaction it may bring to family and friends, the recovery of a limited degree of awareness may be worse than total loss of cognitive function for the patient.

There have been a number of legal cases regarding the cessation of treatment of patients in PVS. Initially these were requests to withdraw ventilation as in the Quinlan case of 1976 (Hannan et al 1994), but more recently, actions have been brought to stop nasogastric tube feeding (Tribe & Korgaonkar 1992). The findings in these cases have confirmed that these are legitimate and ethically acceptable options that the family and doctors of some patients may consider (Jennett 1992).

For patients in PVS where there is little or no hope of functional recovery it may be recommended that all active treatment should cease. The implications of such a decision may have a devastating effect on patients and their carers. Optimal care may be considered to be the maintenance of the patient's bodily functions, joint and muscle range of movement, and tissue viability, and stimulation of cognitive awareness. Withdrawal of active treatment usually refers to the more dynamic intervention such as that which may be carried out by the physiotherapist. Maintenance of joint and muscle range, considered by many to be the remit of the physiotherapist, is difficult and potentially damaging where there is excessive spasticity (Ada et al 1990). Changes of position are frequently utilised to minimise or control the effects of this stereotyped posturing. The provision of

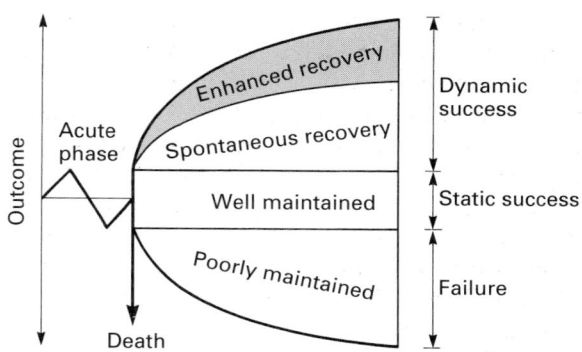

Figure 9.1 Range of possible outcomes following brain trauma (reproduced from Pope 1988 by kind permission).

appropriate support in sitting and in standing the patient, may prove effective in reducing the influence of spasticity. This type of intervention may be considered inappropriate by the medical staff where there is little hope of functional recovery. However, if outcome is measured by the prevention of deterioration as opposed to the attainment of function, active treatment can be viewed as a key component within the management process rather than as a waste of resources on a patient who may be considered to be a hopeless case (Fig. 9.1).

It must be recognised that this dynamic intervention may make the difference between the patient being 'manageable' and the patient deteriorating with the development of gross contracture leading to deformity (Pope 1988).

A diagnosis of PVS should be used with caution. Applied too soon following trauma, it may lead to the denial of further therapy and appropriate management. The effect can be catastrophic for the patient, emotionally devastating for the family and financially demanding for the community (Freeman 1992).

Most importantly, the person in PVS must be recognised as an individual, albeit with little or no cognitive awareness. Communication is a two-way process and where there is no response or recognition from one party, inevitably this will affect the approach of the other. Where there is little or no response over a protracted period of time, it is often difficult for carers, be they professional staff, family or friends, to remain positive in their approach towards that person. It is all too easy to treat patients in PVS on a routine basis with little thought as to how a particular intervention may affect them.

Physiotherapy intervention

The diagnosis of PVS should not preclude treatment. Prevention of secondary complications is essential to optimise potential function and management. The principles of treatment as described in Chapter 5 are of as great an importance to this patient group as to those with a more optimistic prognosis. The majority of patients will demonstrate increased tone, the most common type being that of spasticity. The extent, severity and distribution of this abnormal tone will depend upon the site and extent of the area of damage and on the environmental influences to which the patient is subjected (Bach-y-Rita 1990, Finger & Almli 1985).

The speed at which therapy intervention is carried out is of vital importance; patients in PVS often have difficulty in accommodating to change in respect of movement or position. The proprioceptive input provided by the physiotherapist should ensure appropriate support to facilitate a feeling of stability and security, allowing time for the patient to respond to the movement. Sudden movements, for example attempting to stand the patient without adequate preparation, may lead to an increase in tone which may preclude attainment of this position.

Physiotherapy for people with severe brain injury is part of a 24-hour management process and cannot be viewed in isolation. The remit of the physiotherapist caring for patients in PVS is to maintain and, where appropriate, increase range of movement to enable the optimal level of care. Orofacial treatment as advocated in Chapter 5, in conjunction with the speech therapist, is of particular value for these patients. Full or improved range of movement throughout the body will enable more appropriate seating, positioning in bed, washing, dressing and, perhaps, the ability to stand the person with suitable support. It is only by constant reinforce-ment of correct positioning and handling that deterioration may be prevented.

Positioning should be considered a dynamic aspect of treatment. Prior to moving the patient from one position to another, an explanation should be given of the proposed manoeuvre. Staff and/or carers should inform the patient that, for example, the pillows are going to be removed and request assistance from the patient to accomplish the movement. Mobilisation of the trunk on the pelvis may be used to influence the prevailing tone in an attempt to facilitate the change of position (Davies 1994). At all times, patients must be stimulated to maximise any recovery in both their physical and cognitive status. Being unable to move themselves, they readily accommodate to their enforced patterns of spasticity.

The use of splinting for maintaining and regaining joint range is of great value in the management of patients in PVS. For patients with severe spasticity it is often difficult to maintain full muscle and joint range without using some form of splintage. The types of splints which may be used and the situations in which to use them are described in detail in Chapter 8. However, splinting should not be viewed as a static intervention replacing the need for physiotherapy, but as a dynamic adjunct to treatment. The splinted part must accommodate to the splint in order for the splint to have an inhibitory effect on tone. Any evidence of increased tone or agitation may be indicative of discomfort and potential pressure sores. In this situation, the splint must be removed without delay in case it is the splint that is giving rise to these adverse symptoms.

Summary

Many patients may be diagnosed as being in PVS, often only a short time after their injury or illness. Jennett & Plum (1972) describe the clinical features: '[patients] have periods of wakefulness when their eyes are open and move, their responsiveness is limited to primitive postural and reflex movements of the limbs, and they never speak ... Few would dispute that in this condition the cerebral cortex is out of action'. This state may prevail for years with no tangible change in the patient's condition but Berroll (1986; cited by Freeman 1992) found that a significant number of patients diagnosed as vegetative became conscious within 12 months of trauma.

Every effort should be made to ensure that each patient receives appropriate stimulation and sensitive management to maximise recovery. Many patients diagnosed as being in PVS are maintained in a state of gross sensory deprivation with the utilisation of scarce resources on active treatment being considered inappropriate. The brain is exquisitely responsive to the environment (Delgado 1977; cited by Freeman 1992) and as such is dependent upon the management of the patient and the variety offered by the patient's environment for any positive change in outcome. The use of a gastrostomy as opposed to a nasogastric tube and a leg bag for urine collection as opposed to a mounted catheter bag are examples of sensitive management, respecting the dignity of patients in spite of their lack of awareness.

Active intervention such as that described above need not necessarily mean a great increase in expenditure. Education and involvement of family and friends and other health care workers in patient management promotes stimulation of both cognitive and physical function. Prevention of loss of joint and muscle range provides not only easier nursing care but also greater comfort for the patient. The management of complications such as pressure sores and contractures, which may arise following severe brain injury, may prove to be expensive; prevention of these complications inevitably reduces the ultimate cost of care.

Cerebral palsy in adulthood

Introduction

Cerebral palsy is the result of a lesion or maldevelopment of the brain which is non-progressive in character and exists from earliest childhood (Bobath 1974). The management of children with cerebral palsy is generally recognised as an on-going process from birth, or when the condition is first diagnosed, to adulthood. By this time the individuals should be fully equipped for their needs in life, such as communication aids, wheelchairs and splints. Physiotherapy for those with physical disabilities is an accepted part of management. However, for many people with cerebral palsy, problems may intensify over time when, in many instances, physiotherapy is no longer available. Poor quality of management and treatment of patients who have chronic and often more severe disabilities is becoming increasingly widespread. These patients may not experience an acute episode which would, at least, bring them into contact with the existing services (Condie 1991).

The paediatric services are used to dealing with what are often diverse and complex problems. Maintenance of range of movement and prevention of postural deformity are recognised as key principles of physiotherapy throughout the period of growth. While at school, regular standing, ongoing review of seating and postural supports, and provision of appropriate footwear are examples of components of a physiotherapy programme which is supported by all personnel. However, when the child becomes an adult, such intervention often ceases in spite of the fact that many people show signs of physical deterioration when routine care is withdrawn (Bax et al 1988).

The term 'management' can be used to refer to the entire process whereby patients' problems are identified and their needs analysed, as a result of which they are subsequently admitted to an individually tailored programme of treatment and review which continues for as long as their disability persists (Condie 1991). Unfortunately, this is rarely the case, in spite of people with physical disability being designated a priority group in *Care in Action*, the Government's handbook of policies and priorities for health and social services in the UK (DHSS 1981). Services for disabled people remain confused and extremely variable with a distinct lack of good practice (Beardshaw 1988). In a study looking into the health care of handicapped adults (Bax et al 1988), many subjects with cerebral palsy reported that their physical condition had deteriorated after leaving school; they had become less mobile and their contractures more fixed.

Where there is diffuse brain damage, the whole body may be involved. Symptoms may include quadriplegia, visual and hearing deficits and intellectual dysfunction. The inability to communicate needs, thoughts and feelings is perhaps the most serious defect and one which may lead to an individual being labelled mentally retarded. Many people who were unable to communicate verbally were found to have normal intelligence once taught alternative means of communication (McNaughton 1975; cited by Bleck 1987). 'Because these persons present an almost overwhelming number of problems, efforts toward rehabilitation are apt to be truncated, individuals relegated to the wastebasket category of medical care and their potential as persons neglected' (Bleck 1987). It is essential to make resources available which enable the individual to achieve an optimal level of functional independence consistent with the limitations imposed by the neurological and musculoskeletal impairment.

Physiotherapy intervention

Many people with cerebral palsy maintain an independent lifestyle and do not want or need regular therapy intervention. They may be wheelchair dependent or ambulant, albeit with an abnormal gait, but they cope with their disability and are content with their situation. Indeed, professional overtreatment and striving to remedy deficits rather than compensate for them may be the cause of 'mental distress', which was identified as a predominant disability in adolescents and adults with spastic diplegia (Bleck 1987).

Many people with spastic diplegia walk independently, often with flexion, adduction and medial rotation of the hips, flexion of the knees and plantar flexion and equinus of the feet. The pelvis is usually anteriorly tilted with a marked lumbar lordosis. The arms, which often have

minor motor deficits, are constantly active in maintaining balance. The abnormal stresses and strains imposed on the musculoskeletal system by this posture may lead to arthritic changes in joints. Some of the problems which may arise include:

- Poor alignment of the hip joint during stance phase of gait results in damage to the joint surfaces. The constant pull into adduction and medial rotation may, in severe cases, cause displacement of the joint (Bleck 1987).
- The constant flexion of the knees causes 'alta patella' through overstretching of the patella ligament (Sutherland & Cooper 1978). Effective action of the quadriceps muscle group is never developed and, as the child becomes older and heavier, joint changes are almost inevitable.
- The feet may be severely deformed with breakdown of the medial arch and plantar fascia through the constant forces imposed on these structures with toe walking (Fig. 9.2).
- The anterior tilt of the pelvis may lead to contracture of the psoas muscle, further increasing the lumbar lordosis.

These problems may increase in severity over the years and yet, in adulthood, when they are often compounded by increased weight and reduced mobility, therapy is withdrawn. Although many people remain ambulant, in more severe cases, the individual may become wheelchair dependent. This is obviously a critical time from both a physical and emotional perspective. Provision of a wheelchair should involve not only a thorough assessment as to the most appropriate chair, but should also include physiotherapy to advise and instigate an exercise programme to prevent physical deterioration. In many cases there will already be some shortening of the flexor muscles, and prolonged sitting will exacerbate this problem. A regimen of standing and appropriate stretches should be devised for the individual, to guard against this possibility.

The structural and functional problems of people with cerebral palsy are often neglected and viewed as an integral part of the condition. This is not always the case. For example, pain,

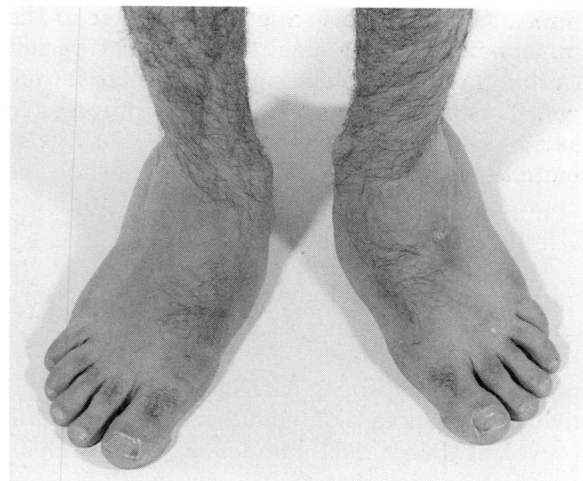

A

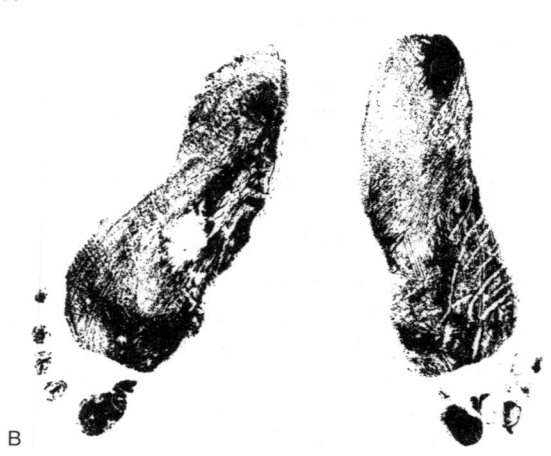

B

Figure 9.2   (A) Collapse of the medial arch in an adult patient with cerebral palsy; (B) weight-bearing surface.

which may result from musculoskeletal changes arising from the abnormal postures and movements, requires treatment just as it does in the able-bodied population. A detailed assessment may be able to identify a specific cause of the pain, which may respond to treatment.

Summary

For those with chronic residual physical disability, the danger of secondary complications, such as respiratory problems, contracture and postural deformity, remains throughout the course of their lives. The more severe the abnormal postures and movements, the greater is the danger. Regular assessment and treatment intervention as indicated is essential to prevent their occurrence. However, it must be recognised that many people cope adequately, even with gross disability and deformity, and do not desire ongoing therapy.

Currently, very few specialist health and coordinated services are organised for people who are only physically disabled, and the development of such services is recommended in each district health authority (Bax et al 1988).

PROGRESSIVE NEUROLOGICAL AND NEUROMUSCULAR DISORDERS

Patients with progressive neurological and neuromuscular disorders will require ongoing treatment and management to ensure optimum function and the prevention of secondary complications. Examples of these disorders include multiple sclerosis, muscular dystrophy, Friedreich's ataxia, spinocerebellar degeneration and the hereditary motor sensory neuropathies (HMSN). The changing neurological and/or muscular status usually affects the clinical signs and symptoms and thereby the patient's functional capability. These conditions are often associated with a multiplicity of symptoms, the management of which require a coordinated, multidisciplinary intervention.

Some people, for example those with multiple sclerosis, may experience exacerbations and remissions as part of the disease process, whereas others, such as those with muscular dystrophy, show a steady deterioration of varying severity. The aim of physiotherapy is to maximise function and prevent secondary complications. To date, there is little that can be done to halt the progression of many of these diseases, but an understanding of the expected complications and compensations from the primary impairment will enable the physiotherapist to intervene more appropriately.

Multiple sclerosis (MS)

Introduction

Multiple sclerosis is an inflammatory, demyelinating disorder which is the most common cause of neurological disability in young adults (Thompson & McDonald 1992, Barnes 1993). A relapsing and remitting course is common but the condition may subsequently become progressive, this being termed secondary progressive. Between 15 to 20% of all MS patients have benign MS where there are few attacks early on and little if any residual disability (Weinshenker 1994). Less than 10% show a primary progressive course (Thompson & McDonald 1992). Over the past decade there has been a significant increase in the survival time, resulting in an almost normal life expectancy for the 'average person' with MS (Mertin 1994).

A diagnosis of MS is dependent upon the clinical demonstration of lesions disseminated in time and space and the exclusion of other conditions which may produce the same clinical picture (Thompson & McDonald 1992). Magnetic resonance imaging (MRI) may support the clinical diagnosis by identifying multiple lesions which indicate dissemination in space, but these do not always correlate with the clinical status (Thompson et al 1991).

The disease is characterised by multiple lesions (plaques) of demyelination with differing degrees of inflammation. There is a predilection for the optic nerve, periventricular areas and the cervical cord but all parts of the brain and spinal cord may be involved. The functional deficit is ultimately due to abnormalities in conduction. Demyelination causes an impairment of the ability of the nerve fibres to transmit impulses. Both demyelination and inflammation contribute to the conduction block and clinical deficit (Thompson & McDonald 1992).

The outstanding characteristic in the early stages is the patient's capacity for clinical recovery from individual episodes, primarily through the resolution of oedema and inflammation with some remyelination. With partial demyelination, some functional recovery takes place. This is mediated by the surviving fibres, either of the same system or of other systems, that permit learning of new strategies to compensate for the deficit. However, compensation for progressive axonal loss continues to become less effective as more fibres subserving a particular function are impaired, leading to permanent disability (Thompson & McDonald 1992).

The clinical manifestations of the disease are varied but often include optic neuritis, sensory and motor disturbance of the limbs and symptoms relating to brain stem and cerebellar dysfunction (Thompson & McDonald 1992). Cognitive disturbances and emotional problems are prevalent (Poser 1980, Minden & Schiffer 1990). Psychiatric disturbance is seen in 40–50% of patients and there is a greater incidence of suicide in the MS population (Weinshenker 1994). Fatigue is common and frequently disabling (Krupp et al 1988). Pain is often associated with MS (Barnes 1993) and bladder symptoms occur in between 50 and 75% of patients (Thompson & McDonald 1992).

Pseudobulbar and respiratory symptoms may occur and respiratory muscle weakness, particularly of the diaphragm, is the most common cause of respiratory distress (Howard et al 1992). Bronchopneumonia is the leading cause of death in MS and may be related to swallowing difficulties with resultant aspiration (Barnes 1993).

The course of MS is extremely variable in terms of the frequency and severity of attacks, the degree of recovery and the development of progressive disability. Progressive onset of symptoms, secondary progression after a remitting phase, older age of onset and motor symptoms at onset generally indicate a poor prognosis (Miller et al 1992, Weinshenker 1994).

Physiotherapy intervention

Given the complexity and variability of the clinical signs and symptoms which may present in MS, a full and accurate assessment is essential to determine the primary problems resulting from the disease pathology. Compensatory strategies, adopted by the patient in an attempt to achieve function, may then be analysed as to their effectiveness, not only in the short term but also over a protracted period of time.

The initial interview between the patient and the physiotherapist must be handled with great sensitivity. It is essential that the physiotherapist is fully aware of information already given to the patient. Has the patient been told of the diagnosis? The majority of people with MS wish to know their diagnosis at an early stage, wish their family to be informed at the same time and wish to be given adequate background information on the disease and a chance to ask their own questions (Barnes 1993). However, in spite of this, doctors occasionally delay giving a definitive diagnosis and patients may learn of their diagnosis in an inappropriate manner.

Referral to physiotherapy in the early stages of disability can be of great benefit, both in planning a long-term management strategy and for instigating preventive therapeutic regimens. Continued monitoring with intervention as required is essential to cater for the changing needs of the patient (DeSouza 1990, Mertin &

Paeth 1994). Unfortunately many patients do not receive this on-going care, and additional problems arising, either from the disease pathology or secondary to imposed abnormal movement strategies, are not addressed. An exercise programme that was designed in the early stages may, over time, become not only ineffective but possibly detrimental.

The patient must be an active participant in the planning of treatment. The patient's priorities may differ from those of the therapist, and discussion is essential to determine effective intervention which meets the requirements of both parties (DeSouza 1990). Multidisciplinary clinics are recommended which facilitate inter-disciplinary cooperation (Fig. 9.3). This professional cooperation is of benefit to all personnel, not least the patients and their relatives (Barnes 1993, Mertin 1994). The aim should be to ensure that there is consistency in approach to treatment and mutually agreed goals.

Although the physiotherapist is often the key player in the management of motor disorders,

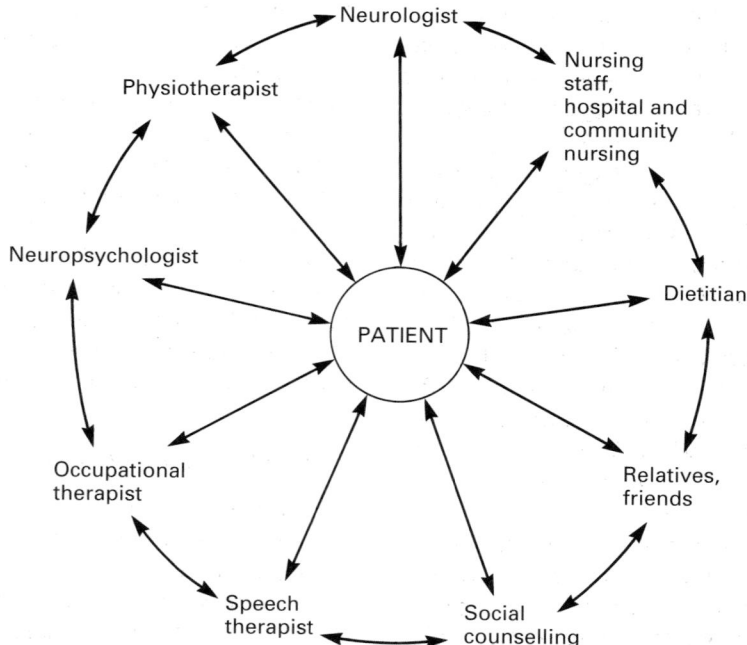

Figure 9.3 The interdisciplinary rehabilitation team (adapted from Mertin 1994).

the management of motor problems cannot be viewed in isolation from the other aspects of disability which may prevail. It is important that the physiotherapist has an understanding of the pathophysiology of MS in that the prognosis is so variable. Physiotherapists may themselves view MS as a progressive disease which ultimately leads to wheelchair dependence and perhaps death. This pessimistic attitude is not generally appropriate. Although consideration must be given to the mode of onset and type of MS, physiotherapy intervention should be geared towards the presenting signs and symptoms.

In many instances, a period of rehabilitation may be of value in ensuring optimal function following any change in the level of disability. Not only is this beneficial in terms of reassessment and restructuring of therapy intervention, but of equal importance is the often dramatic remission after hospitalisation. However, it must be recognised that psychological factors such as anxiety over financial difficulties, marital discord and academic pressures play an important role in the patient's ability to cope with the disease. When the patient is removed from his normal, possibly stressful environment, this in itself may have a therapeutic effect (Poser 1980).

Treatment of patients with MS is determined by the presenting signs and symptoms, those affecting posture and movement being of greatest relevance to the physiotherapist. The most common forms of movement deficit are associated with spasticity and/or ataxia with the secondary effects of fatigue, disuse, pain and sensory impairment (Barnes 1993). The primary aims of physiotherapy treatment are:

- to maintain and increase range of movement
- to encourage postural stability
- to prevent contractures
- to maintain and encourage weight-bearing (Ashburn & DeSouza 1988).

To this end, therapy should not be restricted to passive intervention such as stretching and mobilisations of specific parts. The patient must be involved as an active participant by the promotion of purposeful movements which are part of everyday function (Mertin & Paeth 1994). Exercise programmes are particularly useful in enabling patients to take responsibility for their own management and are often effective in maintaining range of movement and maximising muscle power.

Mertin & Paeth (1994) advocate approaches that differ according to the patient's level of impairment/disability as measured on the Kurtzke Disability Status Scale (DSS). Patients are stratified as having mild (DSS grade 0–2), moderate (DSS grade 3–5) or severe (DSS grade 6–9) disability (Miller et al 1992).

For those with a score of less than 5, the emphasis should be on the normalisation of postural control and inhibition of compensatory strategies. Facilitation of normal movement patterns, particularly those of standing and gait, and an individual home programme of exercises are recommended. For those with increasing levels of impairment/disability, with a DSS score of greater than 6, compensatory strategies should be utilised and refined to improve functional independence with appropriate selection of aids and training in their usage. Maintenance of muscle and joint range, improving postural control, facilitation of normal movement patterns as appropriate, and maintenance of standing posture should be continued as before. Adaptation of the home exercise programme and the training of carers are necessary to respond to the changing functional status of the patient (Mertin & Paeth 1994).

Difficulty in walking is one of the most frequent symptoms of MS, and analysis and treatment of these mobility problems provides perhaps the greatest challenge in MS management (Barnes 1993). Standing is of value for virtually all patients with abnormal tone and movement. This is effective in both maintaining and regaining range of movement, stimulating extensor activity (Brown 1994) and in improving the body's spatial orientation. Assessment of the primary cause of the gait impairment is essential in determining the most appropriate intervention. For those who are mobile without aids, facilitation of a normal gait pattern is recommended. Those requiring mobility aids should receive appropriate training to ensure that these aids are used effectively.

For example, an ankle–foot orthosis (AFO) to control loss of adequate dorsiflexion, may assist in the prevention of unnecessary proximal compensation. Without such support, the patient must inevitably use excessive knee flexion or circumduction at the hip to clear the foot during swing phase of gait. The AFO may allow for a more fluid and efficient walking cycle. For those with ataxia, the use of a rollator walking frame, may prove of benefit in enabling the patient to gain improved stability. However, it is important that the patient uses this aid as a means of balance as opposed to fixation (see Ch. 4).

Hydrotherapy is considered to be effective for patients with MS (Barnes 1993) but treatment in a hydrotherapy pool, where the temperature of the water is often quite high, may increase fatigue. The temperature of the water is important, with increased temperatures potentially slowing nerve conduction (Poser 1980). Patients who enjoy exercise in water may derive more benefit from the cooler temperatures of general swimming pools.

Weights are considered to be effective in the management of ataxia (Morgan et al 1975). They are attached to the affected limb to provide a constant resistance which may dampen the tremor. A weighted cap may be used to control titubation of the head. However, the application of weights in this way may cause fatigue and often does not have a lasting effect. The patient may accommodate to the weights over a period of time with the ataxia remaining relatively unaltered. Following removal of the weight, the ataxia may be greater than before and postural stability further compromised (DeSouza 1990). Weights may be of value as a temporary aid to compensate or dampen tremor, prior to or during performance of a functional task.

Appropriate seating, particularly for those with severe neurological deficit who are wheelchair dependent, is essential. Detailed description of postural control and specialised seating is provided in Chapter 7.

Splinting may be effective in maintaining range of movement, or can be used as a correc-

tive measure for regaining range (Barnes 1993, Mertin 1994).

The management of respiratory complications, particularly in the advanced stages of MS, raises ethical issues. It is important that patients who are at risk of acute respiratory complications, associated with bulbar and spinal cord relapses, are identified early, since provision of appropriate support during the period of respiratory insufficiency reduces the incidence of sudden death and reduces distress (Howard et al 1992). The finding that some patients improve significantly with remission and not all require continued mechanical assistance justifies this intervention.

Summary

The likely progressive nature of multiple sclerosis makes it imperative that regular multidisciplinary assessment, including physiotherapy, continues for so long as patients demonstrate changes in their clinical signs and symptoms. Wherever possible, this monitoring should be undertaken by staff who are familiar with the patient. All too frequently, patients with MS whose condition is being regularly reviewed are seen by different therapists at each assessment. This makes it very difficult to plan and monitor long-term treatment strategies and to evaluate the functional consequences of the changing neurological status. It will inevitably happen, however, when staff are on rotation through different specialities and spend only a limited period of time in any one department.

Standardised testing with the use of appropriate outcome measures is essential to monitor any change in function and effectiveness of intervention.

Hereditary motor and sensory neuropathy (HMSN)

Introduction

This term is used to describe a group of conditions which give rise to progressive weakness and wasting of the distal muscles of the legs and of the hands (Harding 1993). Other names which may be used to describe HMSN include Charcot–Marie–Tooth disease, after the three neurologists who first described the condition, and peroneal muscular atrophy. Most people with HMSN have a dominantly inherited disorder associated with a duplication of chromosome 17 (Malcolm 1993).

There are many different types of HMSN, the most common forms being referred to as types I and II (Geurts et al 1992a). Type I is characterised by a demyelinating neuropathy causing slow nerve conduction whereas type II is the result of axonal degeneration. The clinical signs and symptoms are similar in both type I and type II, the main difference being the age of onset. Type I usually produces symptoms earlier, most commonly between the ages of 5 and 15. In type II, although symptoms may develop in childhood they occur more commonly between the ages of 10 and 20 and often not until much later (Harding 1993).

The sensory symptoms are usually less severe than the motor and generally occur later in life (Medhat & Krantz 1988). However, impaired proprioception is seen in many older patients and may contribute to the balance problems associated with HMSN (Harding & Thomas 1980, Geurts et al 1992b). Postural and intention tremor may be associated with type I HMSN (Harding 1984).

Clinical signs and symptoms

HMSN, although showing great variability in the severity of symptoms, has a predictable course, affecting the feet and legs and much later than the hands and forearms (Harding & Thomas 1980).

Lower limb muscle impairment and functional deficit

The lower limb weakness initially affects the intrinsic foot musculature and peroneus brevis, followed by tibialis anterior, peroneus longus and the long toe extensors, later progressing to affect the plantar flexors (Mann & Missirian 1988, Geurts et al 1992a). This creates an imbalance of activity at the foot and ankle that may result in deformed, unstable and often painful feet, which interferes with gait (Wetmore & Drennan 1989). Pes cavus, equinus and clawing of the toes are typical aspects of the foot deformity (Medhat & Krantz 1988). Contracture of the posterior crural muscle group is common (Mann & Missirian 1986) and ankle sprains are frequently reported (Bacardi & Alm 1986).

The progressive atrophy and the resulting deformity and functional loss are described by Mann & Missirian (1988).

The weakness of the tibialis anterior permits the peroneus longus to function relatively unopposed, which accounts for most of the marked plantar flexion of the medial side of the foot. The lack of function of peroneus brevis permits the tibialis posterior to function without significant opposition, which results in the hind foot being brought into inversion (varus) and the forefoot into a certain degree of adduction. The deformity is further enhanced by the progressive contracture of the intrinsic muscles and plantar aponeurosis, which further brings the forefoot into an adducted and plantar-flexed position. The normal long toe flexors contribute to the adduction of the forefoot because their normal antagonists, i.e., the extensor digitorum longus and the extensor hallucis longus muscles, are weakened by the disease process.

Geurts et al (1992b) demonstrated a decreased postural control in patients with HMSN, even when there was full perceptual information. This was attributed to the lower limb paralysis and the ankle–foot deformities impairing postural sway. For those with no restriction of range of movement of the plantar flexors, a few degrees of forward body inclination was noted.

Difficulties with walking arising from the progressive muscle imbalance are typically those of a high-stepping gait to compensate for the lack of dorsiflexion (Geurts et al 1992a), weight-bearing over the lateral border of the foot (Bacardi and Alm 1986) and lateral instability of the ankle (Wukich et al 1989).

Physiotherapy intervention

Assessment and appropriate intervention by a physiotherapist is of vital importance for patients with HMSN. One of the major problems is that the insidious onset of the disease is often missed both by the patient and the clinician (Geurts et al 1992b) and unless there is a family history of the disease, patients may not present for treatment before symptoms become established.

Harding (1993) stresses the importance of suitable footwear and, particularly for those with sensory impairment, the need to examine both the feet and the inside of the shoes on a regular basis to reduce the risk of ulceration. Splints are advocated to control the foot in the plantigrade position to reduce ankle instability and to allow for a more economic gait pattern (Medhat & Krantz 1988, Harding 1993, Geurts et al 1992a).

There is little literature regarding specific physiotherapy intervention. However, with the relative stereotyped picture which emerges as a result of the disease process, physiotherapy treatment and management can be instrumental in preventing or minimising the expected deformity. For example, the progressive contracture of the intrinsic foot musculature and the plantar aponeurosis may be reduced by an early programme of massage and mobilisation of the feet to maintain flexibility within these structures. This intervention may also prove effective in maintaining range of movement within other muscles affected in the disease process.

The relatively unopposed action of the gastrocnemius has particular consequences which may be managed effectively with appropriate physiotherapy intervention. Shortening of gastrocnemius restricts dorsiflexion and may cause hyperextension of the knee in standing and walking, due to its action over the two joints – the ankle and the knee. The weight tends to be displaced backwards, due to the inability to transfer the weight over the full surface of the foot during stance phase of gait. Maintenance of the centre of gravity within the base of support can only be effected by flexion at the hips. Flexion at the hips produces an anterior tilt of the pelvis creating an excessive lordosis if the individual is to maintain an upright posture.

Regular stretching of gastrocnemius and other affected muscle groups may go some way towards preventing the onset of contracture. However, stretching must be used with caution, particularly where there is substantial somatosensory impairment, with special attention paid to the correct alignment of bony structures.

The imbalance of muscle activity caused by the progressive weakness can be best managed by earlier rather than later use of insoles and AFOs. Insoles may prove effective in the redistribution of weight across the full surface of the foot (see Ch. 8).

The main advantage of the polypropylene AFO is that it is moulded to each individual's foot. It therefore supports the medial arch and the toes, in addition to maintaining the foot in a plantigrade position and preventing lateral instability. The disadvantage of this type of splint is that it does not permit talocrural mobility, particularly dorsiflexion which would redress the varus deviation (Geurts et al 1992a). The use of a hinged AFO may be of benefit to allow this movement into dorsiflexion, but the bulk of these splints often makes them aesthetically unacceptable. A below-knee caliper with heel socket and outside T-strap may be more effective, but these are more obtrusive. The choice of orthosis should be discussed between the patient, the physiotherapist and the orthotist. Whichever type of orthosis is provided, it is essential that the patient be given a structured programme of stance and gait training (Geurts et al 1992a). Monitoring the continued efficacy of the splint or insoles should be carried out on a regular basis and, where the patient is dependent on the splints for ambulation, an additional pair should be provided in case of breakage. The different types of orthoses are described in Chapter 8.

Documented treatment of the foot deformities usually relates to surgery, particularly that of tendon transfer (Medhat & Krantz 1988, Wetmore & Drennan 1989). This would still appear to be appropriate early intervention in redressing the muscular imbalance (Mann & Missirian 1988). Triple arthrodesis was commonly carried out in the past but is now considered to be a 'salvage' procedure limited to those with severe rigid deformity (Wetmore & Drennan 1989, Wukich & Bowen 1989).

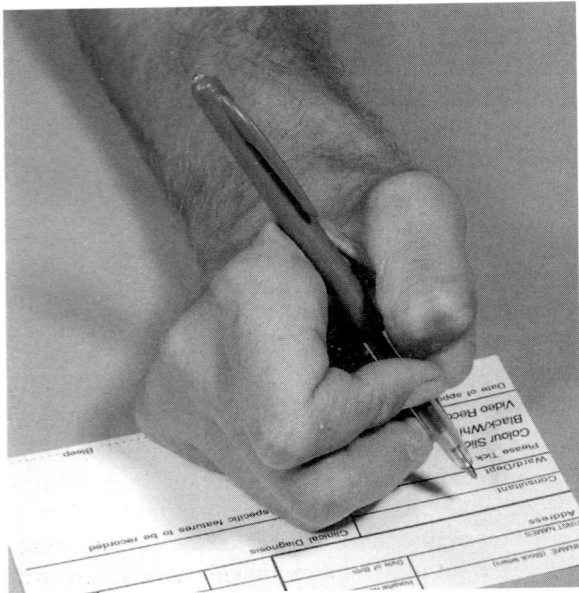

Figure 9.4 Writing without splint.

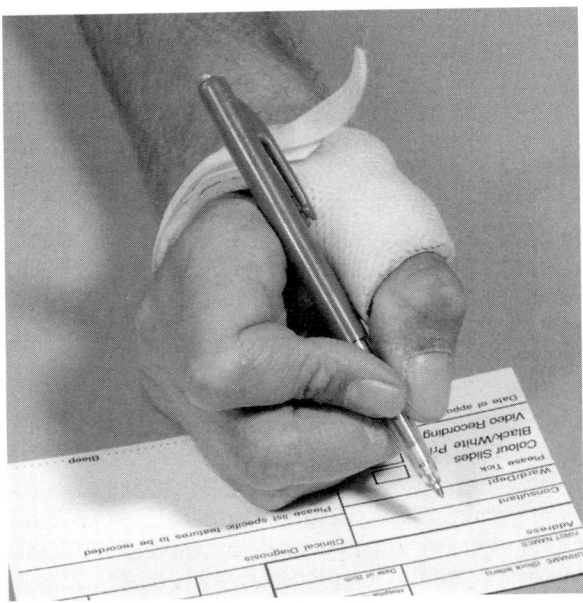

Figure 9.5 Writing with splint.

Upper limb problems associated with HMSN

The weakness of the hands is characterised by wasting of the intrinsic hand muscles, which may progress to the forearms (Harding 1984). Sensory impairment is variable but in severe cases the numbness of the hands may result in injury such as burns to the hands (Harding 1993).

The thenar and hypothenar muscles become progressively weaker and opposition of the thumb to the fingers is impaired. Functionally, these people adapt by using gross flexion for tasks requiring a pinch grip. This is illustrated by the manner in which they write (Fig. 9.4).

Overuse of the affected muscle groups seems to compound the weakness, many people giving personal accounts of how they have never recovered from a bout of strenuous exercise such as painting and decorating. Being so dependent on the hands for function, it is unrealistic to expect people not to use them.

Physiotherapy intervention

The use of a thumb opposition splint may serve to maintain more normal function of the hand by facilitating opposition of the fingers to the thumb without overuse of opponens pollicis. This splint is compact, easy to make and readily applied or removed as the situation demands. People with early signs of hand weakness should be encouraged to use this support to maintain normal hand function with opposition of the thumb to the fingers. Its use is illustrated in Figure 9.5 as a means of improving writing. See Chapter 8 for further details.

Patients with more severe weakness may demonstrate signs of diaphragmatic weakness. This is often characterised by the patient complaining of morning headaches, interrupted sleep and daytime somnolence. The physiotherapist should be aware of this complication and, if it appears to be a problem, check the patient's vital capacity in both sitting and supine positions. Sleep studies may be necessary to determine the extent of the problem, and ventilatory support may be required.

Summary

The fairly clear-cut and progressive nature of this disease makes its course relatively easy to predict and thus appropriate interventions can be instigated.

One of the major problems facing this group of patients is the comparative rarity of the disease. Many therapists, particularly those working in neurology, may have heard of Charcot–Marie–Tooth disease or HMSN but see very few people with this condition. The literature is scarce regarding physiotherapy intervention. Provision of splints is often delayed until there is established deformity and, when provided, they are ill-fitting, causing additional problems of pressure and skin breakdown (CMT International, HMSN Self-Help Group 1995, personal communication).

By identifying the potential problems, appropriate stretching to maintain range of movement, exercise to improve postural alignment and provision of suitable orthoses may markedly reduce the onset of structural deformity. Early and continuing management of patients with HMSN may substantially reduce the need for what is often painful, expensive and, in many cases, preventable surgical intervention. If surgery is deemed necessary, physiotherapy is essential postoperatively to ensure a good functional outcome.

DISCUSSION

The management of these patient groups raises several issues that relate to many with chronic or progressive disability:

- the timing, extent and duration of therapy
- surgical intervention
- the most effective use of finite resources.

The timing, extent and duration of physiotherapy intervention

This is of particular concern, especially for those with severe residual disability such as may arise following severe head injury. These patients may require physiotherapy over a period of many years in order to achieve and maintain the optimal level of function.

Early treatment and management is rarely disputed, but the duration of this intervention is

increasingly questioned (Condie 1991, Bax et al 1988). Adults with cerebral palsy illustrate this point. These people may receive ongoing care throughout childhood and adolescence but, on leaving school, the therapy input is reduced, and this may lead to a deterioration in their condition with resultant loss of function.

The prevention of secondary complications such as contracture, and maximising function is the main remit of the physiotherapist (Pope 1992). Treatment to this effect should be instigated in the immediate aftermath of injury or at the onset of disease. This may involve a period of intensive rehabilitation or merely advice to the patient regarding appropriate maintenance. The timing and duration of rehabilitation is of special concern.

For example, some patients such as those with cervical cord injuries may benefit from an interim period, to come to terms with their disability, prior to undertaking intensive rehabilitation. Their time in hospital may be affected by problems such as respiratory tract infections and autonomic dysfunction. This affects their ability to participate in an intensive rehabilitation programme and, in some cases, they may not realise their full potential prior to discharge from hospital. In the majority of cases, the level of function attained by discharge is that which is assumed to be optimal. Patients who have been managed in a spinal injuries unit will usually be 'followed-up' on a regular basis to ensure there are no medical complications. However, it is rare for patients to be offered an additional period of rehabilitation even though their capability to benefit from this may have significantly improved.

The timing of physiotherapy intervention has been questioned in the management of stroke (Partridge 1994). Providing the patient is not at risk of deterioration, consideration should be given to delaying intensive rehabilitation following sudden onset of disability. Although it is crucial to ensure correct maintenance by instructing carers in appropriate methods of positioning, handling and exercise, patients must be assessed individually to determine the most appropriate timing for intensive rehabilitation.

Surgical intervention

With some conditions, surgical intervention may be necessary to restore range of movement in a contracted limb, stabilise a joint or transfer a tendon to improve function.

The risk of contracture is greatest for those with impaired cognition and spasticity (Ough et al 1981) and increases with prolonged duration of coma (Yarkony & Sahgal 1987). Contractures are best treated by prevention (Frank et al 1984, Cherry 1980) and joint management should be based on the assumption that the patient will make a good neurologic recovery (Yarkony & Sahgal 1987).

It is important to distinguish between spasticity, biomechanical changes of muscle and joint contracture (Ough et al 1981, Garland & Keenan 1983). Treatment using temporary paralysing agents such as phenol or botulinum toxin may be effective in determining the extent of contracture as opposed to the effects of hypertonus. These agents may also be of value in determining the effects of surgical intervention. For example, children with spastic diplegia, characteristically demonstrate predominant flexion of the lower limbs. Plantar flexion at the ankle provides an extensor component which may be essential to keep them upright against gravity. Surgery to elongate the Achilles tendon may permanently take away this extensor component, and further flexion may ensue which can lead to progressive crouch gait (Sutherland & Cooper 1978).

Extensive procedures have been described for the management of residual limb deformities following head injury (Garland & Keenan 1983, Ough et al 1981). Surgical intervention should be considered on a holistic basis and not purely in respect of elongating a contracted muscle or decreasing muscular activity. The functional implications of surgery, particularly of muscles acting over more than one joint, must be considered. It is important to remember that surgical procedures are a means to an end and not the end in itself. Postoperative management is mandatory if a successful outcome is to be achieved and must continue until such time as is necessary to prevent reversal (Pope 1991).

Heterotopic ossification is a recognised complication in patients following spinal cord injury (Silver 1969, Daud et al 1993) or head injury (Garland & Keenan 1983, Yarkony & Sahgal 1987, Davies 1994). It occurs predominantly around proximal joints. Surgical excision of heterotopic bone has had variable results (Garland & Keenan 1983) and conservative management is recommended (Andrews & Greenwood 1993). The incidence of recurrence following surgery is high, particularly in patients with spasticity. Surgical excision should not be performed until at least $1\frac{1}{2}$ years after injury when calcification is no longer an active process. A bone scan should demonstrate a decrease in activity (Garland & Keenan 1983).

The surgical management, such as tendon transfer and joint stabilisation, for patients with progressive neuromuscular disorders has been discussed in relation to patients with HMSN. Similar principles apply for others with muscle imbalance. In all instances, if surgery is deemed necessary, physiotherapy is essential postoperatively to ensure a good functional outcome (Pope 1992).

The most effective use of finite resources

Resources for health care provision are finite and it is therefore essential that further research is undertaken in the field of chronic neurological disability to ensure that there is appropriate use of these resources. There is an approximate ratio of 1 chartered physiotherapist to 86 severely disabled people in the United Kingdom (Condie 1991) and clearly, no matter how well manpower resources are deployed, there will be a continuing problem.

Prevention of secondary complications is of primary concern and physiotherapy intervention may be required for an indefinite period of time to ensure optimal function. Ongoing assessment for people with progressive neurological disorders is essential to contend with any deterioration in their physical status. However, those with non-progressive impairment, such as patients with cerebral palsy or following stroke, brain damage or spinal cord injury, may also deteriorate over time. Abnormal tone may lead to progressive disability due to the impoverishment of movement. People who are restricted to a limited array of postures and movements are as vulnerable to the development of secondary complications as are those with progressive disorders.

Therapists must produce evidence that ongoing treatment for the more severely disabled may significantly improve their level of function, with a consequent reduction in resources being required in the longer term. Given that these resources are limited, the timing of intervention as discussed above is of primary concern. This is an issue of great importance from all viewpoints and demands the urgent attention of physiotherapy researchers.

REFERENCES

Ada L, Canning C, Paratz J 1990 Care of the unconscious head-injured patient. In: Ada L, Canning C (eds) Key issues in neurological physiotherapy: physiotherapy foundations for practice. Butterworth-Heinemann, Oxford

Andrews K, Greenwood R 1993 Physical consequences of neurological disablement. In: Greenwood R, Barnes M P, McMillan T M, Ward C D (eds) Neurological rehabilitation. Churchill Livingstone, London

Ashburn A, DeSouza L H 1988 An approach to the management of multiple sclerosis. Physiotherapy Practice 4: 139–145

Bacardi B E, Alm W A 1986 Modification of the Gould operation for cavovarus reconstruction of the foot. Journal of Foot Surgery 25(3): 181–187

Bach-y-Rita P 1990 Brain plasticity as a basis for recovery of function in humans. Neuropsychologia 28(6): 547–554

Barnes M 1993 Multiple sclerosis. In: Greenwood R, Barnes M P, McMillan T M, Ward C D (eds) Neurological rehabilitation. Churchill Livingstone, London

Bax M C O, Smyth D P, Thomas A P 1988 Health care of physically handicapped young adults. British Medical Journal 296: 1153–1155

Beardshaw V 1988 Last on the list: community services for people with physical disabilities. King's Fund Centre, London

Bleck E E 1987 Orthopaedic management in cerebral palsy. Blackwell Scientific Publications, Oxford

Bobath K 1974 The motor deficit in patients with cerebral palsy. Clinics in Developmental Medicine. No. 23. Spastics International Medical Publications, William Heinemann Medical Books, London

BMA Medical Ethics Committee 1992 Discussion paper on treatment of patients in persistent vegetative state. BMA, London

Brown P 1994 Pathophysiology of spasticity. Journal of Neurology, Neurosurgery and Psychiatry 57: 773–777

Cherry D B 1980 Review of physical therapy alternatives for reducing muscle contracture. Physical Therapy 60(7): 877–881

Condie E 1991 A therapeutic approach to physical Disability. Physiotherapy 77(2): 72–77

Daud O, Sett P, Burr R G, Silver J R 1993 The relationship of heterotopic ossification to passive movement in paraplegic patients. Disability and Rehabilitation 15(3): 114–118

Davies P M 1994 Starting again. Springer-Verlag, London

Department of Health and Social Security 1981 Care in action. HMSO, London

DeSouza L 1990 Multiple sclerosis: approaches to management. Chapman & Hall, London

Finger S, Almli C R 1985 Brain damage and neuroplasticity: mechanisms of recovery or development? Brain Research Reviews 10: 177–186

Frank C, Akeson W H, Woo S L-Y, Amiel D, Coutts R D 1984 Physiology and therapeutic value of passive joint motion. Clinical Orthopaedics and Related Research 185: 113–125

Freeman E A 1992 The persistent vegetative state: a 'fate worse than death'. Clinical Rehabilitation 6: 159–165

Garland D E, Keenan M-A E 1983 Orthopaedic strategies in the management of the adult head-injured patient. Physical Therapy 63(12): 2004–2009

Geurts A C H, Mulder T W, Nienhuis B, Rijken R A J 1992a Influence of orthopaedic footwear on postural control in patients with hereditary motor and sensory neuropathy. Journal of Rehabilitation Sciences 5(1): 3–9

Geurts A C H, Mulder T W, Nienhuis B, Mars P, Rijken R A J 1992b Postural organisation in patients with hereditary motor and sensory neuropathy. Archives of Physical Medicine and Rehabilitation 73: 569–572

Gordon J 1990 Disorders of motor control. In: Ada L, Canning C (eds) Key issues in neurological physiotherapy: physiotherapy foundations for practice. Butterworth-Heinemann, Oxford

Hannan C, Korien J, Panigraphy A, Dikkes P, Goode R 1994 Neuropathic findings in the brain of Karen Ann Quinlan – the role of the thalamus in the persistent vegetative state. New England Journal of Medicine 330(21): 1469–1475

Hardie R 1993 Tremor and ataxia. In: Greenwood R, Barnes M P, McMillan T M, Ward C D (eds) Neurological rehabilitation. Churchill Livingstone, London

Harding A E 1984 The hereditary ataxias and related disorders. Churchill Livingstone, London

Harding A E 1993 Hereditary motor and sensory neuropathies (HMSN). Fact Sheet HE1. Muscular Dystrophy Group of Great Britain and Northern Ireland, London

Harding A E, Thomas P K 1980 The clinical features of hereditary and motor sensory neuropathy types I and II. Brain 103: 259–280

Howard R S, Wiles C M, Hirsch N P, Loh L, Spencer G T, Newsom-Davis J 1992 Respiratory involvement in multiple sclerosis. Brain 115: 479–494

Jennett B 1992 Letting vegetative patients die. British Medical Journal 305: 1305–1306

Jennett B, Plum J 1972 Persistent vegetative state after brain damage – a syndrome in search of a name. Lancet i: 734–737

Klein F C 1982 The silent epidemic. Wall Street Journal 24 November

Krupp L B, Alvarez L A, La Rocca N G, Scheinberg L C 1988 Fatigue in multiple sclerosis. Archives of Neurology 45: 435–437

Malcolm S 1993 CMT: clearing up a mystery. Muscular Dystrophy Group of Great Britain and Northern Ireland, London

Mann R A, Missirian J 1988 Pathophysiology of Charcot–Marie–Tooth disease. Clinical Orthopaedics and Related Research 234: 221–228

Medhat M A, Krantz H 1988 Neuropathic ankle joint in Charcot–Marie–Tooth disease after triple arthrodesis of the foot. Orthopaedic Review XVII(9): 873–880

Mertin J 1994 Rehabilitation in multiple sclerosis. Annals of Neurology 35(S): 130–133

Mertin J, Paeth B 1994 Physiotherapy and multiple sclerosis: application of the Bobath concept. MS Management 1(1): 10–13

Miller D H, Hornabrook R W, Purdie G 1992 The natural history of multiple sclerosis: a regional study with some longitudinal data. Journal of Neurology, Neurosurgery and Psychiatry 55: 341–346

Minden S L, Schiffer R B 1990 Affective disorders in multiple sclerosis. Review and recommendations for clinical research. Archives of Neurology 47: 98–104

Morgan M H, Hewer R L, Cooper R 1975 Application of an objective method of assessing intention tremor – a further study on the use of weights to reduce intention tremor. Journal of Neurology, Neurosurgery and Psychiatry 38: 259–264

Multi-Society Task Force on PVS 1994 Medical aspects of persistent vegetative state. New England Journal of Medicine 21: 1499–1507; 22: 1572–1579

Ough J L, Garland D E, Jordan C, Waters R L 1981 Treatment of spastic joint contractures in mentally disabled adults. Orthopedic Clinics of North America 12(1): 143–151

Partridge C J 1994 Evaluation of physiotherapy for people with stroke. King's Fund Centre, London

Pope P M 1988 A model for evaluation of input in relation to outcome in severely brain damaged patients. Physiotherapy 74(12): 647–650

Pope P M 1992 Management of the physical condition in patients with chronic and severe neurological pathologies. Physiotherapy 78(12): 896–903

Pope P M, Bowes C E, Tudor M, Andrews B 1991 Surgery combined with continued post-operative stretching and management of knee flexion contractures in cases of multiple sclerosis. A report of six cases. Clinical Rehabilitation 5: 15–23

Poser C M 1980 Exacerbations, activity and progression in multiple sclerosis. Archives of Neurology 37: 471–474

Silver J R 1969 Heterotopic ossification: a clinical study of its possible relationship to trauma. Paraplegia 7: 220–230

Sutherland D H, Cooper L 1978 The pathomechanics of progressive crouch gait in spastic diplegia. Orthopedic Clinics of North America 9(1): 143–154

Thompson A J, McDonald W I 1992 Multiple sclerosis and its pathophysiology. In: Asbury A K, McKhann G M, McDonald W I (eds) Diseases of the nervous system, clinical neurobiology. 2nd edn. W B Saunders, Philadelphia, vol 2: 1209–1228

Thompson A J, Kermode A G, Wicks D, MacManus D G, Kendall B E, Kingsley D P E, McDonald W I 1991 Major differences in the dynamics of primary and secondary progressive multiple sclerosis. Annals of Neurology 29: 53–62

Tribe D, Korgaonkar G 1992 Withdrawing medical treatment: implications of the Bland case. British Journal of Hospital Medicine 48(11): 754–756

Vogenthaler D R 1987 An overview of head injury – its consequences and rehabilitation. Brain Injury 1(1): 113–127

Weinshenker B G 1994 Natural history of multiple sclerosis. Annals of Neurology 36: S6–S11

Wetmore R S, Drennan J C 1989 Long-term results of triple arthrodesis in Charcot–Marie–Tooth disease. Journal of Bone and Joint Surgery 71-A(3): 417–422

Wukich D K, Bowen J R 1989 A long-term study of triple arthrodesis for correction of pes cavovarus in Charcot–Marie–Tooth disease. Journal of Pediatric Orthopedics 9(4): 433–437

Yarkony G M, Sahgal V 1987 Contractures: a major complication of craniocerebral trauma. Clinical Orthopaedics and Related Research 219: 93–96

Index

A

Abduction roll, 181
Affolter, F., 8, 11
AFO *see* Ankle–foot orthoses
Akinesia, 71–72
Alzheimer's disease, 44
Amnesia, 46
Ankle, 34–35
    casting of, 172–177
    movement at, 111
    spasticity and, 67
Ankle–foot orthoses (AFOs), 122, 163
    anterior shell, 167–168, 170
    below-knee calipers, 167, 201
    design, 165–166
    dorsiflexion bandage, 168–169
    for HMSN, 201, 203
    hinged, 166–167
    posterior leaf, 164–166
    splint flexibility, 165
Anxiety, 57, 58, 59
Arterial blood gas, 90
Arthrodesis, triple, 201
Assessment of seating requirements
    information required, 146
    procedure, 146–147
    sequence of, 147–148
Associated reactions, 70
Ataxia
    cerebellar, 80–82
    clinical presentation and, 82–83
    sensory, 80
    support for, 157
    vestibular, 80
    weights for, 199
Athetosis *see* Chorea and athetosis
Attention
    clinical observations of deficits, 48–49
    neurological tests of, 48
    treatment of deficits, 49
Australian lift, 126
Ayres, A. J., 9, 11

B

Back slabs
    application, 175–177
    for elbow, 182–183
    for lower limbs, 105–106, 122
Baclofen, 130, 131, 132
Balance, 19–20
Barthel Index, 12
Beck Inventory of Depression, 57–58
Behavioural Inattention Test, 51–52
Biomechanical properties of muscle, 20–22
Blepharospasm, 74, 75, 76
Bobath, K., 5–6, 11, 12
Botulinum toxin, 75, 204
Boxing glove splint, 186
Bradykinesia, 72

Brain injury, acute, 87–90
    cerebral vasodilatation, 89–90
    effect on lungs, 90
    intracranial pressure, 88–89
    PVS after, 190–193
Brunnström, S., 5, 11, 12

C

Calipers, below knee, 167, 201
Care in action (DHSS 1981), 193
Carr, J.H. and Shepherd, R.B., 6–7, 11
Case histories, 115–133
    head injury, 123–129
    multiple sclerosis, 129–133
    right hemiplegia, 116–120
    spinal lesion, 121–123
Casts
    application, 173–174, 177–178, 182
    back slabs *see* Back slabs
    drop-out, 177–178, 183
    elbow, 181–183
    lower limb, 127–128, 172–178
    materials for, 172, 179
    serial, 175, 177, 182
Cerebellar ataxia, 80–82
Cerebral blood flow, 88, 89
Cerebral palsy, 76, 79
    in adulthood, 193–195
    physiotherapy for, 194–195
Cerebral perfusion pressure, 88, 89–90
Cerebral vasodilatation, 89–90
Chanting, 7
Charcot–Marie–Tooth disease, 200
Chest clapping, 92
Chorea and athetosis, 76–79
    clinical presentation, 77–78
    communication and eating problems, 78
    posture and movement problems, 78–79
Collagen, 21
Collar and cuff support, 180
Communication
    athetosis and, 78
    PVS and, 191–192
Computerised tomography, 63
Conductive education, 7–8
Continuous positive airway pressure, 93
Coughing, assisted, 93–94
Cuff support, 180–181

D

Dementia, 44–45
Depression *see* Emotional distress
Digit Span subtest of WAIS-R, 48
Dopamine, 73
Dorsal splint, 184
Dysdiadochokinesia, 81
Dysexecutive syndrome, 54–55

Dysmetria, 80
Dyssynergia, 81
Dystonia
    clinical presentation, 75
    treatment, 75–76
    types, 74

E

Eating problems of athetosis, 78
Educational programmes, 10
Elbow
    back slabs, 182–183
    casts, 181–183
    movements of joint, 110
    spasticity and, 67
Emotional distress
    clinical observation of, 57–58
    neuropsychological tests of, 56–57
    treatment of, 58–59
Equilibrium reactions, 19–20
Ethics
    multiple sclerosis and, 199
    PVS and, 191–192
Executive functions
    clinical observation of dysfunction, 54–55
    neuropsychological tests of, 54
    treatment of dysfunction, 55
Extensor response, 69–70
Extensor thrust, 140

F

Facial movements, 106–107, 192
Finger spreader, 184–185
Fingers, movements of, 110
Foot, 34–35
    casting of, 127–128, 172–178
    insoles, 163–164, 201
    movements of, 111
    orthoses for *see* Ankle–foot orthoses
    supporting the, 154, 155, 157
Forces, 161–162

G

Gait
    AFOs and, 164–165
    athetosis, 76, 79
    cadence and velocity, 33
    cerebellar ataxia and, 81
    cycle, 32
    foot and ankle, 34–35
    hip, 35
    joint angles and, 34
    knee, 35
    multiple sclerosis and, 198–199
    muscle activity and, 34
    neural control, 35–36
    pelvis, 35

Gait (*Cont'd*)
  rotation, 33–34
  spastic, 67
  step and stride length, 32
  stride width, 32–33
  vertical displacement, 34
Gastrostomy, 193
Glasgow Coma Scale, 90, 173
Graded Naming Test, 49
Grasping, 37–38
  reflex, 69
Ground reaction force, 162
Guillain–Barré syndrome, 91, 95
Gymnastic ball, 70, 99–100, 125

H

Hand *see* Wrist and hand
Hare, N., 9–10
Head injury, case history of, 123–129
Hemiplegia
  case history of right, 116–120
  mobilisation of trunk for, 99
Hereditary motor and sensory
      neuropathy (HMSN), 195,
      199–203
  AFOs for, 201
  clinical signs and symptoms, 200
  footwear for, 201
  lower limb weakness, 200
  physiotherapy for, 200–201, 202
  upper limb weakness, 202
Hip, 35
  reduced flexion of, 153
HMSN *see* Hereditary motor and
      sensory neuropathy
Holmqvist, L.W. and Wrethagen, N.,
      10, 11
Human sandwich, 9–10
Humidification, 93
Hydrotherapy, 199
Hyperinflation, manual, 91
Hyperventilation, 90
Hypotonia, 81

I

Insight
  clinical observation of, 56
  neuropsychological testing of,
      55–56
  treatment of (poor), 56
Insoles, foot, 163–164, 201
Intellectual function, general
  clinical observations of loss, 44
  neuropsychological tests of,
      42–44
  treatment of loss, 44–45
Intermittent positive pressure
      breathing, 93
Intracranial pressure, 88, 89–90
IQ scores, 43

J

Johnstone, M., 10, 11
Joint mobility, 95

K

Kabat, H., 11
Kendall muscle test, 12
Key points of control, 23–24
Knee, 35
  flexion contractures, 154
  hyperextension of, 170
  serial casting for, 177
Knee–ankle–foot orthoses (KAFOs),
      169–172
  for flexor spasticity of lower limbs,
      171
  for paralysis of lower limbs, 171–172
Kurtzke Disability Status Scale, 198
Kyphosis, 154–155

L

Language dysfunction, 49–50
  clinical observation of, 50
  neuropsychological tests of, 49–50
  treatment of, 50
Lesch–Nyhan syndrome, 157
Lower limbs
  casts for, 172–179
  KAFOs for, 171–172
  movements, 110–111
  'windswept', 96, 153–154
Lungs, effect of brain injury on, 90
Lying
  control of posture in, 159
  prone, 25–26, 98–99
  side, 26, 97–98
  supine, 24–25, 29–30, 96–97

M

Magnetic resonance imaging, 63, 196
Mat exercises, 6
Memory dysfunction
  clinical observations of, 45–47
  loss of short-term, 127
  neuropsychological tests of, 45
  treatment of, 47–48
Midline, 24
Moments, 162
Motor learning, 18, 19
  cerebellum and, 81–82
Motor relearning programme, 6–7
Movement, analysis of normal, 15–40,
      94
  balance, 19–20
  biomechanical properties of muscles,
      20–22
  key points of control, 23–24

midline, 24
normal postural tone, 16
positioning
  prone lying, 25–26
  side-lying, 26
  sitting, 26–28
  standing, 28–29
  supine lying, 24–25
postural sets, 22–23
reciprocal innervation, 16–17
rotation of body segments, 22
sensory-motor feedback, 18–19
sequences, 29–38
upper limb function, 36–38
walking, 32–36
Movements,
  asymmetrical, 155
  elbow joint, 110
  foot and ankle, 111
  lower limb, 110–111
  orofacial, 106–107
  passive, 94–95
  shoulder girdle and upper limb,
      107–110
  spasticity and, 156
  wrist and fingers, 110
Multiple sclerosis, 44, 56, 195
  case history, 129–133
  emotional distress and, 57
  high amplitude tremors and, 157
  physiotherapy for, 196–199
  symptoms, 196
Muscles
  activity during gait, 34
  biomechanical properties of, 20–22
  impairment of respiratory, 90–91
  mobilisation of, 95
  stability and, 143–144
  tone *see* Tone
Muscular dystrophy, 195

N

National Adult Reading Test – Revised,
      43–44
Nervous system, mobility of, 95
Neural control, 35–36
Neuropsychology, 41–61
  attention, 48–49
  emotional distress, 56–59
  executive functions, 54–55
  general intellectual function,
      42–45
  insight, 55–56
  language function, 49–50
  memory function, 45–48
  spatial processing, 51–54
  visual perception, 50–51

O

Ontogenetic sequence, 4
Opisthotonus, 74

Orofacial movements, 106–107, 192
Orthoses, 161
  ankle–foot see Ankle–foot orthoses
  casts, 172–179, 181–182
  classification, 163
  elbow casts, 181–183
  for HMSN, 201
  foot insoles, 163–164, 201
  knee–ankle–foot, 169–172
  lower limb, 163–179
  shoulder supports, 179–181
  upper limb, 179–187
  wrist and hand, 183–187
Ossification, heterotopic, 128, 204
Oswestry standing frame, 102–104,
  126, 127, 130
Oxford Scale, 121, 122

P

Paced Auditory Serial Addition Task,
  48
Parkinson's disease, 33
  akinesia and, 71–72
  bradykinesia and, 72
  clinical presentation, 72–73
  exercise and, 72, 73
  rotation in, 33, 72, 73
Pelvis, 30, 31, 33, 35
  obliquity of, 153
Perception, 8, 9
  see also Visual perception
Percussion, 92
Peroneal muscular atrophy, 200
Persistent vegetative state (PVS),
  190–193
  ethical considerations, 191
  physiotherapy for, 192
Petö, András, 7
Phenol, 204
Physical Ability Scale, 9, 142, 151–152
Picture arrangement subtest, 43–44
Plaster of Paris, 172, 182
Positioning, 92, 94, 95–106
  for PVS, 192
  in bed, 96–99
  prone lying, 25–26, 98–99
  side-lying, 26, 97–98
  sitting, 26–28, 99–100
  standing, 28–29, 100–106
  supine lying, 24–25, 96–97
  see also Posture
Positive end expiratory pressure
  (PEEP), 93
Positive support reaction, 66–68
Positron emission tomography, 63
Postural drainage, 92
Postural sets, 22–23
Posture, 135–137
  aesthetics versus efficacy, 158
  areas of deviation, 145
  assessment, 146–149
  biomechanics of seated, 142–145
  body structure, 142–143, 144

  cerebellar ataxia and, 81, 157
  check list for prescription, 158
  client versus carer needs, 158
  complications of bad, 141–142
  compromise, 156–157
  counter-strategies, 158–159
  energy-conserving strategies,
    137–138
  incompetence of, 139–140
  learning control, 138–139
  levels of ability, 151–153
  maximising performance, 140–141
  measurement of competence, 142
  movement and, 138
  objectives of control, 149
  specific problem solving, 153–156
  stability of, 143–145
  step-by-step to stable, 149–151
  support versus freedom of
    movement, 157
  support versus mobility, 158
  supporting the feet, 154, 155, 157
  T-roll for asymmetrical, 97
Prehension, 37–38
Pressure, 162
Problem-solving disorders, treatment
  of, 55
Prone standing table, 104
Proprioceptive neuromuscular
  facilitation, 5, 12
Protective reactions, 20
Psycholinguistic Assessments of
  Language Processing in
  Aphasia, 45–50
Psychology see Neuropsychology
PVS see Persistent vegetative state

R

Reaching, 37–38
Reciprocal innervation, 16–17
Recognition Memory Test, 45, 46
Rehabilitation see Case histories
Respiratory dysfunction, 199
  acute brain injury, 87–90
  physiotherapy for, 91–94
  respiratory muscle impairment, 90–91
Righting reactions, 20
Rigidity
  akinesia, 71–72
  bradykinesia, 72
  clinical presentation of
    parkinsonism, 72–74
Rivermead Behavioural Memory Test,
  45
Rood, M. S., 4–5, 11, 12
Rotation, 22, 33–34
  Parkinson's disease and, 72, 73

S

SAM system, 154, 155
Sarcomeres, 21

Scapula, 36–37, 109
Seating, special, 135–136
  for asymmetrical movement, 155
  for knee flexion contractures, 154
  for kyphosis, 154–155
  for pelvic obliquity, 153
  for reduced hip flexion, 153
  for 'windswept' lower limbs, 153–154
  supporting the feet, 154, 155, 157
  see also Posture
Sensory integration, 9
Sensory-motor feedback, 18–19
Sensory stimulation, 4
Shaking, 91–92
Shoulder girdle
  anatomy, 36
  movements of, 107–110
  relationship between structures,
    36–37
Shoulder supports, 179–181
  abduction roll or wedge, 181
  collar and cuff, 180
  cuff support, 180–181
  pillows or tray, 181
Sitting, 26–28
  clinical application of analysis, 28
  moving from supine lying to, 29–30
  principles of positioning in, 99–100
  supported, 27–28
  trunk mobilisation, 99
  unsupported, 27
  use of gymnastic ball, 99–100
  see also Seating, special
Spasmodic torticollis, 74, 75, 76
Spastic diplegia
  in children, 204
  support for, 157
Spasticity, 64–71
  AFOs for, 165
  aims of physiotherapy, 65–66
  associated reactions, 70–71
  casting of foot and ankle, 172–173
  clinical features, 67–68
  extensor response, 69–70
  flexor withdrawal, 68–69
  grasp reflex, 69
  heel support and, 101
  historical perspective, 65
  positive support reaction, 66–68
  posture and, 156
  prone lying and, 98–99
  retraction of scapula and, 109
  splinting for wrist and hand, 184
Spatial processing
  clinical observation of impairment,
    52
  cues, 53
  neuropsychological tests of, 51–52
  treatment of impairment, 53–54
Spinal lesion at T12–L2 level
  case history, 121–123
Splints, 124
  boxing glove, 186
  clinical application, 162–163
  cone, 185

Splints (*Cont'd*)
  dorsal, 184
  finger spreader, 184–185
  for hypotonic wrist and hand,
    185–187
  for spastic wrist and hand, 184–185
  forces, 161–162
  multiple sclerosis and, 199
  orally inflatable, 10
  PVS and, 192
  taping, 186
  thumb opposition, 187
  volar, 184
  volar resting, 185–186
  see also Orthoses
Stability, factors influencing, 143–145
Standing, 28–29
  back slabs for, 105–106
  moving from sitting to, 31–32
  Oswestry standing frame, 102–104
  principles of positioning in, 100–106
  prone standing table, 104
  tilt table, 101–102
  using two or more therapists,
    104–105
State–Trait Anger Inventory, 57, 58
Stroke, 3, 5, 11
  aims of physiotherapy, 65–66
  associated reactions and, 71
  educational programmes and, 10
  historical perspective, 65
  splints for, 10
  timing of physiotherapy, 203
Subjective Memory Questionnaire,
    56
Surgery, 204
Suctioning, 92–93
Swedish knee cage, 170
Swedish Remedial Exercises, 5

T

T-roll, 97
Taping, 186
Test of Everyday Attention, 48
Tests, neuropsychological, 59–60
  of attention, 48
  of emotional distress, 56–57
  of executive functions, 54

of general intellectual impairment,
    42–44
  of insight, 55–56
  of language function, 49–50
  of memory function, 45
  of spatial processing, 51–52
  of visual perception, 50–51
Thumb opposition splint, 187
Tilt table, 101–102
Tone
  abnormal, 63–86
  associated reactions, 71
  ataxia, 80–83
  chorea and athetosis, 76–79
  dystonia, 74–76
  extensor response, 69–71
  flexor withdrawal, 68–69
  grasp reflex, 69
  low, 99, 108–109
  normal postural, 16
  prone lying and, 98
  rigidity, 71–74
  spasticity, 64–71, 109–110
  supine lying and, 96
Tongue, spasticity of, 106–107
Transport component of prehension,
    37–38
Treatment approaches, 3–10
  Affolter, 8
  Bobath, 5–6, 12
  Brunnström, 5, 11, 12
  comparisons, 10–13
  conductive education, 7–8
  educational programmes, 10, 11
  human sandwich, 9–10
  Johnstone, 10
  motor relearning programme, 6–7, 11
  proprioceptive neuromuscular
    facilitation, 5, 11
  Rood, 4–5
  sensory integration, 9
Tremor, 80
Trunk, 30, 31, 33
  mobilisations, 99
  stability, 17, 144

U

Upper limb

function, 36–38
  movements of, 108–110
  orthoses, 179–187
  problems with HMSN, 202

V

Vari-table, 119
Ventilation, 91, 92
Verbal and Spatial Reasoning Test, 44
Vibrations, 91–92
Visual agnosia, 46
Visual Object and Space Perception
    Battery, 51
Visual perception
  clinical observations of deficits, 51
  neuropsychological tests of, 50–51
  treatment of deficits, 51
Visuomotor incoordination, 81
Volar splint, 184
  resting, 185–186

W

Walking *see* Gait
Wechsler Adult Intelligence Scale –
    Revised (WAIS-R), 42–43, 44, 48
Wedges
  abduction, 181
  heel, 101
  prone lying with, 98, 130
  supine lying with, 97
Weights for treatment of MS, 199
Wisconsin Card Sorting Test, 54
Wrist and hand
  boxing glove splint, 186
  cone, 185
  dorsal splint, 184
  finger spreader, 184–185
  movements of, 110
  splints for, 183–187
  taping, 186
  thumb opposition splint, 187
  volar splint, 184, 185–186
Writer's cramp, 74